Digital Convergence

This book focuses on using analytics and artificial intelligence (AI) to offer a high-quality value proposition to address dementia, a growing and concerning global healthcare problem. By enabling better decision-making support, minimizing medical errors and use of specific treatment strategies, digital technologies are key to effective care for People Living with Dementia (PLWD). By taking a unique triumvirate approach of focusing simultaneously on people issues, technical issues and process issues, the critical success issues are identified.

The first point of concern is the different major stakeholders, including PLWD, their family carer, their challenges and major barriers and facilitators. Next, the vast pool of digital tools is considered, such as the different forms of mobile, platforms, sensors, IoT, chatbots, avatars, robots, augmented reality, virtual reality and mixed reality. This leads next to looking at the important considerations for the design and development of digital health solutions for priority areas of action in the Global Action Plan on Dementia, including co-design and research. By using a global perspective, the international examples help to better appreciate culture and practices, as countries differ significantly regarding many key issues pertaining to healthcare delivery. The editors endeavour to cover all areas pertinent to leveraging digital health solutions to facilitate the realization of value-driven healthcare delivery for all healthcare systems.

This book is a new and comprehensive text, which would serve as an important resource for practitioners and professionals in healthcare and would be beneficial as a supplementary text for students undertaking studies relating to health informatics and public healthcare.

Digital Convergence
Better Solutions for People with Dementia

Edited by Nilmini Wickramasinghe, Thu Ha Dang,
Tuan Anh Nguyen, and Sasan Adibi

CRC Press
Taylor & Francis Group
Boca Raton New York London

CRC Press is an imprint of the
Taylor & Francis Group, an **informa** business

Designed cover image: Shutterstock

First edition published 2026
by CRC Press
2385 NW Executive Center Drive, Suite 320, Boca Raton FL 33431

and by CRC Press
4 Park Square, Milton Park, Abingdon, Oxon, OX14 4RN

CRC Press is an imprint of Taylor & Francis Group, LLC

ISBN: 978-1-032-77978-2 (hbk)
ISBN: 978-1-032-77977-5 (pbk)
ISBN: 978-1-003-48568-1 (ebk)

DOI: 10.1201/9781003485681

Typeset in Palatino
by KnowledgeWorks Global Ltd.

For our families, colleagues, students

and all who want to move the needle

to provide tailored, personalized

quality healthcare delivery for all.

Contents

About the Editors ix
Contributors Bios xi
Foreword xvii
Preface.. xix

1   Digital Solutions for People Living with Dementia:
    Possibilities and Pitfalls..1
    Kate Swaffer

2   Family Carers 18
    James Nicholas Chaousis

3   The Role of Digital Twins Powered/Enabled through AI
    for People with Dementia 38
    Nilmini Wickramasinghe

4   Empowering Patient Care: Leveraging Artificial Intelligence
    and Internet of Things for Enhanced Healthcare Delivery................. 45
    Helena Bahrami and Sasan Adibi

5   Advancing Dementia Care: AI and Machine Learning
    in Diagnosis and Drug Discovery.. 75
    Helena Bahrami and Sasan Adibi

6   Conversational Agents in Healthcare: Leveraging Language
    Models and Chatbots for Patient Interaction......................................126
    Helena Bahrami and Sasan Adibi

7   Artificial Intelligence for Dementia 157
    Olalekan Balongun and Sasan Adibi

8   Mobile and Platforms, Sensors, and IoT (Internet of Things):
    Smart Dementia Networks (SDNs) Devising on Real-Time
    Wearable IoT Platforms 171
    Gurdeep Singh

9   Opportunities for Digital Health Solutions in Dementia
    Care: A Scoping Review..195
    Ayesha Nilashini

10 Using Digital Tools to Detect Spatial Navigation Impairment
    in Early Alzheimer's Disease 215
    Ming-Chyi Pai and Sheng-Hsiang Yang

11 Digital Solutions to Empower Multicultural Families
    Impacted by Dementia 232
    Josefine Antoniades and Joyce Siette

12 Digital Solutions in Dementia Treatment, Care, and Support 243
    Upasana Baruah and Zara Page

13 Incorporating AI with a Multilingual Virtual Helper for
    Dementia Carers in Australia: A Case Study 266
    *Nalika Ulapane, Nilmini Wickramasinghe, Thu Ha Dang,
    Antonia Thodis, and Bianca Brijnath*

14 Co-Design of Digital Health Interventions in Dementia 279
    Ellen Gaffy, Frances Batchelor, Bobby Redman, and Anita Goh

15 The Potential of Digital Solutions for Caregivers
    of Individuals with Dementia 301
    Sara J. Czaja and Laura N. Gitlin

16 Dementia Empowerment with Heart Health Intervention
    and LLM-based Health AI Research Assistant 323
    Luuk P.A. Simons, Pradeep K. Murukannaiah, and Mark A. Neerincx

17 Digital Twins of Dementia Patients for Clinical
    Decision Support..346
    Nilmini Wickramasinghe and Nalika Ulapane

Epilogue 361

Index...363

About the Editors

Nilmini Wickramasinghe: Currently, Professor Wickramasinghe is the inaugural Optus Chair and Professor of Digital Health at La Trobe University. She also holds/has held honorary research professor positions at Epworth HealthCare, the Peter MacCallum Cancer Centre and Northern Health. After completing five degrees at the University of Melbourne, she was awarded a full scholarship to complete PhD studies at Case Western Reserve University, Cleveland, OH, USA, and later she was sponsored to complete executive education at Harvard Business School, Harvard University, Cambridge, MA, USA in Value-based HealthCare. For over 20 years, Professor Wickramasinghe has been actively researching and teaching within the health informatics/digital health domain in the US, Germany and Australia with a particular focus on designing, developing and deploying suitable models, strategies and techniques grounded in various management principles to facilitate the implementation and adoption of technology solutions to effect superior, value-based patient-centric care delivery. In 2020, she was awarded the prestigious Alexander von Humboldt Award for outstanding contribution to Digital Health, the first time this honour has been bestowed on someone in the discipline of Digital Health.

Thu Ha Dang is a Research Fellow at the School of Computer, Engineering and Mathematical Sciences, La Trobe University. Her background is in medicine, public health, and digital health. Her research focusses on applying digital technology in chronic conditions management. Within these areas, she has conducted a number of studies on cancer and dementia prevention, awareness and care. She has extensive experience in co-design, development and evaluation of digital health solutions; mixed-methods research; systematic reviews; and teaching. She has authored over 20 publications and contributed to nearly AU$8.5 million in research funding.

Tuan Anh Nguyen is a distinguished researcher and academic renowned for his significant contributions to dementia research, health equity, digital health and the creation of culturally tailored dementia interventions. His career is marked by a steadfast commitment to enhancing the well-being of vulnerable populations, with a particular focus on low- and middle-income countries (LMICs) and culturally and linguistically diverse (CALD) communities in Australia. He leads three international grants, has authored over 100 publications, presented at more than 70 conferences, and secured over $19 million in research funding.

Sasan Adibi is an expert in digital health innovation, currently serving as founder and CEO of Research Vitality and Director of Digital Health & AI at GENI. With over two decades of experience across healthcare, academia and industry, he specializes in developing strategic solutions that bridge clinical practice and technology. His background includes senior roles at Austin Health and the Department of Health, where he led the Outbreak Management System development and managed frameworks for aged-care centres throughout Victoria. Previously, he served as the program leader and lecturer at Deakin University, and he managed healthcare technology projects at BlackBerry Corp. Dr. Adibi holds a PhD in Communication and Information Systems from the University of Waterloo and is PROSCI certified in change management.

Contributors Bios

Josefine Antoniades is an Associate Professor of Health Communication at La Trobe University. She has a background in psychology and public health, and her research focuses on cultural diversity, dementia, mental health, and community engagement, emphasizing meaningful collaboration to create accessible and impactful outcomes. A key aspect of her work is leveraging technology – both to enhance inclusivity in research and to develop practical resources that drive real change among multicultural communities.

Helena Bahrami, Associate Researcher, Auckland University of Technology – Institute of Biomedical Technology | Founder, Helium AI Solutions | AI & Machine Learning Lead Scientist, AI-powered Market Intelligence Platform. Dr. Helena Bahrami is an AI and Machine Learning Lead Scientist specializing in neurodegenerative disease diagnostics, multimodal AI, and biomedical imaging. With expertise in large language models, computational neuroscience, and quantum-inspired deep learning, she applies AI to healthcare, drug discovery, and precision medicine. She collaborates internationally with scientists and surgeons on dementia, lung, and prostate cancer research. A member of the DEMON (Deep Dementia Phenotyping) Network and the Royal Society Te Apārangi, she contributes to AI-driven advancements in dementia research. A mentor, keynote speaker, and industry leader, she integrates AI, IoT, and NLP to transform healthcare. Dr Bahrami holds a PhD in AI and Machine Learning and actively contributes to AI ethics, responsible AI, and the future of human-AI synergy.

Olalekan Balongun is a graduate of Master of Information Technology (Professional), with a major in cybersecurity from Deakin University Australia. He is a proficient and thorough cybersecurity specialist with a deep understanding of information technology and has knowledge of all aspects of security from denial of service attacks to malwares.

Upasana Baruah is Research Fellow at the National Ageing Research Institute (NARI) in Melbourne, Australia, in the Division of Aged Care and Social Gerontology, and is currently working on the e-DiVA project to adapt the WHO iSupport Program for dementia carers in Australia, Indonesia, New Zealand, and Vietnam. She is a psychiatric social worker with extensive experience in mental health and psychosocial research, teaching, and clinical social work, and specializes in dementia caregiving, family-based mental health interventions, and neuropalliative care with a focus on digital solutions and culturally adaptable approaches.

Frances Batchelor is Associate Professor at National Ageing Research Institute, Parkville, Victoria, Australia, and Faculty of Medicine, Dentistry and Health Sciences, The University of Melbourne. He is the Director of Clinical Gerontology at the National Ageing Research Institute and Senior Principal Research Fellow. As a research and clinical physiotherapist she has over 35 years' experience in community, hospital and aged care services. Since completing her PhD in 2010, Frances has focussed on 4 key research areas: healthy ageing, health conditions associated with ageing, health and aged care systems, and technology in health and aged care. Associate Professor Batchelor's career is focused on collaborative approaches to research, policy and practice to improve the lives of older people.

Bianca Brijnath is Professor of Health Communication in Society at La Trobe University. Her disciplinary training is in medical anthropology and public health, and her research expertise is in cultural diversity, dementia, and mental health. Within these disciplinary and contextual boundaries, she has undertaken several studies on dementia prevention, awareness, diagnosis and care, specific to culturally diverse communities in Australia and internationally. She has authored over 150 publications, has produced more than 70 multilingual films, comics, and animations, and generated over $26 million in research income. In recognition of her research, she was inducted into the State Government of Victoria's Multicultural Honour Roll in 2022.

James Nicholas Chaousis is the former Head of clinical social work in the divisions of mental health with the Northern Adelaide Local Health Network, South Australian Department of Health & Well-being. He retired in 2020 after 33 years of public service. His academic background includes social work and sociology, and he has a master's degree in behavioural and cognitive psychotherapy from the Department of Psychiatry, School of Medicine at Flinders University in South Australia. He is currently affiliated with Dementia Australia as a registered dementia advocate and is involved in several university-based research projects and participates in dementia related local and national consultations.

Sara J. Czaja, PhD, the Gladys and Roland Harriman Professor of Medicine and Director of the Center on Aging and Behavioral Research in the Division of Geriatrics and Palliative Care at Weill Cornell Medicine, has extensive experience in aging research. She is the PI of the NIA-funded multisite Center for Research and Education on Aging and Technology Enhancement (CREATE) and the Co-Director of the Enhancing Neurocognitive Health, Abilities, Networks, & Community Engagement Center, funded by the National Institute on Disability, Independent Living, and Rehabilitation Research. Her research interests include aging and cognition, caregiving, aging and technology interactions, training, and functional assessment.

Ellen Gaffy is a Research Fellow within the Aged Care and Social Gerontology Division at the National Ageing Research Institute. Ellen completed her PhD in 2023, which investigated the experience of people living with dementia and family carers in co-designing a dementia training program for home care workers. Her research is focused on end-of-life care, dementia care provision across community and residential care settings, and improving active consumer and community involvement in research.

Laura N. Gitlin, PhD, FGSA, FAAN, an Applied Research Sociologist and Intervention Scientist, is the Distinguished Professor, and Dean Emerita of the College of Nursing and Health Professions, Drexel University. She is also the inaugural executive director of its AgeWell Collaboratory that oversees Drexel's Age Friendly University international designation, and partners with community organizations serving diverse older adults and families. Dr. Gitlin has >40 years of continuous NIH research support to develop, evaluate, implement, and disseminate novel home and community-based interventions that improve the quality of life of older adults and family members. Some interventions have been translated into different languages and used worldwide. She is also the Chief Scientific Officer of Plans4Care, Inc., a company she co-founded to develop digital solutions to support family caregivers and healthcare providers by providing evidence-based nonpharmacological strategies to manage dementia-related symptoms.

Anita Goh (MAPS, FCCN) is a Clinician-Researcher with expertise in mental health, cognition, ageing, and dementia, and a focus on effective translation of evidence into policy and practice. Anita is a Clinical Neuropsychologist and a Principal Researcher at the National Ageing Research Institute, where she is currently Director of Aged Care and Social Gerontology research. Dr Goh is an Advisory Council member of the Alzheimer's Association International Society to Advance Alzheimer's Research and Treatment, Board Director and Fellow of the Australian Association of Gerontology, and Councillor at the Royal Society of Victoria.

Pradeep K. Murukannaiah is an Assistant Professor in the Interactive Intelligence group, Faculty of Electrical Engineering, Mathematics, and Computer Science, at the Delft University of Technology. Engineering socially intelligent agents is the overarching theme of Pradeep's research. He works on hybrid intelligence (HI) methods, where artificial intelligence (AI) techniques support humans in multistakeholder deliberations and multiobjective decision-making.

Mark A. Neerincx is a Professor in Human-Centered Computing at Delft University of Technology and Principal Scientist at TNO Human-Machine Teaming. He focusses on the socio-cognitive engineering of ePartners in health and safety, which enhance the social, cognitive, and affective processes in human-agent teams.

Ayesha Nilashini is a PhD candidate at the School of Computing, Engineering, and Mathematical Sciences at La Trobe University, Australia. With over a decade of experience as a Business Analyst and Project Manager in the field of information technology and as a certified Scrum Master, Ayesha specializes in leveraging digital technologies to drive innovation in healthcare. Their research, "Digital Transformation in Healthcare: The Case of Personalised Self-Management for Wellness and Healthier Lifestyle Understanding," focuses on designing intelligent, patient-centered systems that promote sustainable healthcare solutions.

Zara Page is a final year PhD candidate at the Centre for Healthy Brain Ageing at UNSW Sydney. Her PhD investigates the impact of linguistic and acculturation factors on the neuropsychological assessment performance of older adults from culturally and linguistically diverse (CALD) backgrounds. She is also a Research Assistant at NARI in the Division of Social Gerontology, working on a digital and culturally adapted support program for dementia carers.

Ming-Chyi Pai is a Professor of neurology and gerontology at National Cheng Kung University (NCKU). He heads the Alzheimer's Disease Research Center (ADRC) at NCKU Hospital and is the Principal Investigator of series of projects on spatial navigation ability of people with cognitive impairment, and many multicentre, randomized, double-blind, placebo-controlled trials involving patients with Alzheimer's disease or related dementias.

Bobby Redman is a Retired Psychologist, living on the Central Coast of NSW. Bobby, who was diagnosed with frontotemporal dementia in 2015, is passionate about her consumer advocacy work. She is the immediate past Chair of the Dementia Australia Advisory Committee, sits on the Central Coast Dementia Alliance Committee and chairs the Central Coast Living with Dementia Advisory Group. She is involved in several research projects, sitting on a range of Steering/Advisory Committees. Bobby is a strong Community Member and is also a Rotarian and Red Cross Volunteer. In 2020, Bobby was nominated for the NSW Senior Australian of the Year award.

Joyce Siette, Associate Professor, is a health services researcher whose mission is to contribute to reducing population-wide dementia risk and cognitive impairment through effective and acceptable dementia prevention public health approaches. She currently leads a program of research to identify how we can best prevent dementia by creating effective lifestyle changes for seniors such as sustained physical activity and healthy diet. Her dementia awareness campaigns (e.g., Brain Bootcamp, Re-Imagine), which uses everyday activities of cognitive training, socialisation and physical activity have supported more than 6000 older adults' brain health and wellbeing.

Luuk P.A. Simons, Founder and Director of *Health Coach Program*, helping employers with long-term health and productivity of their employees. Besides, he is a senior research fellow at Delft University of Technology. He focusses on ICT-enabled coaching and bioinformatics feedback for effective health self-management and tooling for improving the health literacy of health professionals.

Gurdeep Singh is associated with the Humanise Lab of Laureate Prof. John Grundy (IEEE Fellow) at FIT Monash University and ITTC Centre for Optimal Ageing. His research is a collaboration with Future Wellness Group, working alongside Innovation Director Mark Foley to develop machine learning (ML) and AI-driven solutions for personal and future health predictions, utilizing wearable IoT technologies for dementia care and delivering real-time and semantic solutions for patient monitoring. His interests are in wearable IoT, data science, ML, AI frameworks, IT services, and software-oriented solutions for healthcare and activity monitoring including sports management. Affiliation-HumaniSE Lab, ITTC Optimal Ageing, Monash University.

Kate Swaffer is a PhD Candidate at the University of South Australia, School of Justice and Society, investigating human rights in post diagnostic dementia care. Her other research includes dementia rehabilitation, and reparations and redress for harm to people living in residential aged care. Swaffer is an highly published author and award-winning disability rights global campaigner. She has been a major catalyst for rehabilitation for people with dementia, and for dementia to be managed as a disability, including equal access to the CRPD. She has a MSc (Dementia Care), Bachelor of Psychology, Bachelor of Arts in Professional and Creative writing, Graduate Diploma in Grief Counselling, and is a retired nurse and retired chef.

Antonia Thodis is a Research Fellow at The George Institute for Global Health with Nutrition Science and Food Policy. She is a trained clinical and research dietitian with expertise in behavioural change strategies, stakeholder and participant engagement, mixed methods research including randomized clinical dietary intervention trials, and culturally responsive digital health interventions for successful ageing and prevention and management of chronic diseases such as dementia and type 2 diabetes in vulnerable and ethnically diverse communities in Australia and internationally.

Nalika Ulapane is a researcher who integrates mathematical modelling, engineering systems design, data analytics, and design science research principles to address challenges in complex systems, including healthcare. He has held various research and teaching positions at several institutions, including the University of Technology Sydney, the University of Melbourne, La Trobe University, Swinburne University of Technology, and the Olivia Newton-John Cancer Wellness & Research Centre. Additionally, Dr. Ulapane serves in several editorial roles for books and academic journals that focus on the application of artificial intelligence in healthcare.

Sheng-Hsiang Yang is a Neurologist at Chi-Mei Medical Center, with clinical and research interests in neurodegenerative diseases and behavioural neurology. Department of Neurology, Chi Mei Medical Center, Tainan, Taiwan.

Foreword

In this timely, forward looking and optimistic book, **Digital Convergence – to provide Better Solutions for People with Dementia, edited by Professor Nilmini Wickramasinghe, Dr Thu Ha Dang, Associate Professor Tuan Nyugen, and Dr Sasan Adibi,** the editors lay out, in a series of crisply written chapters, a series of diverse digital health solutions that seek to address the challenges of diagnosing, managing, and empowering people living with dementia as well as offering novel approaches to supporting caregivers and health professionals in their dementia management roles.

The wide range of digital health solutions examined and expounded in the 17 chapters covers key issues pertaining to the rationale, design, development, deployment, and safe and effective uptake of both conventional and emerging digital health technologies applicable to addressing dementia diagnosis and management. By seeking to ensure that each of the chapters delves into the problems, opportunities, and potential solutions, but also the risks, enabling requirements and further work to be done to achieve their full potential, the editors have assembled a rich and highly informative collection of fascinating and promising advances.

Above all, the book provides the reader with a grounded perspective on the types of digital technologies presently in development, and especially the science underpinning the rationale for the approach to each of them.

This outstanding book provides the reader with a rich understanding of how such technologies offer the potential to deploy new, highly effective tools for ways of diagnosing and managing dementia, significantly improve the quality of life for people living with dementia, and, above all, offer hope and support for their caregivers and loved ones.

I wholeheartedly recommend the book to all readers who are interested to learn about leading edge digital technology trends that hold the promise of significantly improving dementia management and quality of life for people living with dementia.

John Zelcer
La Trobe University

Preface

Dementia is a deeply personal, challenging, and complex experience for people living with the condition and for their families, loved ones, and communities providing care. Moreover, it can be complicated and challenging for healthcare practitioners to treat people living with dementia due to the inherent nuances of the condition and often lack of full and complete information. Given our rapidly increasing aging population, the presence of dementia is also, as to be expected, exponentially increasing. Currently, while there appears to be no cure for all sufferers of dementia, we are able to slow down its progress in many instances and enable people with dementia to have a better quality of life for longer as well as support their loved ones, family, and friends.

Pushing the frontiers of science and technology could hold the key and serve to reshape and reimagine the future of dementia care – and have a profound and dramatic human impact. This book then explores the opportunities and possibilities that technology, most especially all varieties of digital health solutions, can play in this regard. While dementia is a sad and debilitating condition, advances in digital health solutions hold the promise of a light at the end of the tunnel.

The 17 chapters serve as a miscellany of critical issues with respect to the opportunities for digital health solutions to ameliorate the situation for the person living with dementia and/or their loved one or carer. Specifically, they cover the following topics:

Chapter 1, Digital Solutions for People with Dementia: Possibilities and Pitfalls by Kate Swaffer, Discusses the advances in digital solutions which provide the opportunity for addressing needs and supporting people living with dementia. This chapter presents both the possibilities and the pitfalls of such digital solutions for people with dementia.

Chapter 2, Family Carers: A Personal Journey Recounted by Chaousis, provides much illumination and insight into the challenges and issues faced by family carers of people living with dementia.

Chapter 3, The Role of Digital Twins Powered/Enabled through AI for People with Dementia by Wickramasinghe, serves to outline how by incorporating digital twins, it is possible to provide simultaneously more personalized and precise care for people with dementia as well as have a better idea of the likely progress of the disease.

Chapter 4, Empowering Patient Care: Leveraging Artificial Intelligence and Internet of Things for Enhanced Healthcare Delivery by Helena Bahrami and Sasan Adibi, examines the dynamic interplay between artificial intelligence (AI) and the Internet of Things (IoT), and their profound impact on healthcare, especially in enhancing care for patients with Alzheimer's disease and related dementias. It delves into the role of IoT devices, equipped with various sensors, in advancing a more sophisticated approach to healthcare delivery by enabling continuous, real-time monitoring in both clinical and home settings.

Chapter 5, Advancing Dementia Care: AI and Machine Learning in Diagnosis and Drug Discovery by Helena Bahrami and Sasan Adibi, presents an in-depth exploration of how artificial intelligence (AI) and machine learning (ML) are transforming the diagnosis, treatment, and drug discovery processes for dementia, including Alzheimer's disease (AD) and other forms such as Lewy body, frontotemporal, vascular, and mixed dementia. It begins with a detailed examination of dementia's complexity, outlining its various forms and the unique pathological and clinical characteristics distinguishing them. The narrative then delves into the crucial role of clinical and demographic data in refining diagnostic precision, discussing essential diagnostic tools like neuroimaging (PET, fMRI, MRI, EEG) and biological markers from blood tests, alongside factors such as smoking, alcohol use, education, and socioeconomic status.

Chapter 6, Conversational Agents in Healthcare: Leveraging Language Models and Chatbots for Patient Interaction by Helena Bahrami and Sasan Adibi, provides a detailed examination of the application of Natural Language Processing (NLP) and conversational agents, such as chatbots, in the healthcare sector, with a particular focus on supporting patients with dementia and Alzheimer's disease (AD). It delves into how these AI-driven technologies are utilized to develop user-friendly interfaces that not only improve patient engagement but also bolster communication and enhance therapeutic interventions. The chapter scrutinizes the effectiveness of these tools in fostering social interaction, supporting mental health, and reducing caregiver burdens through sustained patient engagement and interactive dialogue.

Chapter 7, Artificial Intelligence for Dementia by Balongun and Adibi, underscores the pivotal role for artificial intelligence in developing digital health solutions to diagnose and treat people living with dementia more effectively, efficiently, and efficaciously.

Chapter 8, Mobile and Platforms, Sensors, and IoT (Internet of Things): Smart Dementia Networks (SDNs) Devising on Real-Time Wearable IoT Platforms by Gurdeep Singh, presents, Smart Dementia Networks (SDNs) or solutions with high-level architecture, use-cases or scenarios to counter and promote healthcare with the use of wearable IoT dementia frameworks, in comparison to other disorders rectified or monitored on these frameworks, especially corresponding to Human-Computer Interaction (HCI) in the form of respective and responsive Graphical User Interfaces (GUIs).

Chapter 9, Opportunities for Digital Health Solutions in Dementia Care: A Scoping Review by Ayesha Nilashini, explores key opportunities and challenges in implementing and adopting these technologies, including barriers such as data privacy, digital literacy, and integration into existing healthcare infrastructures. The findings highlight the transformative potential of digital health innovations to enhance early diagnosis, personalized care, and continuous monitoring through sustainable user engagement. However, to fully experience these benefits, significant challenges in accessibility, trust, scalability, and effectiveness must be addressed. By identifying these gaps, this chapter outlines strategies for advancing the widespread adoption and sustainability of digital health solutions in dementia care.

Chapter 10, Using Digital Tools to Detect Spatial Navigation Impairment in Early Alzheimer's Disease by Pai and Yang, highlights the opportunities afforded by digital tools to enable early detection of Alzheimer's.

Chapter 11, Digital Solutions to Empower Multicultural Families Impacted by Dementia by Antoniades and Siette, unpacks many of the critical and yet at times subtle nuances multicultural or CALD populations face in the context of dementia and getting the required assistance.

Chapter 12, Digital Solutions in Dementia Treatment, Care, and Support by Upasana Baruah and Zara Page, explores the role of digital solutions in enhancing dementia treatment, care, and support. It examines a range of technologies, including digital cognitive assessments, telemedicine, wearable devices, mobile applications, and AI, highlighting their potential to improve diagnosis, monitoring, and personalized care.

Chapter 13, Incorporating AI with a Multilingual Virtual Helper for Dementia Carers in Australia: A Case Study by Ulapane et al., describes the unique role of an intelligent agent or chatbot for supporting CALD populations, who consist of people living with dementia and who currently experience great helplessness and vulnerability.

Chapter 14, Co-Design of Digital Health Interventions in Dementia by Gaffy et al., focuses on co-design, which involves bringing together people with professional and lived experience in design processes to collaboratively identify problems and develop solutions, and the importance of incorporating co-design principles when designing and developing solutions to support people living with dementia.

Chapter 15, The Potential of Digital Solutions for Caregivers of Individuals with Dementia by Czaja and Gitlin, focusses on the opportunities of digital health solutions to support and assist carers of people with dementia to best navigate the road ahead.

Chapter 16, Dementia Empowerment With Heart Health Intervention And LLM-Based Health AI Research Assistant by Simons et al., proposes a design approach with two empowerment options for patients, caregivers and their health professionals. Firstly, it describes how cardiac health successes in enticing senior citizens to large lifestyle improvements may be used for treating early-stage dementia and cognitive decline. Biologically, this uses causality between blood pressure and cardiovascular health on the one hand and dementia outcomes on the other. Practically, it enables daily success feedback, which empowers patients in their health improvement experiments. Secondly, it describes and user-tests an AI Health Research Assistant to extract the best available lifestyle findings from literature, to keep up with the 100,000s of new health publications flooding us every year. Our user test highlights challenges and opportunities for a Health AI, especially regarding claim transparency, data quality, and risks of hallucinations.

Chapter 17, Digital Twins of Dementia Patients for Clinical Decision Support by Wickramasinghe and Ulapane, provides a cutting-edge application of digital twins to support clinical decision-making in the context of dementia.

Epilogue, We hope that our colleagues, students, fellow researchers, healthcare professionals, families of people living with dementia, and even people living with dementia may find the contents of the following pages inspiring, providing a little ray of hope and perhaps also ignite further research into this much-needed area.

Happy Reading
The Editors
Nilmini Wickramasinghe,
Thu Ha Dang, Tuan Anh Nguyen,
and Sasan Adibi Melbourne, Feb 2025

1

Digital Solutions for People Living with Dementia: Possibilities and Pitfalls

Kate Swaffer

1.1 Introduction

The rapid global increase in dementia prevalence has generated an increasing interest in accessible and affordable solutions to support people living with dementia (PLWD) in managing their disabilities, maintaining independence and mobility and accessing appropriate care. This demand also extends to support for their care partners and family members (CPFM). In parallel, technology and software developers have shown increasing interest in this area, recognising the potential for profits in creating tools and software for this growing population. Neurodegenerative dementia diseases cause progressive cognitive and functional decline. As Olazarán et al. (2010) highlight, the consequences of these symptoms can be mitigated through timely and appropriate interventions. By 2024, many such interventions are delivered via digital solutions, including assistive technologies. This shift raises important questions about both the potential benefits and limitations of digital health tools in improving post-diagnostic care for PLWD and support for their families.

It remains unclear whether digital solutions truly lead to early detection, improved support, better clinical outcomes or greater patient satisfaction. Despite this uncertainty, development in the field continues at pace. A significant concern is the limited and often inequitable involvement of PLWD in the research and development of the widely praised "digital solutions." Their participation is too often tokenistic, more about strengthening grant applications than ensuring their voices shape meaningful outcomes. This issue requires urgent attention.

This chapter explores whether emerging digital technologies can advance, rather than compromise, the human rights of PLWD and the broader community. At first glance, technology presents exciting new possibilities, especially for people receiving care in community or residential aged care settings. Yet there is a real risk that these tools could intrude upon and infringe on

DOI: 10.1201/9781003485681-1

people's human rights. At the same time, everyday technologies, from GPS navigation in cars or smartphones, to tools like ChatGPT for writing, predictive text, or voice assistance tools like Siri, have become increasingly useful and integrated into daily life. These developments show that when thoughtfully designed and implemented, digital tools can enhance independence and convenience and potentially improve quality of life.

1.1.1 Dementia as a Disability

Beyond its biomedical definition, the World Health Organization (WHO) also defines dementia as "a major cause of disability and dependence globally" (World Health Organization, 2023). Each year, about 10 million people develop dementia, and in 2019, an estimated 57 million people were living with the condition (Steinmetz et al, 2019), a number projected to increase to 152.8 million by 2050.

These figures strengthen the growing evidence that dementia poses a significant global challenge, and highlight the need to better support and enable PLWD to maintain independence for longer.

In Australia, an estimated 450,000 people live with dementia, including approximately 30,000 people with younger onset dementia (YOD). Sixty-five percent of people with dementia live in the community, a figure expected to rise as more people want to remain and die in their own homes rather than in institutional settings such as nursing homes. An estimated 1.7 million people provide informal care of PLWD (Dementia Australia, 2023). Dementia is the leading cause of death among women and the second leading cause of death among men in Australia. Additionally, more than 68.1% of PLWD living in aged care facilities have cognitive impairments despite lacking a formal diagnosis. Globally, dementia is the seventh leading cause of death (World Health Organization, 2023).

The biomedical model of dementia focuses on impairments and deficits, framing limitations as intrinsic to the individual and the disease. In contrast, the social model of disability views disabilities as a product of social and environmental barriers, which Longino (2020) refers to as "socially produced dependency" (Longino, 2020). It is an important concept, when we consider the WHO statement that dementia is a major cause of disability and dependence, and then compare the current biomedical model and post-diagnostic pathways for PLWD against the post-diagnostic pathways for people with other neurological conditions, such as traumatic brain injury (TBI), multiple sclerosis and stroke, or indeed with other pathways for critical illnesses such as cancer.

Despite decades of research and advocacy, there has been little global progress in delivering health and social care services that have actually improved outcomes for PLWD. Attitudes have remained negative to and about PLWD (Alzheimer's Disease International (ADI), 2019, 2024; Chang & Hsu, 2020), and stigma has not improved (ADI, 2019, 2024; Chang & Hsu, 2020). Access to timely and accurate diagnosis, as well as comprehensive post-diagnostic support also remains elusive (ADI, 2024; Day et al, 2022).

Crucially, PLWD are often denied recognition that their symptoms constitute acquired cognitive disabilities. As a result, they are frequently excluded from disability assessment and do not receive proactive disability-related supports. Unlike individuals with other degenerative conditions, such as stroke or TBI, those of us living with dementia are not routinely referred to rehabilitation services designed to improve quality of life, maintain independence and agency, and avoid or delay the need for institutional care (Cations et al, 2020). Furthermore, environments, both in the community and in residential care, are often not designed with accessibility or dementia-inclusive principles in mind (Fleming et al, 2020). This lack of inclusive design continues to limit the ability of PLWD to live with independence, agency and self-determination, and a sustained quality of life.

1.1.2 Digital Technology, Assisted Technology and AI

Digital technology (DT), assistive technology (AT) and artificial intelligence (AI) are increasingly being seen as critical tools in the diagnosis of dementia, as well as the provision of the care of PLWD in the community and in institutional assisted living settings, and they even have the potential to improve the lives of people with disabilities due to a diagnosis of dementia. They have also meant there is an increasing "digitisation" of our world, which can feel confronting, but it is often helpful. There are likely as many possibilities as there are pitfalls for society in general. Technologies also claim to improve productivity, and even the "client" experience, but it is important to question whether they are morally appropriate or ethical, and whether they really do improve diagnosis and care of PLWD, or indeed, whether they are doing harm. It is critical to investigate and better understand the pitfalls, not only the possibilities, when developing and implementing technologies claiming to support PLWD and CPFM. They come in many forms and functions, including wheelchairs and white canes to digital solutions such as speech recognition or captioning.

The emergence of technologies which many people with and without dementia already use include video calls using platforms such as Zoom, Google Meet and Teams, voice activated assistance such as Alexa, smart watches for health, falls and exercise monitoring, mobile phone apps for daily reminders, managing photo collections and so on, and safety sensors that monitor food and hydration intake, falls, mobility and so on. These are useful tools, but further investigation is required to assess the potential pitfalls, such as how invasive they are of each individual's privacy, the level of cybersecurity needed to protect individuals, and whether they are being used unlawfully, such as without a person's knowledge or consent to influence decision making, frauds and scams.

Technologies such as these can support PLWD to proactively manage their disabilities, enabling them to maintain independence and continue engaging in productive and meaningful activities, often beyond what they or others believed possible. They support PLWD in pursuing activities that hold personal value, and may help reduce the stigma, shame, apathy, depression, discrimination, isolation and loneliness that frequently accompany a dementia diagnosis. By doing so, they can also help reduce social inequalities stemming from a loss of identity. Importantly, these tools promote meaningful, positive and individualised engagement and offer PLWD a sense of personal achievement and dignity. In addition to digital tools, there are many low-cost, low-risk strategies, which I refer to as "life enhancement strategies," or "soft technologies," such as laminated reminder sheets or reading panels. Despite their simplicity, these approaches can be highly effective yet are often overlooked or undervalued by those providing care.

Digital technologies have transformed nearly every aspect of our lives, from how we live, communicate, and work, to how we play and even how we sleep. Technology developers often promote these innovations as tools to increase profitability, boost speed to market for products and enhance customer satisfaction and loyalty. However, a critical gap remains. Technologies designed specifically for PLWD often exclude them from the research and development process. This disconnect limits the effectiveness and relevance of these tools for the very individuals they are meant to support.

Broadly, DT refers to the application of scientific or engineering knowledge in the creation and practical use of digital or computerised devices, methods and systems. These technologies include electronic tools that generate, store or process data. Examples include social media platforms, online games, multimedia tools and mobile phones. AT is related but distinct concept. It refers to adaptive and rehabilitative devices designed to support with disabilities and the elderly, helping them maintain or improve their functional abilities and quality of life.

Many people say they have a "love–hate" relationship with DT, and some describe it as the 21st-century version of an online "Big Brother." Ironically, it is often said that most people use iPhones, so whether they love or hate it, they are using AI, AT and DT regularly. However, access remains inequitable. According to the United States Census Bureau International Database (IDB) (2025), the global population was estimated at 8 billion in 2022. Nevertheless, the most recent data indicates there are approximately 1.382 billion active iPhone users worldwide (Backlinko Team, 2025). This gap highlights that DT is still far from universally accessible, leaving billions of people not only shielded from its potential downsides but also excluded from its many benefits.

People with disabilities often have difficulty performing activities of daily living (ADLs) independently, or even with assistance. AT can ameliorate the effects of disabilities that limit the ability to perform ADLs. AT promotes greater independence by enabling people to perform tasks they were formerly unable to accomplish, or had difficulty with, either by enhancing their capabilities or by offering alternative ways of interacting with their environment.

In its broadest sense, AI refers to the intelligence demonstrated by machines, particularly computer systems. AI is a branch of computer science focused on developing methods and software that enable machines to perceive their environment, learn from experience, and take actions that maximise their chances of achieving defined goals.

One person living with dementia, whom I spoke to about the possibilities and the pitfalls of AT shared the following insight:

> Well, if researchers and developers took the care and time to ask PLWD who are early in their disease trajectory what they actually needed and wanted, and included us end to end in the development, we might actually make some progress. Currently we are viewed as waking up one day in the very late stages of dementia and being unable to provide meaningful contribution. I can think of a hundred pieces of AT that would help me function and stay (and feel) safe, but instead I'm offered AT for people with physical disability. There is so very much potential, but instead we live in a world where it is still easier to provide AT that might make life easier for our paid and unpaid carers and supporters. Systemic risk aversion also deeply limits creativity and innovation in this space, as well as structural ageism. For example the NDIS refused an OT request for a shower temperature modulator as 'my partner should be showering me before he goes to work at 6am, and I'd be in residential care soon anyway, so it wasn't deemed value for money.
>
> **2024, PLWD**

1.1.3 Possibilities

Technology offers numerous benefits and possibilities, especially for individuals living with disabilities, including those affected by dementia. It can provide vital support for ADLs[1] and promote greater independence by enabling individuals to perform tasks independently. In doing so, it fosters confidence, independence, agency and self-reliance.[2] It can also improve quality of life by facilitating participation in activities, employment and hobbies. Communication devices, such as speech-to-text, text-to-speech, and other assistive platforms, play a crucial role, as the ability to communicate is strongly linked to quality of life.

Mobility aids and home modifications can reduce the risk of accidents and falls, creating a safer living environment for PLWD. In education and employment, technology supports equal and accessible participation by helping individuals with disabilities access resources and accommodations. For care partners, technology can alleviate some of the demands of daily caregiving, reducing stress and freeing up time for other responsibilities, including their own self-care. Finally, technologies and assistive devices can support individuals to engage more fully in activities, social and community, including hobbies, reducing isolation through fostering a sense of community and belonging. These benefits help to emphasise how technologies can positively impact individuals with and without disabilities including those with dementia, and their families and care partners, as well as society as a whole.

While many find it invasive and pervasive, others, both with and without dementia, consider it to be incredibly helpful as an aid to maintain independence, productivity, mobility, and even agency and identity. This is largely due to the increased access it provides to individualised and meaningful engagement. Here I share a personal example of how helpful it has been for me.

About eight years ago, one of my sons offered me some practical advice after overhearing me say how frustrating it was not being able to remember the names of the artists and music I love listening to. He said: "Hey mum, why don't you set up a play list now that you can't remember the names of the music you like?" If only it was that easy. I responded: "I'd love to do that, but I can't remember what music I like." The downloading of an App called Shazam helped me not only find the music I liked, but together my son and I were able to set up some playlists on my phone. It was the best gift he'd ever given me. The added bonus is it was free, and now that AI is more widespread, Sonos and Apple provide me with playlists selected by AI, including my own "channel," with music that is based on what artists and music I play frequently. For me, it is a positive outcome of "Big Brother."

1.1.4 Pitfalls

On the flip side, technologies also have significant potential to do harm and can further deny PLWD their human rights. Their development has largely been exclusive of equitable inclusion of PLWD rather than their proxies, who they are intended to support. The rise of "digital dementia," and of voice cloning, scams, identity theft, deep fakes, financial abuse, prescription hacking and so on, are just a few of the pitfalls facing society, and potentially worse for people with cognitive disabilities that are also progressive, increasing the person's capacity to detect potential fraud or scams. Technology, specifically digital transactions, can also provide challenges. For example, "spoofing" is a tactic used by scammers to disguise their identities and impersonate legitimate senders, often leading to serious financial consequences to individuals who have been spoofed. One concerning trend involves email scams that target families arranging aged care for a family member. Scammers have been known to gain access to personal email accounts, intercept communications and manipulate payment details to redirect significant sums of money into their own accounts. The increasing voice cloning trend also means the increasing misuse of voice cloning. In milliseconds, scammers can clone a voice and then quickly and easily convince people into thinking, for example, that a trusted friend or family member urgently needs money. There are many warnings issued to the public, and these types of scams have the potential to impact millions of people. As technology makes it easier for criminals to invade our personal spaces, staying cautious about its use is more important than ever. The economic cost of scams, spoofing and hacking to

Australians is substantial. For example, the ACCC reported that Australians lost over 3 billion dollars to scammers in 2022.[3]

From the perspective of someone living with dementia, tokenistic inclusion is still the norm, despite proclamations of co-design and collaboration. Too many things that impact PLWDa remain *about us, without us*, and are a global issue on most aspects of dementia research, care and development of services and supports, including technology.

The pitfalls of technology can be broad and far-reaching, encompassing issues such as privacy and security, dependence, health impact, eye strain, poor posture, repetitive strain injury, disrupted sleep and psychological effects including anxiety and depression, social isolation, job displacement, misinformation, environmental impact and the digital divide. Increased data collection, while often necessary, should prompt serious concerns about privacy and security for everyone. These concerns are particularly pressing for individuals with cognitive disabilities, who may be more vulnerable and marginalised due to their diagnosis. Cyber-attacks and data breaches are increasingly common, often with severe consequences.

Dependence and an over reliance on technology make some people more vulnerable, especially when systems fail, such as a server crashing. School children were recently quoted after participating in a school initiative to not use mobile phones or technology, that, "surprisingly, they felt more connected" without their phones. Other pitfalls of technology include the potential for lost employment or job displacement, because automation and AI can lead to job losses in certain sectors creating social and economic challenges. There is an impact on the environment from the production and disposal of electronic devices, which contribute to environmental degradation. The potential for misinformation, and the rapid spread, especially on social media, can lead to the dissemination of false information which impacts public opinion, behaviour as well as political campaigns and elections. Deep fakes are increasingly common. Finally, there is a digital divide between those with and without access to technology, which can exacerbate social, economic and political inequalities.

Many people, both with and without dementia, have strong concerns about personal security and the growing sense of coercive control of technology. These concerns are particularly acute when considering the potential harm to vulnerable populations, such as people with disabilities resulting from a dementia diagnosis.

> I have a love hate technology, I hate that it is breaking down family units, coming in between relationships. I believe it has good and bad and the trick is to use it so it is a good addition or tool, unfortunately it has created a whole new type of addictions. It is in my opinion is taking people's human connections away, creating a more singular focus rather than a community focus, whether that be family, community we live etc. Truthfully as much as I like some of the good, it terrifies me.
>
> **Person living with dementia**

Another example of a potential pitfall is people with addictions or addictive personalities, where the gambling industry in Australia is currently under intense scrutiny for corrupt and coercive marketing practices to problem gamblers. The Australian government and some state governments are considering legislation against gambling advertising, due to the strong link between exposure to betting advertising and riskier gambling behaviour.[4] There are risk factors for everyone, but the risk could be seen as higher in groups of people who are either vulnerable or marginalised, such as PLWD and indeed, living with other forms or causes of disability.

1.1.5 Smart Technology: "If It Is So Smart, Why Can't It Fix Itself?"

Smartwatches have the potential to transform dementia and also delirium care in line with policy shifts towards digital, community-based and preventative approaches. These wearable devices can continuously monitor vital signs, activity levels, sleep patterns and other physiological data, creating a digital record that, with the individual's or guardian's consent, can be assessed remotely by families, healthcare professionals and care providers. This aligns with the move from analogue to digital systems, allowing for more "efficient" and data-driven care. Unexpected changes in body data may indicate early signs of health problems, such as the onset of delirium in PLWD living in the community – and these might be picked up with an AI algorithm.

However, these benefits come with ethical and practical concerns. Continuous monitoring can be seen as invasive, even coercive, particularly when care decisions are based solely on data, leaving little room for individual autonomy, such as the right to choose not to shower or eat on a given day. Having widespread, continuous surveillance across community and care settings raises important human rights questions, especially around consent, privacy and dignity. Advocates for such tracking often argue that it's not the tracking per se which interests them, but the ability to "make decisions." This is a questionable stance, as the cybersecurity of individuals is certainly under threat. These developments call for careful ethical scrutiny and a rights-based approach to the design and deployment of such technologies.

In seeking feedback from PLWD for this chapter, one person with dementia said of "smart technology," using the example of smartwatches: "If smart technology is so damn smart, why doesn't it fix itself when it crashes????!!!!" It is a good point!

1.1.6 Human Rights, People Living with Dementia and Technology

International human rights foundations are applicable to everyone, including people with disability from dementia. The United Nations Convention on the Rights of Persons with Disabilities (UNCRPD) was adopted in 2006 (United Nations, 2006). The Articles of the UNCRPD clearly outline the rights of persons with disability, which include basic human rights to equal access to, for example, the right to health and rehabilitation, support to live independently, equitable access and inclusion and the right to be free from all forms of exploitation, coercion and all other forms of abuse. Legal recognition was given to the UNCRPD through the provision of international standardised frameworks as an essential part of an individual's independence and self-determination. The UNCRPD was developed to advance the human rights of all people with disabilities. It is particularly important in the context of dementia care, as it provides a clear, legally binding framework for ensuring the rights of individuals with dementia are respected. As a formal agreement between a country and the United Nations, the UNCRPD holds countries accountable for upholding these rights in law, policy and practice. It sets out a pathway for that country to improve the lives of people with disabilities by ensuring their human rights are recognised and met. Globally, most countries, including Australia, are falling behind in their human rights obligations as disabled persons, including PLWD, who still do not have equal access to their disability rights or equal access to health and social care.

The Australian Human Rights Commission in their research into technology for people with disability:

> … several applications of the technology created unique human rights risks. In Australia there are 4.4 million people with disability, and many neurotechnologies focus on medical applications. Cochlear implants have been used to restore functional hearing to an estimated 1 million people worldwide. Yet the implantation, or use, of neurotechnologies may unduly impact the human rights of people with disability under the Convention on the Rights of People with Disability. For example, there are no robust protections in place when people with disability's implants are decommissioned or made redundant.

If digital technologies are not developed and deployed ethically, they can pose risks to human rights. According to the Australian Human Rights Commission, three human rights repeatedly raised during consultations are the rights to privacy, non-discrimination and freedom of thought, which are considered in detail here. The right to privacy (protected under Article 17 of the International Covenant on Civil and Political Rights (ICCPR)) is particularly vulnerable. Many digital technologies have the capacity to – and do – collect and process sensitive personal information, creating a significant risk to individuals' privacy. Similarly, Article 18 of the ICCPR protects the right to freedom of thought – yet this right can be undermined by technologies that manipulate thought processes. For example, deepfakes, where AI is used to create fake images, videos and even audio, often involving celebrities[5] or politicians. These are increasingly being used to spread misinformation, abuse individuals and distort public discourse. The right to non-discrimination, protected under Articles 2 and 25 of the Universal Declaration of Human Rights, is also at risk. Without adequate safeguards, digital technologies could develop biases which unduly impact certain groups.

The Australian Royal Commission into Aged Care Quality and Safety (ACRC) framed dementia as a chronic, fatal health condition based on a pathologised, biomedical view and approach to it, rather than using a human rights framework. This approach allows continued human rights violations, and the ACRC found that PLWD and others receiving care have their "basic human rights denied. ... It is a shocking tale of neglect". This is in stark contrast to the approach of the Disability Royal Commission, which is grounded in a human rights framework informed by the UNCRPD. The ACRC failed to adequately consider the prevailing lack of access to justice for PLWD, both in the present and into the future, including their right to redress and reparative justice. Therefore, the ACRC did not sufficiently address existing rights violations and harm or offer recommendations to prevent future abuse of PLWD or older Australians accessing care now or in the future. The recent Australian National Dementia Action Plan consultation paper failed to reflect or even mention human rights for people with dementia and older Australians, or refer to dementia as a cause of disability, further indicating a 20th-century biomedical approach to dementia.

Notwithstanding the WHO defining dementia as "a major cause of disability and dependence among older people" for well over a decade, and recognition of this by the UNCRPD Committee and, for example, the then Special Rapporteur on the UNCRPD (Devandas-Aguilar & Catalina, 2019), no country has yet moved away from dementia as a biomedical chronic health condition, towards providing a post-diagnostic pathway that adequately supports dementia symptoms as disabilities. This gap is particularly relevant to the development of technology. PLWD remain largely excluded from meaningful participation in the design and development of technologies intended for their use. Decisions about what is deemed "best" for them are still predominantly made by those without dementia. Including 1-2 PLWD as advisors or in research projects is, at best, highly tokenistic and fails to reflect true co-design or inclusion.

Treating dementia as a condition causing disabilities could lead to very different treatment options and supports, including access to allied health, rehabilitation, support to equal access in the community, access to the CRPD and support to live at home. This is critical to maintaining a person's independence, quality of life and self-determination for longer as well as reducing the human and economic cost of dementia and is relevant to the discussion about the use of the various forms of AT.

1.1.7 Unequal Access to Technology: A Human Rights Violation

Digital technologies are appropriate and can be useful for both people with and without dementia, but reliable and affordable access to the internet is necessary. Banking, government and disability support, as well as participation in civic life, now require such access. In the United Kingdom, many general practice clinics no longer provide access to telephones to make appointments, insisting all appointments are booked online. This results in unequal access to healthcare for many people. Similarly, technology platforms that rely on stable access exclude large segments of the population from participating in fundamental aspects of life, effectively stripping them of agency. Accessible alternatives must be provided to ensure equitable access to information and promote individual autonomy. Many PLWD have a strong desire to use technology; however, the impediments can be overwhelming.

Generally, dementia and aged care workers and support workers often lack the necessary skills to support PLWD in using technology. This gap is often overlooked in training programs, despite much of the training being provided online. Yet, even if care and support workers were adequately trained, PLWD would still face the difficult trade-off of sacrificing their privacy in exchange for support, particularly in the absence of strong safeguards. This not only puts individuals' personal information at risk but also places the support worker in a difficult position. Hence, the development or review of all digital platforms must include the creation of accessible training modules tailored for people living with disability and their supporters. This training should also be available in multiple formats, not just digitally but also in print and through in-person sessions to ensure true inclusivity and accessibility.

Recognising the human rights of PLWD, both in the community and in long-term institutional care settings, requires ensuring their equal access to the CRPD and other international human rights instruments. This recognition must be accompanied by concrete strategies aimed at deinstitutionalisation and de-segregation, including within residential aged care institutions and secure dementia units. Such facilities should also be subject to regular monitoring as places of detention (Devandas-Aguilar, 2019; Grenfell, 2019). Also, upholding the rights of PLWD includes ensuring access to safe, appropriate and adequate services and supports, including technologies.

In 2016, the Australian government enabled eligibility for access to the National Disability Insurance Scheme (NDIS), if they met age, residency and functioning requirements. This enabled many people with young onset dementia living in Australia to move from aged care services to disability support providers. Importantly, this sets a global precedence by recognising in practice that dementia is a cause of disabilities. It also reinforces the rights of PLWD of all ages to access technologies that are affordable, accessible, usable, ethical and sustainable, and to be meaningfully involved in their development.

An estimated 2.4 billion people globally – 1 in 3 people – need some form of AT. These include hearing aids, wheelchairs, walking sticks, medication dispensing packs, eyeglasses and prosthetic limbs. For people with disabilities, not having access to these vital lifelines means being locked out of education, accessing healthcare and having a full and equitable livelihood compared to people without disability. About 18% of Australians have disability, including from dementia, and people with disabilities face vast discrepancies between health, social and economic outcomes compared to those without disabilities. For example, while 65% of Australians without disability have excellent or very good health outcomes, only 24% of adults with disability experience the same health outcomes (AIHW, 2022).

Many opportunities are taken for granted in developed countries such as the United States of America, Canada, England and Australia. In low-income countries, only 10% of people have the AT they need, in stark contrast to 90% of people in need in high-income countries. In some countries, that access is estimated to be as low as 3%, which is clearly unacceptable (WHO[6]).

Sunstein provides multiple examples of technologies that support functioning and inclusion for our daily lives, such as GPS or alarm clock:

> In daily life, a GPS device is an example of a nudge; so is an app that tells people how many calories they ate during the previous day; so is a text message that informs customers that a bill is due or that a doctor's appointment is scheduled for the next day; so is an alarm clock; so is automatic enrolment in a pension plan; so are the default settings on computers and cell phones; so is a system for automatic payment of credit card bills and mortgages. In government, nudges include graphic warnings for cigarettes; labels for energy efficiency or fuel economy; "nutrition facts" panels on food; MyPlate, which provides a simple guide for healthy eating (see choosemyplate.gov); default rules for public-assistance programs (as in "direct certification" of the eligibility of poor children for free school meals); a website like data.gov or data.gov.uk, which makes a large number of datasets available to the public; and even the design of government websites, which list certain items first and in large fonts.
>
> **Sunstein (2019, p59)**

All change brings with it both possibilities and pitfalls, but perhaps more so when we consider digital technologies. One noteworthy example is the adoption of electronic health records, which affect everyone, not just PLWD, and have brought an increased risk to our private health information. Cybersecurity has become a major concern, and within aged and dementia care, a critical issue is the capacity of the providers to fund and maintain adequate cybersecurity measures. In the USA, 385 billion e-Health records have been breached,[7] with patients' data stolen, and potentially ending up on the dark web, mirroring a recent incident involving the data of 645 NDIS clients in Australia.[8] Yeo and Banfield (2022) suggest "The healthcare sector continues to be the industry suffering one of the highest costs of a data security breach. Healthcare lags behind other industries in cybersecurity preparedness despite advances in cybersecurity technologies." This not only highlights the increased risk to all individuals accessing healthcare but also suggests the urgent need to assess the increased risks faced by particularly vulnerable groups. These include people with cognitive disabilities due to dementia, and people with psychosocial or intellectual disabilities. Notably, university ethics committees place these cohorts into the highest risk category, yet this classification is often overlooked by both technology developers and service providers, who may prioritise efficiency or cost-saving over ethical considerations and data protection.

Assistive technologies can be transformative tools, often essential for enabling people with disabilities to participate fully in society and their communities, on an equal basis with others. Without access to AT, too many people with disabilities are locked out of social, educational and employment opportunities. There is a need to work to support the calls for coordinated AT procurement systems, along with training in maintenance and use, so that both AT users and providers can unlock the benefit of their assistive devices for years to come.

The Paralympic Games are an excellent example of the transformative power of AT to unlock potential. From advanced prosthetics to adaptive wheelchairs, these technologies not only enhance performance but also foster inclusivity and equal participation. They also highlight the reality that people with disabilities due to a diagnosis of dementia are being denied equal access to technology, except, perhaps, for those technologies that align with the business or strategic direction of service providers, healthcare professionals and society more broadly.

In a series published on The Conversation on the great internet letdown,[9] the internet used to be more fun and less invasive in the past. Furthermore, the information was more accurate, more informative, and far less inundated with misinformation and advertisements. It was more user-friendly and populated by real people, not content provided by platforms such as ChatGPT and other forms of AI. Social media was predominantly used for connecting with close family and friends, or for connecting within specific communities, such as academic groups with similar research topics using hashtags to connect and collaborate, and to find information. It was not used so persistently or often for fuelling outrage. As stated in the newsletter from the Conversation promoting this series, "Bizarre AI-generated slop wasn't at the top of everyone's feeds. What happened?" Marc Cheong and Wonsun Shin suggest the biggest problem is that financial motives drive much of the content now[10]; "Between incessant advertising and opaque algorithms fed with surveillance-level user data, we are getting less of what we want when going online." The increased drive for profit has created as many pitfalls and harm as it has created positive opportunities and possibilities.

1.1.8 Alternative Perspectives through Collaboration with People with Dementia

Globally, numerous human rights are routinely denied to the majority of PLWD. These include a lack of access to healthcare, denial of rehabilitation services, exclusion from disability assessments and supports, and broader rights violations linked to poverty, inadequate housing and food insecurity. Such systemic failures also restrict access to ethically developed and implemented AI. Crucially, the voices of those with the living experience of dementia, as well as their CPFM, are frequently overlooked, or more troublingly, heard but ultimately ignored.

What people need from the time of diagnosis of dementia is not only knowledge about dementia and the disabilities the symptoms cause, but involvement in the development of, and equal access to digital technologies, as well as more practical support for the disabilities acquired due to dementia, otherwise referred to as symptoms. People without dementia are proactively supported with disability support, and for example, reasonable accommodations in the workplace or a tertiary institution, such as people born with dyslexia or autism. Everyone has the right to receive disability support throughout their lives.

The list of disabilities listed below, which are caused by or related to a number of the symptoms of dementia, has been revised from one published in 2016 (Swaffer, p. 224). Most can be well managed with disability support for a person with dementia to maintain some level of functioning and independence, and include disabilities such as:

- Apraxia (a motor speech disorder making it hard to speak)
- Acquired dyslexia (difficulty breaking words into sounds or letters when reading)
- Dysgraphia (difficulty with the act of writing)
- Progressive Aphasias, such as Primary Progressive Aphasia (word finding or understanding, expressing thoughts or changes in comprehension abilities)
- Vision impairment (related to changes in the area of the brain that processes visual information coming from the eyes)
- Spatial or other sight impairment (affecting mobility, depth perception, spatial awareness)
- Learning difficulties that require support
- Memory impairment, e.g., retention of new information
- Organisation and planning abilities may be impaired

Highlighting the symptoms of dementia as disabilities is critical to further strengthen the need for a rights-based approach in all aspects of diagnosing and supporting PLWD, and the necessity to be provided with disability support, using all forms of technology, alongside what I refer to as "soft" technology, as referred to earlier. It also highlights the need for equal access to the CRPD, in the same way people with other disabilities have.

In a post on the social media platform X by Neil Crowther[11], he stated in relation to a "Pitch by tech company on LinkedIn 'We have developed a new way to *monitor vulnerable people at home* - it's never 'to support you to live safe and well in the place you call home' is it?" he posts, "I think tech could play a profoundly valuable role in putting more power in people's hands. But it's so curiously paternalistic & the overriding driver is demand management & savings." In "A digital cage is still a cage," Crowther and McGregor ask us to consider how "new and emerging digital technologies advance, rather than put at risk, the human rights of older people who draw on social care?"

Taking a Pollyanna approach to using digital technologies may be doing more harm than is currently evident, as it ignores the very real injustices faced by people with dementia and older persons who often have limited access to digital technologies, and who may be harmed, due to age related access issues (for example, many older people do not have the internet), and the added vulnerability faced by PLWD of all ages. While there is significant anecdotal evidence through their confidential and free peer-to-peer support groups provided by Dementia Alliance International for its members who all live with dementia, that digital technologies have been embraced by people with young onset dementia, PLWD may not have fully understood the negative consequences. The ethical factors, or perhaps the lack of a truly ethical approach to the development of technologies, are less understood.

Using the example of smart watches, by enabling remote monitoring, smartwatches and various other technologies can support the shift from hospital-based care to community-based care, and PLWD can be monitored in their homes or care facilities, reducing the need for frequent hospital visits. This is highly debatable whether it is a positive or negative impact, as reduced face-to-face interaction can intensify feelings of loneliness and social isolation. Devices can alert care partners, family members and paid carers, or healthcare providers to changes in the person's routine, including eating and drinking habits, as well as measurable health markers such as heart rate or falls. Smartwatches can be programmed to provide reminders for medication, hydration and other activities that help maintain independence and mobility such as reminders for exercise routines. Smartwatches can enhance the quality of life and independence of PLWD while reducing CPFM stress. Features like GPS tracking add an additional layer of safety. By providing this support in the community setting, smartwatches help delay the need for more intensive care interventions, aligning with the moving focus by governments, researchers and healthcare professionals towards prevention and community-based care.

Who knows what the future holds, but digital technologies are here to stay, so it is critical we get used to them, as well as ensure they are not only robust, but accessible and ethical for everyone, including people with dementia.

Notes

1 https://www.who.int/news-room/fact-sheets/detail/assistive-technology
2 https://stjudes.com.au/news/what-is-assistive-technology-and-how-is-it-beneficial/
3 https://www.accc.gov.au/media-release/accc-calls-for-united-front-as-scammers-steal-over-3bn-from-australians
4 https://aifs.gov.au/research/research-snapshots/gambling-participation-experience-harm-and-community-views
5 https://www.businesstoday.in/technology/news/story/hollywood-going-the-ai-way-how-the-new-indiana-jones-movie-de-aged-actor-harrison-ford-390481-2023-07-19
6 https://www.who.int/news-room/fact-sheets/detail/assistive-technology
7 https://www.healthcaredive.com/news/cybersecurity-hacking-healthcare-breaches/643821/
8 https://www.itnews.com.au/news/data-of-645-ndis-participants-caught-in-hwl-ebsworth-breach-601806
9 https://theconversation.com/au/topics/internet-letdown-series-163842
10 https://theconversation.com/the-internet-is-worse-than-it-used-to-be-how-did-we-get-here-and-can-we-go-back-236513
11 https://x.com/neilmcrowther/status/1798671056083075454

References

Alzheimer's Disease International. (2019). *World Alzheimer Report 2019: Attitudes to dementia*, Alzheimer's Disease International, London.

Alzheimer's Disease International. (2024). *World Alzheimer Report 2019: Global changes in attitudes to dementia*, Alzheimer's Disease International, London.

Backlinko Team. (2025). iPhone Users and Sales Stats. https://backlinko.com/iphone-users

Cations, M, May, N, Crotty, M, Low, L-F, Clemson, L, Whitehead, C, McLoughlin, J, Swaffer, K & Laver, KE. (2020). Health professional perspectives on rehabilitation for people with dementia. *The Gerontologist, 60*(3), 503–512. https://doi.org/10.1093/geront/gnz007

Chang, C-Y & Hsu, H-C. (2020). Relationship between knowledge and types of attitudes towards people living with dementia. *International Journal of Environmental Research and Public Health, 17*(11), 3777. https://doi.org/10.3390/ijerph17113777

Chen, S. et al. (2019). The global macroeconomic burden of Alzheimer's disease and other dementias: estimates and projections for 152 countries or territories. *The Lancet Public Health, 12*(9), e1534–e1543.

Day, S, Roberts, S, Launder, NH, Goh, AMY, Draper, B, Bahar-Fuchs, A, Loi, SM, Laver, K, Withall, A & Cations, M. (2022). Age of symptom onset and longitudinal course of sporadic Alzheimer's disease, frontotemporal dementia, and vascular dementia: A systematic review and meta-analysis. *Journal of Alzheimer's Disease, 85*(4), 1819–1833. https://doi.org/10.3233/JAD-215360

Dementia Australia. (2023). *Dementia statistics.* https://www.dementia.org.au/statistics

Devandas-Aguilar, Catalina. (2019). *Report of the Special Rapporteur on the rights of persons with disabilities*, UN Doc. No A/74/186, accessed 7 March 2023. https://digitallibrary.un.org/record/1663842?v=pdf

Fleming, R, Zeisel, J & Bennett, K. (2020). *World Alzheimer Report 2020: Design dignity dementia: Dementia-related design and the built environment Volume 1.* London, England: Alzheimer's Disease International.

Grenfell, L. (2019). Aged care, detention and OPCAT. *Australian Journal of Human Rights, 25*(2), 248–262.

Olazarán, J., Reisberg, B., Clare, L., Cruz, I., Peña-Casanova, J., Del Ser, T., Woods, B., Beck, C., Auer, S., Lai, C., Spector, A., Fazio, S., Bond, J., Kivipelto, M., Brodaty, H., Rojo, J. M., Collins, H., Teri, L., Mittelman, M., Orrell, M., Feldman, H. H., & Muñiz, R. (2010). Nonpharmacological therapies in Alzheimer's disease: A systematic review of efficacy. *Dementia and Geriatric Cognitive Disorders, 30*(2), 161–178. https://doi.org/10.1159/000316119

Sunstein, CR. (2019). *How change happens*, MIT Press, p. 59. *ProQuest Ebook Central.* http://ebookcentral.proquest.com/lib/unisa/detail.action?docID=5750437. Created from UniSA on 2024-08-21 02:57:12.

United States Census Bureau International Database. (2025). *International Database: World Population Estimates and Projections.* https://www.census.gov/programs-surveys/international-programs/about/idb.html

World Health Organization. (2023). *Dementia*, accessed 12 March 2023. https://www.who.int/health-topics/dementia/

Yeo, LH & Banfield, J. (2022). Human factors in electronic health records cybersecurity breach: An exploratory analysis, *Perspectives in Health Information Management, 19*(2). Spring, 1–10.

2

Family Carers

James Nicholas Chaousis

*"Someone with Alzheimer's may undergo a regression to a "second childhood",
but aspects of one's essential character, of personality and personhood, of self,
survive – along with certain, almost indestructible forms of memory … it is as
if identity has such a robust, widespread neural basis … that it is never wholly
lost …."*[1]

2.1 The Who Question: Who Are We? – the Family Tribe

Let me introduce myself and my family. I am an Adelaide born Australian
citizen of Greek heritage. I have been married to Linda for 41 years and we
have two adult daughters. Both live and work interstate. Our youngest, a
scientist specializes in the application of real-world data and artificial intelligence to medical innovations, while our eldest works as a safeguarding specialist, an advocate of human rights, and teller of stories with the Transport
Accident Commission in Victoria. We are also the proud grandparents of two
cherished granddaughters aged 18 months and 5 years of age.

I am a recently retired mental health professional having completed
33 years of public service in 2020 with the divisions of mental health in our
State Department of Health and Wellbeing. My years of service there have
given me substantial clinical and senior managerial experience in a complex
field of health and well-being. My initial training was in clinical social work
and sociology, which was later supplemented with training in a clinical
master's degree program specializing in behavioural and cognitive psychotherapy for a range of psychological disorders. This training was completed
through the Department of Psychiatry in the School of Medicine at Flinders
University.

Post retirement, I became a registered dementia advocate with Dementia
Australia. This advocacy role enabled me to participate in numerous local
and national consultations, I was co-opted to be featured in training videos
for dementia researchers and I also narrated our story for the Face Dementia

DOI: 10.1201/9781003485681-2

campaign. In addition, I am participating in dementia related university-based research projects as someone with lived experience expertise.

Linda, an American from Boston, Massachusetts, USA, has a background in economics, psychology, and information technology, and since our marriage in 1983 has resided in Australia. She has always been considered a gifted educator, writer, and public speaker due to her superb communication skills. She retired from an adjunct university lecturing role around 2017 with an American university, following ten years of service at their Adelaide campus as well as undertaking several stints joining the international university faculty to deliver the month-long Summer College Preview Program at their international campus, in Education City in her favourite place on this planet in Doha, Qatar. At the Adelaide campus, Linda instructed international students enrolled in a master's degree program in Public Policy or in Information Technology. Linda's specialty was in the field of Organizational Behaviour.

Additionally, Linda always had high expectations for herself. It was Linda's grittiness and boldness that drove her pursuit of her big dreams – often turning these into reality. As such, Linda was exceptionally enterprising in securing work as an international business consultant to the oil and gas field companies in the middle east and the USA, she worked as a radio broadcaster during the Festival of Arts, during Writers Week, and published at least a dozen textbooks in her field of expertise, was featured in business training videos for the Asian Pacific region, in addition to being an active podcaster. At least a dozen or so of her video podcasts can still be accessed on YouTube.

This is not an exhaustive report of the many things she put her hands to over her wild, 37-year vocational history. Rather these kinds of activities showcase something of her agility, her diverse niches, her creative edge, and cognitive finesse, which she applied to whatever project she undertook. She was therefore a life-long learner who embraced the slogan NO FEAR with a sense of boldness and the mindset of a trailblazer.

Linda's zest and energy for getting things done were contagious to those who had the opportunity to work alongside her.

2.2 The Emerging Perplexing Oddities

Around 2018, Linda complained about feeling fatigued and had difficulty finding appropriate words in conversations. She therefore visited a new general practice with a reputation for an integrated and holistic medical approach. After some investigations, Linda received a provisional diagnosis of hypothyroidism and was started on a new treatment regime.

At this time, our daughters and I started to notice several anomalies such as Linda's writing on her Facebook posts was increasingly plagued with grammatical errors, repetition, and a degree of incoherence. We also noted that other social media communication was slipping. This was unusual as Linda was an accomplished writer and had authored multiple textbooks. We also noticed she was easily distracted or had some odd angry outbursts.

On one occasion, she remained disengaged, almost in a frozen state, during a conversation at a post-movie dinner date. She would gaze at me but not initiate any conversation. This odd behaviour stumped me. She remained quiet for most of the time, and I ended up having a monologue, in part to prompt her to engage with me. This didn't quite work at all. Linda was usually a vibrant and active conversation partner – always a keen observer and intelligent reflector. She was a masterful communicator. And she always enjoyed conversations. Something had stymied her spontaneity to speak freely. This was perplexing for us all.

This lack of spontaneity was also on display following the loss of her handbag, the fraudulent use of her credit cards in her purse, the loss of her house and car keys. The bank fraud line asked her to self-identify as a security requirement and preamble to progressing her claim. She was unable to state her full name, her date of birth, or her home address. We had to pursue this matter in person with the assistance of our local bank manager.

Another matter surfaced. Linda had previously managed our financial affairs, but we started receiving final notices about unpaid bills.

Furthermore, Linda oddly started reverting to American terms for vegetables, such as scallions for spring onions, talking about American public holidays, for example, St Columbus Day, and referencing imperial weights and measures rather than operating with our long-established metric system here in Australia.

Another startling peculiarity was her difficulties pronouncing words. It was as if her masterful communication skills were now being dismantled and undone as she struggled to verbalize the congruent rhythms, tempo, and inflections of speech in day-to-day conversations. Something that Linda herself found perplexing and depressingly exasperating.

The constellation of behavioural and verbal perplexities and oddities had us stumped and scratching our heads.

Our family wanted clarity as to whether these peculiarities were congruent with her provisional diagnosis of hypothyroidism (which could cause temporary cognitive issues and fatigue) or if they were better explained by another condition. So, we went back to her GP for further investigations in February 2019.

Having the support of Linda's GP helped us understand that what she was experiencing was not normal. So, the GP referred Linda to a stroke physician/geriatrician who, after ordering some scans and reviewing the findings of neuropsychological investigations, finally diagnosed Linda in January 2020 with *Logopenic progressive, non-fluent aphasia (LPA)*. This is a type of dementia characterized by language disturbance, including difficulty making or understanding speech.

That specialist referred Linda to a female geriatrician for ongoing care, and we discovered the aphasia was in fact secondary to a frontotemporal dementia.

2.3 Some System Failures

Obtaining a much more precise diagnosis for Linda was only the beginning of a new chapter in our lives as a family. We also needed to gain some further clarity as to what resource systems we could access to assist us on the road ahead in providing the best possible care and support for Linda. Moreover, it seemed as if the medical and allied health specialties were narrowly focused on generating a precise diagnosis with zero time to discuss the meaning of this life-changing event (diagnosis) nor highlighting what kind of adaptations will be required of both the person living with dementia and their carer. It was as if this vital "double aspect" of the "dementia" revelation – the human experience of caring and coping – seemed to fall well outside of the scientific domains and interests of these investigative processes.

All things considered, our experience with medical specialists initially left us in the dark about the road ahead. They did not provide a map, tools, or resources that would help us navigate this new dementia landscape nor this journey of caring and coping with a lot of unknowns. So, the matter of what's the next step was left up entirely to the family to search and discover through persistent investigations via Google searches on the internet.

We had to be proactive and seek more information to better understand the diagnosis and adjust. I recall former colleagues of mine speaking highly of the online unit modules on dementia that were on offer, as a free online program through the University of Tasmania. I completed the online module, Understanding Dementia MOOC with the Wicking Dementia Research and Education Centre at the University of Tasmania.

This training module amounted to a refresher course for me in understanding something of the disease models of dementia, its impact, and the current treatment and care practices. It was an excellent learning experience.

2.4 Seeking Help

Linking in with Dementia Australia was pivotal. Their resource co-ordinator provided us with a handbook of key resources and information about the trajectory of care and support systems Linda and I would need. Furthermore, they linked us to MyAgedCare, and we initially received some funding to have Linda go on social outings with a support worker, as part of a buddying/ respite program for several hours a fortnight.

A support services consultant with Dementia Australia helpfully guided the family regarding which service providers to approach to find a compatible match for Linda.

Following an ACAT assessment we were assigned a Level 4 Home Care Package, which we self-managed. We found care workers for a variety of activities like domestic and gardening services and one-on-one personal support for Linda.

At this time, Linda was both perturbed and perplexed by her daily challenges of conversing fluently and making herself understood. Our inquiries led us to harness the resources and assistance of a Speech Pathologist. Linda did attend a few sessions and was introduced to a range of methods to aid her impaired communication. We did eventually use several communication strategies (the use of Icons – combined with texts – as visual prompts) and even purchased and uploaded a program, Proloquo4Text and urVoice for Linda's iPad as an additional communication aid for her. They were useful tools for a while to bridge the language impairment. Linda became increasingly frustrated and disheartened by her aphasia condition, as it was continually stifling her ability to freely engage in conversations.

Linda found the icon sheets with corresponding texts much easier to use than the uploaded program alluded to above.

It became clear to the family that while Linda had difficulties with language and speech, she was not intellectually impaired. Something of her high intelligence was well preserved, she was acutely aware of and sharply attuned to her environment. But the non-fluent aphasia was increasing the risk of Linda being misunderstood, neglected, and isolated from her extensive social network. All round, the loss of speech and later the loss of mobility was for Linda a devastatingly tragic scenario as it eroded the quality of life she enjoyed at home.

This was the beginning of a succession of losses for Linda. Losses that began to progressively contract her quality of life, as she once enjoyed it. These included the following

- losing her <u>independence</u> (she had trouble finding her way home after going on routine walks) and therefore needed someone to accompany her and guide her home. This was evidence that her spatial cognition was adversely affected by her brain disorder. Despite this obvious impairment to her spatial cognition, she often insisted that she go on her regular beach walks, unaccompanied. This fierce independence was fraught with all kinds of risks and a source of anxiety for the family.

- loss of <u>confidence</u> due to not being able to communicate her location and whereabouts when going on a drive – so discussions with her general practitioner resulted in his recommendation that, for legal and medical reasons, she <u>surrender her driver's license,</u>

- <u>socially isolated</u> (due to not being able to maintain contact with her extensive social network by whatever means, iPhone, or emails), she lost the ability to craft coherent communication in written form and
- <u>socially disengaged</u> (she could no longer participate in her highly valued regular coffee or lunch catch-ups with her former students or circle of professional friends because of her aphasic condition), and her
- <u>diminished powers of communication</u> (precluded her from conducting her own financial/business and related affairs). There were occasions when I sought to assist her with depositing a royalty cheque at her bank by clarifying with Linda which of her three accounts she wanted to deposit the funds into. Not able to stipulate which account the money would go into, she nevertheless physically removed me from the bank, as a measure of wanting to maintain her independence and dignity, while denying her diminished powers of communication. It took a while for Linda to acknowledge that she had nominated me, back in 2010 to take up the responsibility of performing the functions of an enduring power of an attorney, when she no longer had legal mental capacity.

These cumulative losses were quite devastating for Linda as she prided herself on being fiercely independent. They impacted her sense of self-worth, her sense of competence and sense of belonging. Being cut off from her circle of friends and business contacts, and, of course, her extensive network of university alumni, was quite a diabolical matter for Linda. Linda always thrived in social contexts, where she could devote some mentoring time with her former students, or be a listening ear and a source of encouragement whenever they chose to debrief about difficulties and challenges in their professional or personal lives.

The succession of losses meant that in practical day-by-day terms, I needed to step up and take on a larger range of new roles, to support Linda's new reality, and undergird her dignity by working with her and her set of values to buttress the quality of life she cherishes.

2.5 My New Job Description: Carer/Advocate/ Mouthpiece/In-House Comedian

These and many other challenges launched me into the caring and advocacy role. Amongst other functions my role included assisting Linda with

- Communication and social participation
- Advocacy and representation (mouthpiece and substitute decision maker)

- Co-ordination of services and supports
- Primary Health Care and related appointments
- Providing emotional support and coaching/managing stresses
- Managing all our financial affairs (Linda previously did all this)
- Personal safety at home (she's had a couple of falls and could not get up unassisted)
- Overseeing the daily/weekly domestic 101 chores, including exercising our 2 border collies
- Grocery shopping and preparation of all meals

There were a couple of things that enabled me to transition meaningfully into this newly evolving carer role. One was reminding myself that our house was often filled with laughter, especially when our daughters or friends would visit. Whatever the circumstances Linda always found a place to thrive by displaying a great sense of humour and hilarity. So, I naturally tapped into playing the in-house comedian to provide opportunities for laughter, humour, giggling, and chuckling as the occasion opened the opportunity for this light-hearted mood to everyday affairs. Linda responded enthusiastically to my silly gestures. Laughter at home once again continued to be a regular daily event as I put on my Charlie Chaplin persona.

Coupled with the importance of humour and light-heartedness was my keen interest to draw inspiration from the interventions and applications of Martin Seligman's influential contribution to the field of mental health, through his development of Positive Psychology.[2] The school of positive psychology advocates focus on five factors to harness human flourishing and well-being: these are increasing the frequency of positive emotions, engaging with others and one's environment, relationships that foster intimacy and authentic connections, meaning that answers the question, "why are we on earth?", and accomplishments based upon goals and informed by one's values.

I subsequently organized our social routines around three key values, informed by Seligman's emphases and considering our companionship and social history. These routines gravitated around people, places, and activities that potentially could generate positive and strong emotions for Linda and me.

It became clear to me that while Linda's language and fluency difficulties were imposing certain constraints on her socializing experiences, this also presented us with the ongoing challenges of the undesirable contraction of her quality of life. I felt it was imperative for us to work together and try and maximize the opportunities for enhancing and maintaining mental, visual, ecological, and relational stimulation – for generating positive emotions, joy, delight, laughter, and so on.

They centred on what Linda (and I) prized and cherished. Our marriage was characterized by a wonderful companionship and togetherness.

The home-based period spans the years 2018–2023, when she still was fully ambulant. The Supported Residential Care Facility (SRCF) period 2023–2025 signalled the loss of her mobility, confinement to a Princess Chair and the dependence on the quantum of carers and support staff for her daily needs. This was a huge lifestyle transition for Linda, in stark contrast with what she had previously enjoyed at our home.

2.6 People

2.6.1 Home-Based Phase

We maintained regular contact with a very small circle of long-established friends – by inviting them over for BBQs or dinners or attending some of their dinner invites. These friends had known Linda over many years and understood empathically something of Linda's constraints. They were not put off by the fact that her communication/conversational fluency was stymied by her aphasia. They purposefully engaged with her in ways that enabled her to feel included, valued, and esteemed as a person.

Our daughters would visit from interstate several times a year for short blocks of time and maintain communication with us by phoning us on a regular basis. I would place the call on speaker mode, so Linda was included in the conversation and ensuing discussion – all in the service of maintaining the important family connection.

We would occasionally FaceTime our daughters in the Gold Coast and Melbourne and have a virtual catch-up with the opportunity to say hello to our granddaughters, too. Those occasions provided avenues for strengthening emotional and social support for Linda and me.

My walking buddies would often call in to see me and visit Linda. This was also the case with their partners. One Autumn, they invited us to join them on tour of the famous wine growing region Clare Valley, over a long weekend. We did take up the invite and accompanied them on this weekend adventure, exploring the wineries and other historic sites within the region.

Without doubt the FaceTime connections were stimulating and special times for Linda, while she could not make conversation, she nevertheless was able to say "hello" and wave. These events often put a smile on her face and her eyes would twinkle and light up.

The video call technology via the FaceTime app allows Linda to use her body language to express herself and thus overcome the constraints imposed by her aphasia.

Many of Linda's video podcasts and digital photographs were accessed at times to provide both me and Linda with some reminiscence therapy –to remind us of her vibrant, extraverted personality and to listen to her unique Bostonian accent and sweet sonorous voice.

Additionally, Linda enjoyed accessing and scrolling through her family photo albums stored on her iPad to check out photos of our grandchildren, daughters, and their partners, and so on.

2.6.2 Supported Residential Care Facility-Based Phase

Linda's Smart TV enabled her to enjoy watching programs featuring some of her favourite US talk show hosts such as Oprah Winfrey, Jimmy Fallon, Stephen Colbert, and Jimmy Kimmel. These shows were often a highpoint because she liked their intelligibility, quick wit, and sense of humour. These TV personalities provided her with an occasion to become engrossed in their storytelling and share somewhat in their humour.

The Smart TV technology served to remind Linda of her familiar American roots and culture via these talk show programs.

One of Linda's closest and long-term friends, Peggy from Maine, USA, would maintain regular contact with Linda via sending four postcards a month and often sharing various stories of the cheeky and devilish things they got up to when they both lived and worked together in Washington, DC. I would read these old familiar stories to Linda, and she would affirm their veracity by nodding her head or grinning and affirming with a "Yea!"

Peggy would supplement the card communication with FaceTime sessions/or WhatsApp video chats with Linda and me. These were thrilling moments for Linda for she often recognized her dear friend's face and voice and often expressed delight at the face-to-face video chats. Sometimes in the winter Peggy would send photos snaps of the state of her property following a snowstorm, to my mobile phone – Mainly to remind Linda that she has escaped these severe New England winters by residing in Australia!

Our daughters also prioritized visiting Linda several times a year with our grandchildren in tow – Linda's face would light up during these visits – human connection and encounters were thrilling times for us all.

2.7 Places

2.7.1 Home-Based Phase

We frequently visited the places that brought her great joy. The Art Gallery of South Australia, Glenelg or Brighton Beaches, and the CIBO Café (coffee and gelato) or Henley Square. Other regular places included the nearby Westfield

Shopping Centre, seaside townships like Port Elliot and Victor Harbour. We also occasionally travelled up to the Gold Coast, Melbourne, and Sydney for short getaways. These were some of Linda's favourite places.

While the local beaches were one of her favourite places to go to, living in the Southern Adelaide hills also offered some fantastic scenery in our nearby national park or along the Sturt linear walking trails, or even up at the Mount Loft Lookout and botanic gardens. She loved the brilliant colours on display in the hills together with the abundance of birdlife like the rainbow-coloured Lorikeets.

Other times we would check out videos and photos of some of her favourite places on the planet that included Qatar, Hawaii, California, and New England, and cities such as Washington DC, Gold Coast, Cairns, and Sydney.

During the period 2020–2021, while Linda was still driving, we resorted to using the Find my friends App on my iPhone to locate her whereabouts, or on other occasions, we used the Bluetooth smart tile tracker when she was unable to give us her location.

Sitting on a bench watching the evening sunset at one of her favourite beaches was always a sensationally, awe-inspiring experience. So, visiting beaches during the summer months was sometimes an all-day affair, because Linda was ravished by the tranquillity and beauty of the ocean and our pristine sandy beaches.

2.7.2 SRCF-Based Phase

Being confined to a Princess chair limited the freedom she previously enjoyed at home, where she was ambulant and relatively independently active. In the residential setting, I frequently wheeled her out to one of the two main spacious courtyards to enjoy some sunlight, explore the tropical plants and gardens, rockeries, and small fountains. Here too she was drawn to the colourful gardens with a variety of roses, crepe myrtle trees, magnolia trees, and sight the brilliant Birds of Paradise. In this setting digital technology enabled me to show her recent photos or video clips of our granddaughters on my mobile phone or play Linda some of her favourite music.

There were often benches and armchairs located within the courtyard. We would frequently find a secluded spot so I could park her Princess Chair, take a seat and play some of her favourite tunes or songs (Beach Boys or the Beatles), with the volume turned up loud. The music often induced a deeply emotional response, a sense of delight and joy. It was a wonder to witness as it often put a smile on my face too.

I also took advantage of the Access Cab subsidized scheme and had Linda transported several times to Glenelg, her favourite beach, to wheel her around the esplanade, ending up with a visit to her beloved Italian cafe for a latte and gelato.

2.8 Activities

2.8.1 Home-Based Phase

While she was still ambulant Linda loved visiting either the Mount Lofty Botanic Gardens or the Southern Adelaide hills township of Stirling to photograph the flowers and colourful plants lining the street or gardens.

Linda particularly loved the music of Simon & Garfunkel, and so when a tribute show was performing at a local theatre, I made it a priority for us to see the show. The music performed in this tribute show touched Linda deeply.

Similarly, when she heard about a one-off Beach Boys concert in Darling Harbour in Sydney, we got tickets and attended this show – their characteristic bopping rock vibe and heavenly harmonies generated some good vibrations that prompted Linda to turn to me to signal with her hands, seeking my permission to go forward and dance near the stage with several other Beach Boys fans. My thumbs immediately went up, signalling that she should join in and have some fun.

We were regular cinema goers, and a regular tradition included combining seeing a film at The Event Cinema's or Palace Nova, with a late dinner at Betty's Burgers or Grill'd Healthy Burgers joints.

Breakfast and long walks in the hills township of Stirling were a favourite thing on Saturday mornings. Alternatively, long walks at one of our favourite beaches were followed by a long, lingering breakfast. These kinds of activities formed new and varied routines for us and were something we both relished.

At home Linda enjoyed watching some of her favourite American sitcom shows on our Smart TV, in the evening her favourite talk shows. But she also watched her favourite drama series NCIS, BULL, or Hawaii 50. Smart TV technology kept Linda engaged with talk shows and TV series.

Sometimes Linda enjoyed searching for and watching interesting documentaries on all sorts of topics on one of the streaming platforms. Additionally, she particularly enjoyed accessing her iPad (she could still recall her six-digit password), playing her favourite songs, listening to these songs on her wireless Bose headphones, going through her photo albums, and watching the American news reports on NBC, CBS, and so on. The iPad kept Linda up to date with American news and some reminiscence therapy.

I sometimes found her going through a collection of photos that included the high school and university she attended and some of the historic sites that were a feature of Topsfield, a town 20 miles north of Boston, where she grew up.

Technology provided a vehicle for Linda's need for multi-sensory stimulation including watching, listening, touching keyboards or remote controls, avenues of understanding for her inquisitive mind, and her intelligibility.

All these routines provided her with the kind of mental, visual, environmental, and relational stimulation that she yearned for and compensated for her cumulative losses.

2.8.2 SRCF-Based Phase

My twice daily activities with and for Linda included assisting her with her meal, wheeling her around the corridors, or out to explore any one of the courtyards and the gardens, reading, e.g., James Herriot's collection of dog stories, Mary Oliver's poetry or playing some of her choice music videos featuring her favourite artists on my mobile phone or her iPad. My approach was to check-in with Linda (blink once if you would like this activity today) and sense what activity she might enjoy. My visits also included bringing in a small tub of tiramisu, chocolate mousse, or a Greek yoghurt. I was keen to expose her to multi-sensory experiences.

Some friends of mine, a husband-and-wife pastoral team called in once a fortnight and taking a personal care approach, would do some of the following

- They shared something of their lives and family with Linda, compiling a playlist of videos and hymns they thought Linda would like. (Linda had a long history with the Christian tradition and communities) and playing these on her Smart TV.
- Linda particularly enjoyed a video of Doha, Qatar, and a video of her hometown in Boston – she recognized these beloved places.
- There were several familiar Christian hymns that they played, and which brought tears to her eyes. She was visibly moved.

The in-house Coordinating Chaplin reported the following observations regarding Linda's participation in the weekly ecumenical church service.

- During the services Linda would often *mouth* the words to popular hymns which were sung, and she would often have a tear in her eyes, also when the Lord's Prayer was shared.
- Linda would also have a tear in her eye after the service because of something connecting with and touching her within.

These reports from the Pastoral and Chaplaincy ministries regarding Linda's exposure to familiar hymns, melodies, and worship songs, evoking poignant responses in Linda and prompting her to *mouth* the lyrics, are startling observations. And they should not be glossed over! Why not? Because, as reported by Oliver Sacks,[3] these kinds of familiar activities may astonishingly shine a light on her identity and her rich fund of memories that in turn enable her to gush congruent responses – such as adoration, consolation, and assurance. How remarkable for Linda's diagnosis of Logopenic progressive, non-fluent aphasia!

Here, too, technology was engaged in the ecumenical worship services as a means to facilitate some reminiscence therapy for participants like Linda.

2.9 My Coping and Caring?

2.9.1 Home-Setting Phase

The routines I alluded to above buoyed me and kept my daily momentum going, performing a wide range of domestic tasks, while I simultaneously grieved for Linda. The diminishing of her cognitive powers to engage in conversations, my long-time conversation partner tragically silenced by aphasia – coupled with her loss of independent living skills, I sensed all these losses very deeply here. The grieving came in waves. It was often triggered by a memory of some kind at home or in a particular place that was special for us. The ruminations of losses and coming to terms with our current reality were countered by a profound sense of gratitude for the decades of life we shared together. The pre-eminent memory I have of Linda is the twinkle in her eye and her cascading and contagious laughter.

My early morning walking routines at a local beach with my walking buddies provided an enjoyable physical activity and an avenue to discuss some of my feelings with my male friends. Although I often chose not to share what my life as a carer entailed, as I didn't want to burden my friends with my challenges and showcase our set of circumstances. But at the same time, I was disappointed that no-one asked me questions like, "what does your typical week look like, now?" and 'how are you coping with this new situation that you and Linda find yourselves in?" – and perhaps, ask "Is there anything I/we can do to support you and Linda?". Nothing like this kind of probing was forthcoming. I found this lack of empathy and imagination by "some" of my friends more than a little disconcerting.

One rather surprising source of support came from a couple of female ex-colleagues and friends, in that they not only inquired about my health and well-being but also cooked meals for me and kept in regular contact with me. That made the world of difference for me – these friends cared for me, and what Linda and I were going through in this dementia landscape.

A couple of other close buddies accompanied me and Linda on our difficult journey into the darkness of the dementia landscape by remaining steadfast in their friendship by making themselves available to me in times of crisis.

I did access a counsellor at Dementia Australia, attended three or four sessions then she abruptly discharged me from "therapy/support" as she sized up that I was effectively channelling my grieving into my broad-based advocacy work – and therefore I did not need her ongoing support. I reluctantly accepted her perspective and ploughed myself into the advocacy work that was an integral part of my role as a carer of Linda.

Listening to music on my iPod with earphones was a soothing and comforting experience that sometimes brought on tears and weeping. But these tears were often about a deep sense of gratitude in sharing life with Linda these past 41 years and the privilege of caring for her following the deterioration in her health.

Digital technology was utilized here as a means of reducing some of the anxious and stressful moments I had been experiencing during my taxing, daily caring routines.

2.9.2 The SRCF Phase

Over the past two years, since Linda moved to the SRCF, I have been visiting her twice a day, seven days a week – to assist her with her mealtimes – totalling around 45 hours per week. From the outset of her placement in the SRCF, I wanted to maintain the high continuity of care that I was able to deliver to Linda (in our home setting) by actively partnering with the care team, to extend the personalized care activities to Linda and informed by my personal knowledge of her likes and dislikes.

I describe my involvement as adding some "colour to her otherwise grey nursing home routines." My regular presence has enabled me to forge a positive working relationship with senior management, nursing staff, regular team of carers, and allied health staff. This networking has been a richly rewarding experience as it has provided me with a vehicle for giving constructive feedback based on my direct observations of care, and an avenue to flag when something was awry or substandard regarding Linda's care.

2.10 The End of Home Care and the Transition to Supported Residential Care Facility

In October 2021, Linda had two episodes of muscle weakness and functional decline (inability to mobilize), on the same day, she was unable to get off the toilet seat. This led to an Emergency Department admission for investigations, where she was diagnosed with Rhabdomyolysis.

Linda had a further episode in February 2022 of muscle weakness and functional decline and was once again diagnosed with Rhabdomyolysis, requiring a brief admission to the Emergency Department. It was hypothesized that these presentations were precipitated by the COVID-19 Vaccine boosters' number 2 and 3, as there had been reports in the medical literature of this rare, adverse side-effect of a non-exertion muscle injury. After a few weeks Linda was once again able to mobilize unaided.

In the main, Linda was able to shower and dress herself and mobilize unaided prior to these admissions. However, she was having continence issues (urinary) and so, in consultation with Linda's new female general practitioner, it was suggested the need to link into a service that could conduct a home assessment. Our daughter conducted an internet search, which then led us to a continence service. Following an assessment and recommendations by a continence nurse, a continence management plan was enacted, and we were able to source several continence aids that made a difference in our home setting.

There was a further acute deterioration in her mobility on Boxing Day 2022, which warranted a lengthy admission into a rehabilitation ward at our local medical centre. Rehabilitation physiotherapists worked extensively with Linda to help her regain her full mobility.

Following a series of investigations and workups by the rehabilitation team it was hypothesized that Linda had a rare muscle atrophy in her legs for which there is no restorative treatment available. The medical team therefore made the overriding decision that Linda could not return into my care, at home. Rather, Linda now required full nursing care in a Supported Residential Care Facility (SRCF). That revelation was devastating news for me and for Linda.

Up until the December 2022 admission, we were going for 35-minute walks each evening prior to sitting down for dinner. Walking along walking trails in various linear parks and botanic gardens was always a highpoint of the day for Linda and me – as this routine was followed by coffee and a delicious serving of carrot cake at our favourite local café.

It took about 3 weeks before we found a suitable SRCF, in March 2023, some 20 minutes' drive from our residence in the Southern Adelaide Hills.

Of course, her allocated room was spartan with a bed and a built-in wardrobe and en suite. Our family and I quickly transformed her room, personalizing it with a huge collage of family photos virtually taking up one wall. On another wall we placed a Smart TV with a Blu-ray player, a bookcase with stacks of DVD's movies & musical concerts. Plus a few books like James Herriot (the Yorkshire Vet) favourite dog stories. We had a string of border collies and German Shepherds over the years. We also plastered the walls with various pieces of information, snapshots about Linda's background identity, her preferred TV channels, and am and pm, listing the TV shows she likes to watch. We also hung up a painting of a beach scene. Overall, it helped tone down the cold clinical feel of the room by creating a more homely ambience for Linda.

2.11 My Personalized Care Activities

My twice-daily presence at the SRCF, during a two-hour block of time centred on assisting Linda with her meal. On any given day, I might bring in Linda's iPad and assist her in accessing several programs (her bundles of songs and music, her photo albums and video clips of our family, and perhaps her Kindle library of books). We sometimes would watch a movie from the large collection of DVDs that she has in her bookcase. A regular feature was to read a chapter from James Herriot's favourite dog stories and then watch YouTube video clips of border collies doing extraordinary things on my Android mobile phone.

Early on in her admission to the SRCF, I had stumbled upon Oliver Sacks's chapter Speech and Song: Aphasia and Music therapy in his book Musicophilia.[4] Sacks suggests that people with the non-fluent type of aphasia, those who have lost the feeling of the rhythm and inflections of speech, seemingly do well with music therapy. He reports that this non-fluent cohort feel excited when they can sing (some) lyrics to a familiar song. Playing Linda's favourite and iconic songs became a daily staple of our time together. It was an activity that animated and engaged her at a deeply emotional level.

I mention Sacks's chapter on the place of music therapy here, as I too have observed Linda becoming emotionally expressive (delighted), in fact quite joyous at times as she responds to some of her favourite Beatle's tunes – this was especially evident when Linda watched a video clip of Paul McCartney performing the classic hit song, Let It Be.

Linda is confined to a princess Chair. Weather permitting, I would wheel her out to the outdoor garden area before lunch or dinner to experience some warmth, sunlight, and check out the tropical gardens. We would often hunt for a golden leaf to pluck from the Magnolia trees or clip a flower from the Crepe Myrtle tree.

Every few weeks, I would organize for an Access Cab to transport us to Linda's favourite beach where we could wheel around for a couple of hours taking in the ocean and beach scenes, enjoy a latte and gelato before our return journey to the SRCF.

The 41-year partnership Linda and I have shared helps me know something of what brings her delight and enjoyment in her daily life and social routines, and conversely, what she usually finds distressing and unsettling. While pushing forward day by day and enduring losses, I allow the process of grief to take its natural course. But I still hold on to a profound sense of gratitude and privilege for sharing a life together over four decades. This includes my time as Linda's full-time carer, anchor, and the resident comedian.

2.12 My Coping and Caring? – Following Her SRCF Placement

In early 2023, the medical team in the rehabilitation ward advised me that Linda's unresponsive muscle atrophy meant that she now had to be placed in an SRCF, as she required ongoing nursing care. The news that we were going to be separated due to her immobility was a hard one to digest. One that plunged me further into a process of grieving as everything would be different without Linda at home, the home we have shared these past 30 years.

In fact, it amounted to the uncoupling of a 41-year companionship. She has been at the core of my life and world for a long time. This was one of the most painful relational ruptures I have ever experienced in my life. I imagined that the move into the SRCF would also be devastating for Linda, and a tragic one for her due to impaired speech and immobility as she was an exceptionally personable extrovert and loved connecting with others.

During this phase, I had to slowly acclimatize to coming home to an empty house, not having a conversational partner present to welcome me, and adjust as all the things that Linda and I did together have to now be done on my own.

Connecting with an older friend who had lost her husband to dementia enabled me to have meaningful conversations with someone who understood something of this kind of personal loss for myself (and to grasp something of what it might mean for Linda too). Grief and gratitude were held together. I celebrated and cherished the 41 years we had together, and I continue to grieve the loss of my vibrant life companion and often imagine what it must be like for her being in a strange environment, with a bunch of strangers – a place that's not home for her.

The SRCF staff frequently ask me, "Do you live nearby and why you come twice a day?" My best response to this probing is the greatest gift I can give Linda, at this time of her life and under these circumstances, is my faithful presence.

2.13 Technology: An Invaluable Adjunct to Personalized Care

The story I have just shared spans the period 2018–2025, from home care to the transition to an SRCF is punctuated with many examples of the way in which technology has played a significant adjunct role in the process of delivering personalized, compassionate care to my wife, Linda – all in the service of maintaining her connections with all our family members, her circle of friends and the places that were important to her.

We can clearly see here the benefits of technology for crafting personalized care in a variety of settings. However, I would like to table some of the challenges I experienced in using digital technology in the SRCF setting:

- Utilizing Wi-Fi networks that were unsecure (privacy was not guaranteed) was limiting.
- Sometimes international calls were timed out.
- Sometimes interstate and international calls were hampered by poor picture and audio quality.

- Sometimes the person phoning or calling in on a video chat apps had intrusive distractions at their end that hampered the conversations.
- In some areas of the SRCF there were dead spots, and I was unable to maintain my internet connections.

I have emphasized the primacy of personal face-to-face encounters and connections with others. Why? Because I have found that being personally present to Linda allows me to be singularly attuned to whatever she may be expressing or sensing in the moment, focusing much on her non-verbal gestures, and occasionally noting one-word expressions – this allows for some deep resonance to be experienced between us. Being personally present also provides unique opportunities for physical contact – a kiss, a hug, holding or touching her hand, and indeed the importance of eye gaze. These are deeply meaningful human forms of communication that express the beautiful bonds of companionship.

This is the context into which digital technologies play a wonderfully supportive role in maintaining her connection with the people, places, activities, and her cultural roots that have shaped her identity and membership to her valued community.

Let me summarize in dot point form the variety of ways specific technologies have been utilized in our caring journey from home to residential-based care.

- Internet-accessed online educational modules with the University of Tasmania
- Internet –searches to screen the most suitable SRCF for Linda and identify specific service providers
- Smart TV – for educational and entertainment purposes for Linda and accessing YouTube video podcasts (Linda's) for reminiscing therapy for her and family
- Speech Therapy recommended Software program- uploaded onto Linda's iPad to assist with communication
- iPad – for Linda to access her photo albums, music, and Netflix American sitcom soap operas, and Kindle library to connect with her American roots
- iPod – Jim's device to listen to his music and other uploaded programs – soothing and therapeutic activity
- S21 Samsung mobile phone – primary for communication with family and friends, local, interstate, and overseas via FaceTime and WhatsApp chat modes, Google searches – to play Linda's favourite artists or compositions (music) and other documentaries, to find her current location via Bluetooth smart tile tracking technology
- The use of the wireless Bose headphones when listening to her choice music or documentaries from her iPad tablet

2.14 Human Connections and Technology Are Transcending the Limitations of Distance

There is no substitute for human face-to-face encounters in delivering personalized, compassionate, and person-centred care and in bolstering personal connections. All the verbal and non-verbal forms of communication need to be fully engaged and attuned to in the caring process and with a view to accurately comprehending their meaning. How does a masterful communicator like Linda, who has long had her capacity to speak and write impaired by a non-fluent aphasia, communicate some final messages to those she loves?

The Friday before she was admitted to the Emergency Department of our local hospital, for an assessment and treatment of a deep pressure wound and suspected sepsis infection, the following happened ....

It was a beautiful, poignant thing.

I had spent well over an hour just trying to assist Linda with her main course (dinner) and a double serving of ice cream for dessert (she usually polishes off all this in 35–45 minutes), but she didn't want to eat. She just wouldn't open her mouth wide to take in a teaspoon of protein or vegetables – remember everything is minced up and it must be moist with gravy because of her swallowing difficulties. I tried every little manoeuvre I could think of, but nothing worked.

So, in my exhausted state at about 6:30 pm I placed (rested) my right hand on her chest. I turned my head for a moment and watched the news report on the TV regarding Cyclone Alfred heading towards Queensland. A moment later I felt Linda's finger running up and down my right hand, I turned back and watched as she did this action a couple of times, tracing my fingers up and down with her index finger. And I caught her glancing at me with her piercing, beautiful blue eyes.

It was getting late, so I kissed her goodnight and went home. All the way home I was wondering what that gesture was all about. What did she mean by touching my hand?

Bone tired, I went to bed around 10 pm. At midnight I woke up, as it dawned on me with utter clarity what Linda's tactile message was to me that evening.

Linda – the masterful communicator could still trace out a message of love with her index finger to her carer/husband. This was her message to me ....

"These loving hands have cared for me for such a long time, and I now want you Jim to rest your hands, - to rest them, now!"

Ten days later, as I sat in a room beside my wife Linda, listening and watching her breathing became slower, her gurgling noisily as her breathing became more laboured, with longer pauses between breaths, my phone rings. I answer. It's Peggy, Linda's best friend, who resides in a small seaside town in Maine, USA. Peggy is very direct in her instructions to me. "Put the speaker mode on, I want to speak to Linda – place your phone near her ear". She then spoke to Linda a personal message of love and affection, their cherished friendship, which had endured 60 years, across continents. Maine, USA, is 17,000 km from Adelaide!

Here, when the minutes are quickly ticking by, everything counts, and technology in the form of a mobile phone transcended the limitations of distance and provides a platform for a vital personal message to be delivered to a dying friend.

Notes

1 Oliver Sacks, *Musicophilia: Tales of Music and the Brain*, New York, Alfred A. Knop Inc, 2007, p336.
2 Martin Seligman, T*he Hope Circuit: A Psychologist's Journey from Helplessness to Optimism*, Sydney, Penguin Australia, 2018. Corey L. M. Keyes & Jonathan Haidt, eds., *Flourishing: Positive Psychology and the Life Well-Lived*, Washington, DC, American Psychological Association, 2003.
3 Oliver Sacks, *Everything in Its Place: First Loves and Lost Tales*, New York, Alfred A. Knoff, 2019, pp 144–154.
4 Sacks, 2007, 214–223.

3

The Role of Digital Twins Powered/Enabled through AI for People with Dementia

Nilmini Wickramasinghe

3.1 Introduction

Dementia is a fairly common neurodegenerative disease that affects the brain and includes gradual cognitive and memory deterioration and a decrease in the ability to perform daily tasks. The global population is aging and it is projected that the number of dementia patients will rise owing to the fact that about 2 billion people will be aged over 60 years by 2050 (World Health Organization, 2021). This growth presents great implications for future healthcare delivery, caregivers, and society as a whole. The current practice in managing dementia is inadequate in addressing the diverse and dynamic needs of patients, which means new approaches are required. Digital twins that are exact replicas of physical objects have become one of the most disruptive technologies in the healthcare industry. With the help of artificial intelligence (AI), digital twins can offer tailored, immediate supervision and management recommendations for those with dementia. This chapter discusses the use of digital twins in dementia care, as well as how innovative technologies such as sensors can be implemented in order to improve the lives of both patients and caregivers.

3.2 Digital Twins: An Overview

Digital twin definition is a simulation of a physical object or a process in a digital environment. In the context of healthcare, therefore, a digital twin can refer to a single patient, meaning a digital model that is continuously updated as the patient progresses through the course of their treatment. These are virtual models that operate based on AI and machine learning (ML) algorithms from data acquired from different sources such as wearable

DOI: 10.1201/9781003485681-3

devices, electronic health records, and environmental sensors. It enables predictive analysis, individualized care plans, and constant monitoring, making digital twin valuable in the management of dementia.

Digital twin technology was initially used in the manufacturing domain to monitor manufacturing processes and to predict equipment failures. In the medical field, digital twins have been applied to mimic internal organs, mimic operations, and monitor some diseases. For dementia care, there is no better tool than digital twins that depict the mental and physical state of the patient in real time, making the care offered unique and proactive.

3.3 The Role of AI in Digital Twins for Dementia Care

AI is a critical element for enhancing the capabilities of digital twins. Big data can be analyzed to make timely and customized treatment plans based on the results predicted by data science tools. For instance, AI can analyze the data collected by wearable gadgets to predict early signs of dementia, including aggression. By so doing, the caregivers are able to check or even prevent the likelihood of such outcomes, thus enhancing the patients' well-being.

The unstructured data, along with sensor information, can be processed through Natural Language Processing (NLP) applications that include caregiver notes and patient diaries. The digital twin recommendations become more precise through this approach because it allows adjustments to drug dosages and environmental parameters and exercise prescriptions (Wickramasinghe et al., 2022). The use of AI technology allows for uniting multiple data sources into a unified understanding of patient health status. The proposed digital twin can represent an accurate patient health condition by combining data from wearable sensors with environmental sensors and EHRs through methods like Kalman filtering and Bayesian networks (Sun et al., 2023).

3.4 Sensor Technologies in Dementia Care

Different benefits emerge from incorporating sensor technologies into dementia patient care and management systems. AI digital twins together with other technologies enable both ongoing and real-time physical and mental assessment of patient health conditions. Wearable gadgets and home appliances alongside clothing integrated with multiple sensors allow health practitioners and caregivers to monitor patient activities thus enabling timely care during irregularities. The following sections explain primary dementia care sensors alongside their applications.

3.4.1 Wearable Sensors

Wearable sensors have become one of the most popular innovations in dementia care. Smartwatches, fitness trackers, and biosensors keep track of pulse, physical activity, and sleep. These sensors can be particularly useful in helping a patient monitor his or her health and well-being. For instance, a sharp reduction in physical movement or disturbances in sleep can be a sign of cognitive deterioration or the development of conditions such as depression or agitation, which are typical of dementia (Palmese et al., 2024).

Also, the wearable sensors are capable of identifying falls, which are common in dementia patients. Fall detection algorithms monitor the movements of the residents and send an alert to the caregivers in case of a fall. Other wearables also come with geofencing functionality that alerts caregivers if the patient goes beyond a certain vicinity. These functionalities offer a timely patient monitoring system, which makes the task less stressful for caregivers.

3.4.2 Environmental Sensors

The installation of environmental sensors within smart home systems ensures both safety measures and comfort for the residents including individuals with dementia. Temperature sensors along with humidity and air quality detectors help create optimal living environments for the building inhabitants. The monitoring capabilities of environmental sensors include detection of potential problems together with indicators of harmful events that need immediate intervention (Moyle et al., 2021). Motion sensors detect long periods without movement, which could signal either a fall or cognitive decline or confusion among residents. The installation of proper door and window sensors helps dementia patients by alerting caregivers if the patient attempts to leave through an open door. Smarter lighting technology combined with environmental sensors enables better confusion management by automatically controlling room illumination according to daily time cycles for enhanced human circadian rhythm regulation.

3.4.3 Biometric Sensors

Biometric sensors provide a better understanding of the physical and emotional condition of a dementia patient. These sensors track parameters like the pulse, blood pressure, and skin conductivity to help the caregivers and health practitioners detect the levels of stress, anxiety, and agitation (Xefteris et al., 2016). Fluctuations in biometrics might be due to emotional upset, which may be triggered by environment, side effects of medication, or lack of needs fulfillment. For instance, elevated baseline heart rate and electrodermal activity may indicate distress or discomfort to ward off anyone away, which can be useful to caregivers. Digital twins allow for the inclusion of biometric data in the model, which allows caregivers to predict behavioral changes and adjust treatments.

3.4.4 Location Tracking

GPS and indoor positioning systems play a critical role in the safety of dementia patients. These tracking systems enable the caregivers to easily identify the position of the patient at any given time since the movement of the patient is being monitored in real time and this is especially important since wandering is one of the major causes of harm for patients with dementia (Bartlett et al., 2019). Advanced locative media employ geofencing, whereby the caregivers set restricted areas. When the patient strays from these zones, signals are sent to the caregivers to enable them to attend to the patient and do something accordingly. It also can be helpful to know when a particular patient is apt to roam and measures to prevent it can be instituted. Personal GPS monitoring devices, shoes with built-in location tracking systems, and mobile applications enhance security and minimize stress for the patient and the care provider.

3.4.5 Voice and Speech Analysis

AI in the form of voice and speech analysis in the context of dementia care has turned out to be useful diagnostic indicators as well as monitors. These technologies analyze speech rate, tone, and content for possible signs of degenerative diseases and depression (Huang et al., 2024). It is worth noting that speech and language difficulties, increased pausing, and word finding difficulties may be indicative of neurodegenerative diseases like Alzheimer's disease. Another advantage of speech analysis tools is that they can also consider the feelings of the speaker depending on the tone of the patient, and therefore, the caregiver can tell whether a particular patient is feeling anxious, frustrated, or depressed. In applications with digital twins, such tools can give warnings on a patient's microstates or cognitive and emotional conditions for timely intervention.

3.5 Integration of Sensor Data in Digital Twins

The major concern when it comes to integrating data from multiple sensors into a digital twin is using AI algorithms, which can process and analyze data of different forms. Some of the modern methods for data fusion include Kalman filtering and Bayesian network that can be used to combine data from different sources and, therefore, get a more complete picture of the overall condition of the patient (Sun et al., 2023).

NLP enables AI algorithms to examine unstructured data including caregiver notes alongside patient diaries that contain additional information about sensor readings. The perspective enables the digital twin to generate personalized recommendations about medicine dosage adjustments as well as environment modifications or exercise protocols (Wickramasinghe et al., 2022). Digital twins become more effective when they incorporate sensor data for the development of prediction models. AI algorithms provide predictions about health complication deterioration through their combination of historical and current data processing capabilities. Risk assessment models determine the fall likelihood of patients, which healthcare providers use to prevent falls through home environment changes and physiotherapy (Thapa et al., 2022).

3.6 Predictive Analytics and Personalized Interventions

Digital twins employed with AI produce predictions about systems through their capabilities. The predictions made by AI algorithms become possible because these algorithms analyze historical and real-time data to identify when health complications will worsen. Risk assessment tools help forecast when patients are likely to fall so home modifications and physiotherapy treatments can be implemented to prevent such incidents (Thapa et al., 2022).

Digital twins also provide the advantage of delivering customized healthcare services to patients. In this, digital twins enabled by patient data allow AI to recommend suitable therapeutic approaches including cognitive exercises and dietary modifications or physical activities. Healthcare professionals use patient-specific factors to evaluate recommended interventions, which need to demonstrate durability for the long run according to Vallée (2024). Digital twins use real-time sensor data to modify patient scheduling within their virtual model. The collected patient data showing increased morning activity levels leads the digital twin to recommend increased mental tasks for that time period. The collected data indicates increased evening agitation so the digital twin system suggests performing specific activities together with home environment modifications including noise and light controls (Jones et al., 2021).

3.7 Ethical Considerations and Challenges

Despite its potential benefits, there are ethical and practical concerns about using AI-enabled digital twins. Still, the greatest weakness that cannot be turned a blind eye to is privacy, as digital twins require constant surveillance and data collection. To this end, it is important to protect data and obtain permission from the patient and their caregivers (Huang et al., 2022).

Another challenge is that algorithms applied in ML are often followed by bias. This is because algorithms are simply formalized data and if the data fed into the formula is prejudiced, then the conclusion will also be prejudiced.

To eliminate such discrepancies, it is crucial that the data used in training and developing AI models is a true representation of the population (Rakshit et al., 2024).

The last but not the least is that digital twins incorporated into dementia care require the application of technology and infrastructure. The healthcare providers who are going to implement these systems should be trained, and the patients and caregivers should understand the pros and cons of using those systems (Andargoli et al., 2024).

3.8 Conclusion

Digital twins represent a modern approach to dementia care, which implements AI to deliver individualized monitoring and prompt intervention. The digital twin models accept multiple sensor integration to create a real-time and comprehensive awareness of patient conditions and necessary actions. Digital twins in dementia patient care and caregiver support bring advantages through their implementation although privacy issues and algorithmic bias require attention. The future application of this technology in dementia care should bring about additional opportunities to enhance patient experiences according to current developments.

In summary, digital twins are an emerging technology that builds on in silico representations of an individual that can be used for the purposes of therapy, preventative care, and enhancement (Bruynseels et al., 2018). Such predictive technology has the ability to better estimate an individual's potential likelihood of developing dementia as well as the rate of progression of the disease. Given that with DT modeling it is possible to dynamically recognizes molecular status, physiological status, and lifestyle over time, this provides an opportunity to review the records of people with dementia to better predict various factors of dementia; thereby, making it possible to develop a personalized and precise, person-centered treatment that will minimize risk to patients, while improving their quality of life and supporting family members.

References

Andargoli, A. E., Ulapane, N., Nguyen, T. A., Shuakat, N., Zelcer, J., & Wickramasinghe, N. (2024). Intelligent decision support systems for dementia care: a scoping review. *Artificial Intelligence in Medicine*, *150*, 102815. https://doi.org/10.1016/j.artmed.2024.102815

Bartlett, R., Brannelly, T., & Topo, P. (2019). Using GPS technologies with people with dementia: a synthesising review and recommendations for future practice. *Tidsskrift for omsorgsforskning*, *5*(3), 84–98.

Bruynseels, K., Santoni de Sio, F., & Van den Hoven, J. (2018). Digital twins in health care: ethical implications of an emerging engineering paradigm. *Frontiers in Genetics*, *9*, 31. https://doi.org/10.3389/fgene.2018.00031

Huang, P. H., Kim, K. H., & Schermer, M. (2022). Ethical issues of digital twins for personalized health care service: preliminary mapping study. *Journal of Medical Internet Research*, *24*(1), e33081.

Huang, L., Yang, H., Che, Y., & Yang, J. (2024). Automatic speech analysis for detecting cognitive decline of older adults. *Frontiers in Public Health*, *12*, 1417966.

Jones, C., Jones, D., & Moro, C. (2021). Use of virtual and augmented reality-based interventions in health education to improve dementia knowledge and attitudes: an integrative review. *BMJ Open*, *11*(11), e053616.

Moyle, W., Murfield, J., & Lion, K. (2021). The effectiveness of smart home technologies to support the health outcomes of community-dwelling older adults living with dementia: a scoping review. *International Journal of Medical Informatics*, *153*, 104513.

Palmese, F., Druda, Y., Benintende, V., Fuda, D., Sicbaldi, M., Di Florio, P., ... & Domenicali, M. (2024). Wearable sensors for monitoring caregivers of people with dementia: a scoping review. *European Geriatric Medicine*, *16*(2), 473–483. https://doi.org/10.1007/s41999-024-01113-8

Rakshit, P., Saha, N., Nandi, S., & Gupta, P. (2024). Artificial Intelligence in Digital Twins for Sustainable Future. In *Transforming Industry Using Digital Twin Technology* (pp. 19–44). Cham: Springer Nature Switzerland.

Sun, T., He, X., & Li, Z. (2023). Digital twin in healthcare: recent updates and challenges. *Digital Health*, *9*, 20552076221149651.

Thapa, R., Garikipati, A., Shokouhi, S., Hurtado, M., Barnes, G., Hoffman, J., ... & Das, R. (2022). Predicting falls in long-term care facilities: machine learning study. *JMIR Aging*, *5*(2), e35373.

Vallée, A. (2024). Envisioning the future of personalized medicine: role and realities of digital twins. *Journal of Medical Internet Research*, *26*, e50204.

Wickramasinghe, N., Ulapane, N., Andargoli, A., Ossai, C., Shuakat, N., Nguyen, T., & Zelcer, J. (2022). Digital twins to enable better precision and personalized dementia care. *JAMIA Open*, *5*(3), ooac072.

World Health Organization. (2021). "Global Status Report on the Public Health Response to Dementia." Geneva: WHO Press. https://www.alzheimer-europe.org/sites/default/files/2021-11/Global%20status%20report%20on%20the%20public%20health%20response%20to%20dementia.pdf

Xefteris, S., Doulamis, N., Andronikou, V., Varvarigou, T., & Cambourakis, G. (2016). Behavioral biometrics in assisted living: a methodology for emotion recognition. *Engineering, Technology & Applied Science Research*, *6*(4), 1035–1044.

4

Empowering Patient Care: Leveraging
Artificial Intelligence and Internet of
Things for Enhanced Healthcare Delivery

Helena Bahrami and Sasan Adibi

The chapter details how the integration of artificial intelligence (AI) and
Internet of Things (IoT) technologies is revolutionizing patient care. It
illustrates how sensor-based IoT solutions not only enable comprehensive
monitoring but also integrate smoothly with existing healthcare frameworks to improve the management of dementia. This synergy enhances
the capabilities of caregivers and healthcare professionals by providing
them with accurate, real-time data, thus enhancing patient safety and
quality of life. Furthermore, it discusses how machine learning (ML) algorithms utilize this data to predict health deteriorations and dynamically
customize care plans, promoting a shift towards proactive and preventative care models.

Focusing on the refinement of patient care delivery, the narrative highlights the critical role of wearable devices and smart home technologies.
These tools provide ongoing health monitoring and generate valuable
data that improve patient management. This real-time data is essential for
enhancing patient safety, particularly for those with the unpredictable progression of dementia-related conditions. ML algorithms analyse this data
to foresee potential health declines and appropriately adjust care plans,
marking a significant move towards more proactive and personalized care
strategies.

Additionally, this chapter discusses both the technological advancements and practical implementations of AI and IoT in dementia care. It
also addresses potential challenges such as data privacy, system interoperability,
and the need for scalable solutions to meet the needs of an aging population. The chapter aims to underscore how cutting-edge technologies can be
effectively harnessed to support caregivers and improve the lives of those
affected by dementia and Alzheimer's disease. We propose the "Integrative
AI-Enhanced Health Monitoring Ecosystem for Elderly and Dementia Care:
A Unified Approach to Real-Time Safety and Medical Response." This

DOI: 10.1201/9781003485681-4

section provides a comprehensive overview of the current capabilities and future prospects of AI and IoT in healthcare, detailing how these innovations can be synergistically integrated to enhance patient care and support systems.

4.1 Introduction

The convergence of the IoT, ML, and Data Analysis heralds a new era in the management and care of dementia, focusing on precision, efficiency, and personalization. IoT devices play a pivotal role in continuous patient monitoring, with wearables tracking vital signs and activities, thereby ensuring patient safety and timely intervention (Chen, Wan, & Li, 2012; Rashidi & Mihailidis, 2013). Smart home systems extend this monitoring to the residential environment, automating tasks and securing the living spaces of dementia sufferers, thus preventing common accidents (Chimamiwa et al., 2022; Moyle, Murfield, & Lion, 2021).

ML amplifies the capabilities of dementia care by providing predictive analytics for early detection and progression of the disease, thus facilitating early and tailored interventions (Ding et al., 2019). ML algorithms also analyse behavioural patterns through data from IoT devices, enhancing the understanding of patient needs and behaviours over time. This integration allows for the development of highly personalized care plans that adapt to the evolving conditions of the patient.

Data analysis synthesizes information from diverse sources, creating a holistic view of each patient's health status. This integration supports enhanced decision-making through Clinical Decision Support Systems (CDSS), optimizing treatment plans and predicting potential complications, thereby improving outcomes for patients (Koutsouleris et al., 2021; Salvi et al., 2024). The combination of IoT, ML, and advanced data analytics creates a dynamic framework for supporting dementia patients and their families, ensuring a higher quality of life and more effective management of the disease (Nebeker, Torous, & Bartlett Ellis, 2019).

To build on the insights from the initial exploration of AI and ML models in "Advancing Diagnosis and Drug Discovery: AI and Machine Learning Models for Dementia and Alzheimer's Disease," this chapter extends the discussion into the practical applications of these technologies within IoT-enhanced environments for real-time patient care. As we transition to the next chapter, "Conversational Agents in Healthcare: Leveraging Language Models and Chatbots for Patient Interaction," we will explore how conversational AI can further personalize and enhance the patient experience, bridging the gap between technological innovation and practical, everyday applications in dementia care. This progression underscores the journey towards our comprehensive proposal for a globally integrated AI-powered framework that promises to revolutionize the approach to dementia diagnosis, treatment, and ongoing care.

4.2 IoT Devices and Sensors in Healthcare for Alzheimer's Disease and Dementia

The integration of IoT technologies with healthcare systems has revolutionized the management and care of Alzheimer's disease and other dementias, becoming increasingly crucial as the global prevalence of dementia rises (World Health Organization, 2020). IoT devices, equipped with a plethora of sensors, enable continuous, real-time monitoring of patients, providing caregivers and healthcare professionals with essential data to navigate the complexities of dementia care (Jeon, Chae, & Kim, 2022).

These technologies not only improve patients' quality of life through precise and timely interventions but also encourage the adoption of more proactive and personalized healthcare approaches (Li et al., 2024). The data harvested from IoT devices are analysed using advanced ML algorithms, allowing for predictions about health deteriorations and the tailoring of care plans to individual needs (Ahamed, Shahrestani, & Cheung, 2020; Alsharif et al., 2020; Doraiswamy, Narayan, & Manji, 2018). Furthermore, the seamless integration of these technologies within existing healthcare frameworks enhances communication among various care providers, thereby streamlining the efficiency and effectiveness of service delivery (Abdulmalek et al., 2022; Oskouei et al., 2020; Sheikhtaheri & Sabermahani, 2022).

This transformative potential of IoT in healthcare is highlighted in "IoT-Based Healthcare-Monitoring System towards Improving Quality of Life: A Review," which meticulously catalogues advancements in IoT-based systems and the integration of wireless and wearable sensors in monitoring health (Abdulmalek et al., 2022). The paper discusses the significant benefits of IoT in healthcare, such as enhanced patient care efficiency, cost reduction, and improved outcomes through continuous monitoring and immediate data accessibility. It also addresses challenges such as security, privacy, and data integrity, advocating for robust protocols to ensure the safe use of sensitive health data.

Consequently, the application of IoT technologies in dementia care presents a promising avenue for enhancing patient autonomy, reducing caregiver burden, and improving the overall quality of healthcare services. Future advancements in IoT for healthcare could revolutionize care strategies for Alzheimer's and dementia, making them more proactive, patient-centred, and efficient.

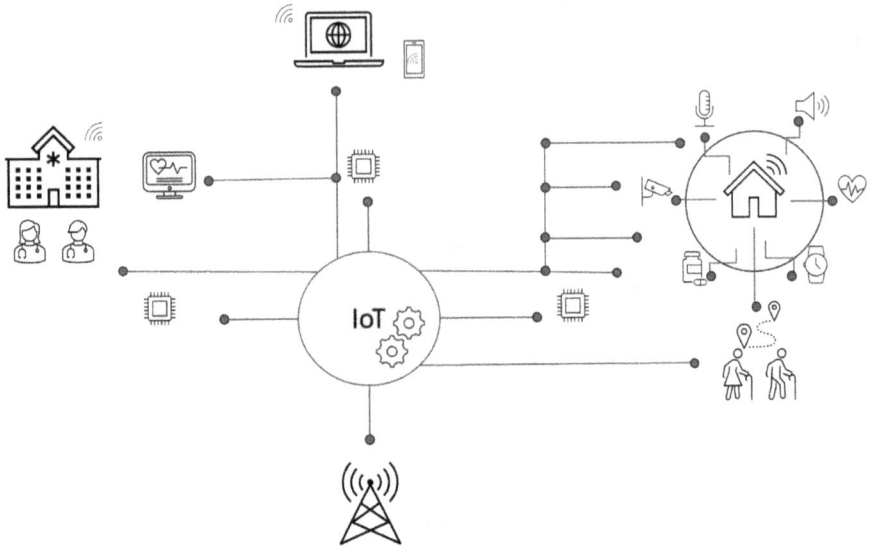

FIGURE 4.1
Harnessing IoT devices and sensors for advanced dementia healthcare solutions.

Figure 4.1 shows an array of IoT devices and sensors, seamlessly integrated into healthcare systems, specifically designed to monitor and support Alzheimer's disease and dementia patients.

Building upon the promise of IoT technologies, the following sections delve into specific applications that further the capabilities of personalized healthcare for dementia patients, starting with wearable devices for continuous health monitoring.

4.2.1 Wearable Devices

4.2.1.1 Smartwatches and Wearable Sensors

Wearable technologies, including smartwatches, fitness trackers, and specialized health monitors, are designed to continuously monitor a variety of physiological parameters. Devices such as the Apple Watch and Fitbit are renowned for their reliability and comprehensive tracking features. These wearables can measure heart rate, blood pressure, skin temperature, sleep patterns, and physical activity levels (Bächlin et al., 2010; Piwek et al., 2016).

For instance, smartwatches are pivotal in healthcare for their ability to detect changes in gait or sudden drops in physical activity, which could indicate an increased risk of falls or mobility issues. These signs are particularly relevant in the early stages of dementia. By providing continuous health data, these devices facilitate the early detection and management of various health conditions, potentially including dementia. The continuous data collection enables timely interventions and supports proactive healthcare management, enhancing patient outcomes and improving quality of life.

4.2.2 In-Home Sensors

4.2.2.1 Motion Sensors

Devices like infrared motion detectors and smart floor mats play a crucial role in monitoring movement within the home. These sensors help track activity levels and detect falls, significantly contributing to the safety and well-being of dementia patients (Rashidi & Mihailidis, 2013).

4.2.2.2 Smart Home Systems

Comprehensive smart home systems integrate various interconnected devices, including motion detectors, smart lighting, smart thermostats, door sensors, and appliance usage monitors. These systems create adaptive environments tailored to the needs of dementia patients by continuously observing daily routines and behaviours. For instance, motion detectors monitor the frequency and duration of room usage, while smart lighting adjusts based on activity levels to provide appropriate illumination. Smart thermostats maintain comfortable temperatures, and appliance monitors detect irregular usage patterns, such as leaving the stove on for an extended period or not using the refrigerator, ensuring a safer living environment (Chan et al., 2008; Majumder et al., 2017).

By combining these technologies, smart home systems can provide a comprehensive, responsive environment that enhances the safety, comfort, and overall well-being of dementia patients, facilitating better care and management within their homes.

4.2.3 Location Tracking Devices

4.2.3.1 GPS Trackers

Devices such as GPS-enabled bracelets and shoe inserts are invaluable tools for monitoring the location of dementia patients who are at risk of wandering. These devices provide real-time location tracking, which is crucial for ensuring the safety of patients and offering peace of mind for caregivers (Morris et al., 2013; Shoval et al., 2008).

4.2.3.2 Functionality and Benefits

GPS trackers offer several significant benefits for monitoring dementia patients, ensuring their safety and providing peace of mind for caregivers. These devices continuously transmit the patient's location in real-time to caregivers or monitoring centres, enabling immediate intervention if the patient strays beyond predefined safe zones. Many GPS tracking systems also include geo-fencing capabilities, allowing caregivers to set virtual boundaries. If the patient crosses these boundaries, alerts are sent to caregivers, prompting quick action to ensure the patient's safety.

Additionally, GPS trackers often store historical location data, which caregivers and medical professionals can review to analyse movement patterns. This historical data is crucial for identifying frequent wandering episodes or specific areas the patient repeatedly visits, aiding in understanding behaviour and planning appropriate interventions. Modern GPS devices are designed to be discreet and comfortable, often integrated into everyday items like bracelets, watches, or shoe inserts. This discreet design ensures that patients are more likely to wear the devices consistently, providing continuous monitoring without causing discomfort or stigma.

Moreover, GPS trackers can be integrated with broader smart home systems, enhancing the overall monitoring and safety infrastructure. For instance, if a smart home system detects that a patient has left the house unexpectedly, the GPS tracker can provide continuous location updates until the patient is safely returned. This integration creates a comprehensive safety net, ensuring that caregivers can quickly respond to potential risks and maintain the well-being of dementia patients.

GPS trackers have several critical applications in the care of dementia patients, with case studies highlighting their effectiveness in various scenarios. One of the primary uses is in preventing wandering, a common and dangerous behaviour among dementia patients. These devices provide caregivers with real-time location data, enabling them to quickly locate and return wandering patients, thereby preventing potential harm (Edelstein & Staats, 1998; Klein et al., 1999; Rolland et al., 2003). Additionally, GPS trackers offer peace of mind for caregivers by significantly reducing the anxiety and stress associated with not knowing the exact location of their loved ones. This constant reassurance allows caregivers to attend to other tasks or take needed breaks, confident that they will be alerted if any issue arises (Pot, Willemse, & Horjus, 2012).

Furthermore, GPS tracking enhances patient autonomy by providing a safety net that allows dementia patients to enjoy greater freedom. Patients can move about within predefined safe zones without requiring the constant physical presence of a caregiver, which can significantly improve their quality of life and sense of independence (Rowe & Kahn, 2015). These applications demonstrate the profound impact of GPS tracking technology in ensuring the safety, reducing the stress of caregivers, and promoting the autonomy of dementia patients.

By integrating GPS tracking into the care routines for dementia patients, caregivers can significantly enhance the safety and quality of life for these individuals. The ability to monitor location in real-time, combined with features like geo-fencing and historical data analysis, makes GPS trackers an essential component of modern dementia care strategies.

4.2.4 Health Monitoring Sensors

4.2.4.1 Blood Pressure Monitors and Glucose Monitors

Wearable devices that track blood pressure and monitor blood glucose levels are indispensable for managing chronic conditions in elderly patients, including those with dementia (He, Goodkind, & Kowal, 2016; Moore et al., 2021; Teixeira et al., 2021).

Wearable blood pressure monitors can track patients' blood pressure throughout the day, offering a comprehensive view of their cardiovascular health. Consistent monitoring helps in detecting hypertension or hypotension early, allowing for timely interventions. In dementia patients, who may have difficulty communicating symptoms, continuous blood pressure monitoring ensures that fluctuations are promptly identified and managed. This proactive approach can prevent complications such as strokes or heart attacks, which are particularly detrimental to elderly individuals with cognitive impairments.

Continuous glucose monitors (CGMs) are essential for patients with diabetes, a common comorbidity in the elderly population. These devices track glucose levels throughout the day and night, providing critical data for managing diabetes effectively. For dementia patients, who may forget to check their blood sugar or fail to recognize symptoms of hypo- or hyperglycaemia, CGMs are lifesavers. The real-time data and alerts for abnormal glucose levels enable caregivers and medical professionals to intervene swiftly, ensuring that blood sugar levels remain within a safe range. This continuous monitoring helps prevent severe complications like diabetic ketoacidosis or hypoglycaemic comas, which can be fatal (Savoy et al., 2024).

Both blood pressure and glucose monitors can be integrated into broader health management systems. These systems aggregate data from various wearable devices, providing a holistic view of the patient's health. For instance, combining data from blood pressure monitors, glucose monitors, and other wearable sensors can help identify patterns and correlations between different health metrics. This integrated approach facilitates personalized care plans and more accurate adjustments to medications and lifestyle interventions.

For caregivers, these wearable monitors alleviate the constant need for manual health checks, reducing their workload and stress. They can receive alerts and updates through connected apps, ensuring they are always informed of the patient's health status. Medical professionals benefit from access to detailed health records over time, which aids in making informed decisions about treatment plans. The continuous data stream allows for better tracking of the effectiveness of treatments and timely modifications based on the patient's current condition.

Wearable blood pressure and glucose monitors improve patient compliance by simplifying the monitoring process. Patients are more likely to adhere to health monitoring protocols when the process is seamless and non-intrusive.

This increased compliance leads to better management of chronic conditions, resulting in improved health outcomes. For dementia patients, who may struggle with complex health routines, the simplicity and reliability of wearable monitors are particularly beneficial.

4.2.5 Communication Aids

4.2.5.1 Smart Speakers and Tablets

Devices like Amazon Echo and Google Home, along with tablets and smartphones, facilitate communication, provide medication reminders, and support cognitive exercises through telehealth consultations (Chang, Chen, & Huang, 2011; Peek et al., 2014).

Smart speakers and tablets are particularly valuable in facilitating communication between dementia patients, caregivers, and healthcare providers. Devices like Amazon Echo and Google Home use voice-activated commands, which can be especially beneficial for patients who may have difficulty using traditional interfaces. These devices can be programmed to make hands-free calls, send messages, and even provide visual communication through video calls. This capability ensures that patients can maintain regular contact with their caregivers and medical professionals, reducing feelings of isolation and enhancing their overall well-being.

One of the critical challenges in managing dementia is ensuring that patients take their medications correctly and on time. Smart speakers and tablets can be programmed to provide timely medication reminders. These devices can announce reminders audibly and display them visually, helping to ensure that patients do not miss their doses. For example, an Amazon Echo can be set to remind a patient to take their morning medication at a specific time each day, while also providing instructions on dosage. This functionality is crucial in preventing medication errors, which are common in dementia care due to memory lapses (Paul et al., 2024).

Cognitive exercises are essential in slowing the progression of dementia and maintaining cognitive function. Smart speakers and tablets support a wide range of cognitive training applications and programs. These devices can guide patients through brain games, puzzles, and other cognitive activities designed to stimulate the mind. Applications available on tablets and smartphones can be personalized to the patient's cognitive level and preferences, making the exercises engaging and effective. Additionally, smart speakers can facilitate interactive activities, such as storytelling or question-and-answer games, which can help improve cognitive skills and provide mental stimulation.

The integration of telehealth services with smart speakers and tablets has revolutionized healthcare access for dementia patients. These devices enable virtual consultations with healthcare providers, allowing patients to receive medical advice and care without the need to visit a clinic. Telehealth consultations are particularly beneficial for patients with mobility issues or those living in remote areas. Tablets and smartphones equipped with video call capabilities can connect patients with doctors, therapists, and other healthcare professionals, ensuring continuous and comprehensive care. This approach not only enhances convenience but also ensures that patients receive timely medical attention, which is crucial in managing dementia effectively.

Smart speakers and tablets provide an interactive and engaging way to deliver care. For instance, these devices can be programmed to play music, audiobooks, or favourite radio stations, providing entertainment and relaxation for patients. They can also be used to set routines, such as morning greetings, reminders to hydrate, or notifications for exercise times, helping to establish a structured daily routine that can be comforting for dementia patients (Shu & Woo, 2021).

In case of emergencies, smart speakers can be programmed to contact emergency services or caregivers immediately. Devices like Amazon Echo can recognize distress signals or commands such as "help," triggering an emergency response. This feature provides an added layer of security for patients living independently or with minimal supervision.

Tablets and smartphones can also serve as educational tools for caregivers. They provide access to a wealth of information, including care tips, training videos, and resources on dementia management. Caregivers can use these devices to stay informed about best practices and new developments in dementia care, improving their ability to provide effective support.

4.2.6 Medication Management

4.2.6.1 Smart Pill Dispensers

Devices such as MedMinder and Hero Health dispense medication at prescribed times and alert patients, ensuring compliance and reducing errors in medication administration (Gargioni, Fogli, & Baroni, 2024; Hero Health, 2023; Holden et al., 2020; Jeon, Chae, & Kim, 2022; Mann et al., 2005; Nasir et al., 2023; Shahani et al., 2022).

In addition to automated dispensing, smart pill dispensers provide reminders and alerts to ensure patients take their medication on time. These reminders can be in the form of audible alarms, flashing lights, or even notifications sent to a patient's smartphone or smartwatch. For example, Hero Health can be programmed to send alerts to both the patient and their caregiver, ensuring that medication adherence is maintained even if the patient misses the initial reminder (Gargioni, Fogli, & Baroni, 2024; Shahani et al., 2022).

One of the standout features of smart pill dispensers is the ability to connect to mobile apps or cloud-based systems, allowing caregivers and healthcare providers to monitor medication adherence remotely. This connectivity ensures that caregivers are immediately informed if a dose is missed, enabling them to take timely action. This feature is particularly beneficial for caregivers who may not live with the patient or who need to manage multiple patients simultaneously (Gargioni, Fogli, & Baroni, 2024; Holden et al., 2020).

Many smart pill dispensers come with locking mechanisms to prevent patients from accessing the medication outside of the prescribed times. This feature is essential for preventing accidental or intentional misuse of medication, ensuring that patients only take their medication as directed by their healthcare provider. Devices like MedMinder are equipped with secure compartments that can only be opened when it is time to take the medication (Mann et al., 1999; Mann et al., 2005).

Smart pill dispensers can be programmed to accommodate complex medication schedules, including multiple medications taken at different times of the day. This capability is crucial for dementia patients who often have complicated medication regimens. By providing a personalized schedule, these devices help manage polypharmacy, reducing the cognitive load on patients and caregivers (Gargioni, Fogli, & Baroni, 2024).

Advanced smart pill dispensers can integrate with electronic health records (EHRs) and other healthcare systems, ensuring that medication data is accurately recorded and accessible to healthcare providers. This integration facilitates better coordination of care, as providers can easily track medication adherence and make informed decisions about treatment plans (Mann et al., 2005; Walling et al., 2023).

Research has shown that smart pill dispensers significantly improve medication adherence rates among elderly patients. By ensuring that patients take their medication as prescribed, these devices help manage chronic conditions more effectively, leading to better health outcomes. For dementia patients, consistent medication adherence can slow the progression of the disease and improve overall quality of life (Gargioni, Fogli, & Baroni, 2024; Holden et al., 2020; Shahani et al., 2022).

Some smart pill dispensers also offer educational resources and training support for patients and caregivers. These resources can include instructional videos on how to use the device, information about the medications being taken, and tips for managing side effects. This support helps patients and caregivers feel more confident and informed about their medication regimen (Gargioni, Fogli, & Baroni, 2024; Mann et al., 1999; Mann et al., 2005).

By automating medication management and providing reliable reminders, smart pill dispensers reduce the anxiety and stress associated with managing multiple medications. This reduction in cognitive burden allows patients to focus more on their daily activities and enjoy a better quality of life. For caregivers, the assurance that their loved ones are taking their medication correctly provides peace of mind and reduces the time and effort required to oversee medication management (Gargioni, Fogli, & Baroni, 2024; Holden et al., 2020; Jeon, Chae, & Kim, 2022; Nasir et al., 2023; Shahani et al., 2022).

Smart pill dispensers like MedMinder and Hero Health play a crucial role in enhancing the safety and efficacy of medication management for dementia patients. By ensuring timely and accurate medication adherence, these devices help mitigate the risks associated with medication errors and support better health outcomes. Their integration with modern healthcare systems and remote monitoring capabilities further extends their benefits, making them an indispensable tool in the proactive and personalized care of the aging population (Hero Health, 2023; Mann et al., 1999, 2005; MedMinder, 2023).

IoT devices and sensors significantly enhance healthcare delivery by enabling continuous monitoring and real-time intervention. These technologies provide essential data that improve the management of dementia, increasing safety and improving the quality of life. By integrating IoT devices into healthcare routines, providers can develop more proactive and personalized healthcare solutions for the aging population (Botsis et al., 2008; Holthe, Halvorsrud, & Lund, 2022; Milligan, 2010; Moore et al., 2021; Teixeira et al., 2021; Uddin, Khaksar, & Torresen, 2018).

IoT devices such as wearable sensors, smart home systems, and smart pill dispensers enable continuous monitoring of physiological parameters, environmental conditions, and medication adherence. This continuous data collection allows for the early detection of health issues and timely interventions, which are critical in managing chronic conditions and ensuring the well-being of dementia patients (He, Goodkind, & Kowal, 2016).

The real-time data provided by IoT devices allows healthcare providers to intervene promptly when potential issues are detected. For example, if a wearable sensor detects abnormal heart rate patterns, an alert can be sent to both the patient and their healthcare provider, enabling immediate action. This capability is particularly important in preventing severe health events and managing acute conditions (Botsis et al., 2008; Holthe, Halvorsrud, & Lund, 2022; Milligan, 2010; Uddin, Khaksar, & Torresen, 2018).

The data collected by IoT devices can be analysed to develop personalized healthcare solutions tailored to the specific needs of each patient. By understanding individual health patterns and behaviours, providers can create customized care plans that address the unique challenges faced by dementia patients. This personalized approach improves the effectiveness of treatments and enhances patient outcomes (He, Goodkind, & Kowal, 2016).

By providing continuous monitoring and real-time interventions, IoT devices help improve the quality of life for dementia patients. These technologies enable patients to live more independently and safely while ensuring that caregivers and healthcare providers have the information they need to provide optimal care. This balance between independence and support is crucial in enhancing the overall well-being of dementia patients (Botsis et al., 2008; Holthe, Halvorsrud, & Lund, 2022; Milligan, 2010; Uddin, Khaksar, & Torresen, 2018).

IoT devices and sensors significantly enhance healthcare delivery by enabling continuous monitoring and real-time intervention. They provide essential data that improve the management of dementia, increasing safety and improving quality of life. These technologies are integral to developing more proactive and personalized healthcare solutions for the aging population.

4.3 IoT Systems Supporting People with Dementia, Caregivers, and Medical Professionals

Dementia, a progressive neurodegenerative disorder characterized by cognitive decline and behavioural issues, affects approximately 50 million people worldwide, a number expected to triple by 2050 (World Health Organization, 2020). This substantial increase underscores the urgency of innovative solutions to support individuals with dementia, their caregivers, and medical professionals. The IoT, which connects physical objects to the internet, offers a promising avenue for addressing various challenges associated with dementia care (Atzori, Iera, & Morabito, 2010).

4.3.1 Support for People with Dementia

IoT systems have been proposed to assist people with dementia in numerous ways. These include aiding in daily activities (Rashidi & Mihailidis, 2013), supporting cognitive and physical therapies (Ahamed, Shahrestani, & Cheung, 2020; Alsharif et al., 2020; Doraiswamy, Narayan, & Manji, 2018), and enhancing safety through monitoring and alert systems (Jovanov et al., 2003). IoT devices such as smart home sensors, wearable devices, and GPS trackers can provide real-time data to monitor the physical and cognitive status of people with dementia, thereby enabling timely interventions and enhancing the quality of life for these individuals (Chan et al., 2009).

4.3.2 Support for Caregivers

Caregivers, both formal and informal, play a crucial role in the management of dementia. IoT systems can alleviate the burden on caregivers by providing tools for remote monitoring, real-time alerts, and automated assistance (Ahamed, Shahrestani, & Cheung, 2020; Cahill, Begley, & Faulkner, 2007; Esquer, Rodríguez, & Gutierrez-Garcia, 2023; Sokullu, Akkaş, & Demir, 2020). For instance, IoT-enabled smart home environments can detect unusual behaviours such as wandering or falls, notifying caregivers immediately and potentially preventing harm (Cahill, Begley, & Faulkner, 2007). Additionally, IoT solutions can facilitate communication between caregivers and medical professionals, ensuring coordinated care and timely updates on the condition of people with dementia (Moyle et al., 2017).

4.3.3 Support for Medical Professionals

Medical professionals benefit from IoT systems through enhanced diagnostic tools, continuous patient monitoring, and data-driven decision-making support (Islam et al., 2015). IoT devices can collect comprehensive health data over extended periods, providing insights that are not possible with intermittent clinical visits. This continuous data collection helps in early detection of disease progression, monitoring treatment efficacy, and adjusting care plans accordingly (Dimitrov, 2016).

4.3.4 Promising Areas of IoT Devices in Dementia Care

The integration of IoT devices in dementia care has opened several promising avenues for enhancing patient support, caregiver assistance, and medical management. Below are some of the key areas where IoT technologies are making significant strides:

4.3.4.1 Integration of IoT and AI

The combination of IoT and AI presents a significant opportunity for improving dementia care. ML algorithms can analyse data collected from IoT devices to detect patterns and predict health outcomes, leading to more personalized and effective interventions (Islam et al., 2015; Rashidi & Mihailidis, 2013). This integration can enhance the accuracy of diagnoses and the efficiency of care delivery.

4.3.4.2 Comprehensive Data Analysis

Utilizing consolidated datasets from various IoT devices can help identify common features across different dementia categories. Such comprehensive data analysis can reveal insights that are not apparent from isolated studies, potentially leading to breakthroughs in understanding and treating dementia (Esquer, Rodríguez, & Gutierrez-Garcia, 2023; Sheikhtaheri & Sabermahani, 2022).

4.3.4.3 Outdoor IoT Systems

Expanding IoT applications to outdoor environments can provide a more holistic approach to dementia care. Outdoor IoT systems can monitor patients during activities such as walking or gardening, which are known to have therapeutic benefits. This expansion can enhance the quality of life for people with dementia by promoting physical activity and providing caregivers with more comprehensive monitoring tools (D'Cunha et al., 2020; Finnanger Garshol, Ellingsen-Dalskau, & Pedersen, 2020; Mitchell & Burton, 2010).

4.3.4.4 Adaptive IoT Systems

Developing IoT systems that adjust according to the progression of dementia can provide tailored support for patients at different stages of the disease. Adaptive systems can modify their functionality based on the patient's current condition, offering more relevant and effective assistance as the disease progresses (Hallewell Haslwanter, Neureiter, & Garschall, 2020; Moyle et al.,

2017). This adaptability ensures that IoT solutions remain useful and supportive throughout the dementia trajectory.

4.4 Key Objectives in Dementia Care Using IoT Devices

The integration of IoT devices in dementia care serves multiple objectives, each aimed at improving the quality of life for patients and easing the burden on caregivers and medical professionals. The key objectives include disease detection, patient monitoring, patient localization, patient assistance, and cognitive training. Each of these objectives leverages specific IoT devices and AI/ML methods to achieve effective and efficient outcomes.

4.4.1 Disease Detection

IoT devices such as wearable sensors and smart home systems can continuously monitor various physiological and behavioural parameters. AI algorithms can analyse this data to detect early signs of dementia, enabling timely intervention and treatment (Dimitrov, 2016; Domingos et al., 2022).

4.4.2 Patient Monitoring

Continuous monitoring of patients using IoT devices such as smart watches, cameras, and environmental sensors helps track daily activities, vital signs, and potential health risks. ML models can predict and alert caregivers about unusual patterns that may indicate health issues (Islam et al., 2015).

4.4.3 Patient Localization

GPS-enabled wearables and beacon systems can track the location of dementia patients, providing real-time data to caregivers and preventing incidents such as wandering or getting lost. AI techniques can enhance location accuracy and predict potential wandering behaviours (Mitchell & Burton, 2010).

4.4.4 Patient Assistance

IoT devices such as smart speakers and automated home systems can assist patients with daily tasks and provide reminders for medication, appointments, and other activities. AI-driven personal assistants can adapt to the patient's needs and preferences, providing customized support (Moyle et al., 2017).

4.4.5 Cognitive Training

IoT devices can facilitate cognitive training exercises through interactive and engaging applications. AI and ML methods can personalize these exercises

TABLE 4.1

IoT Devices and AI/ML Methods for Dementia Care Objectives

Objective	IoT Devices	AI/ML Methods
Disease Detection	Wearable sensors, smart home systems	Machine learning algorithms (e.g., anomaly detection, supervised learning)
Patient Monitoring	Smartwatches, cameras, environmental sensors	Predictive modelling, pattern recognition
Patient Localization	GPS-enabled wearables, beacon systems	Geospatial analysis, predictive analytics
Patient Assistance	Smart speakers, automated home systems	Natural Language Processing (NLP), reinforcement learning
Cognitive Training	Interactive applications, VR/AR devices	Personalized learning algorithms, adaptive learning models

based on the patient's cognitive level and progress, promoting mental stimulation and potentially slowing cognitive decline (Rashidi & Mihailidis, 2013).

Table 4.1 insightfully categorizes various IoT devices alongside AI/ML methods tailored to enhance dementia care, ranging from disease detection to cognitive training. For disease detection, wearable sensors and smart home systems employ ML algorithms like anomaly detection and supervised learning, enabling nuanced health assessments and early disease identification. In patient monitoring, smartwatches, cameras, and environmental sensors utilize predictive modelling and pattern recognition to meticulously track health metrics, improving the management and timely intervention in dementia care.

Patient localization is significantly advanced through GPS-enabled wearables and beacon systems, which harness geospatial analysis and predictive analytics to ensure precise location tracking, crucial for the safety of dementia patients. For patient assistance, smart speakers and automated home systems integrate natural language processing and reinforcement learning, enhancing daily living assistance and interaction. Lastly, cognitive training is revolutionized by interactive applications and VR/AR devices that apply personalized and adaptive learning models, offering engaging and effective therapeutic activities tailored to individual cognitive needs (Adibi et al., 2024; Al-Ansi et al., 2023; Ermolina & Tiberius, 2021; Shajari et al., 2023; Zhang et al., 2023).

This table underscores the convergence of IoT with advanced AI/ML techniques, offering a spectrum of tools that not only improve the quality of life for individuals with dementia but also push the boundaries of what is possible in proactive health monitoring and personalized care. The comprehensive insights provided in the table and supported by seminal works emphasize the transformative role these technologies play in modern healthcare, marking significant strides toward more integrated, intelligent solutions in dementia care.

4.5 Commercial Tools Using IoT Devices in Dementia Care

Several commercial tools currently utilize IoT devices to enhance dementia care, offering innovative solutions for continuous monitoring, medication management, and patient safety. These tools integrate advanced technologies to provide comprehensive support for patients, caregivers, and healthcare professionals.

- **MedMinder**
  MedMinder is a smart pill dispenser that helps patients manage their medication schedules (Figure 4.2). It features audio and visual reminders and locks to prevent overdosing. It ensures timely medication intake, reduces errors, and allows remote monitoring by caregivers (Gargioni, Fogli, & Baroni, 2024; Mann et al., 2005; Shahani et al., 2022).

- **Hero Health**
  Hero Health offers an automated medication management system that dispenses the correct dosage at the scheduled times and sends reminders (Figure 4.3). It improves medication adherence, reduces caregiver burden, and integrates with mobile apps for remote monitoring (Gargioni, Fogli, & Baroni, 2024; Hero Health, 2023; Shahani et al., 2022).

- **Apple Watch and Fitbit**
  These wearables track various physiological parameters such as heart rate, sleep patterns, and physical activity levels (Figure 4.4).

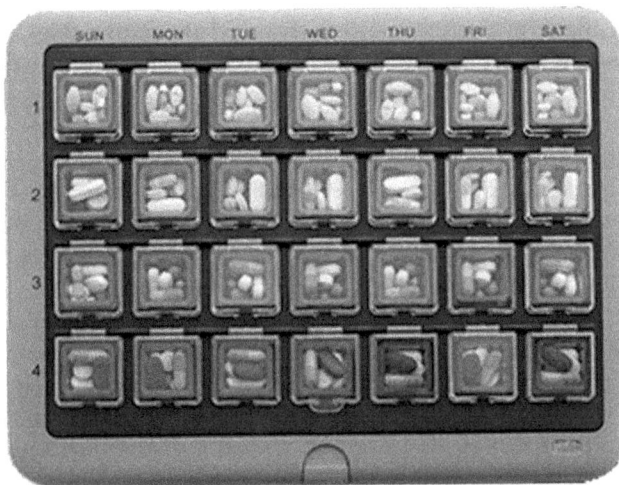

FIGURE 4.2
MedMinder medication dispenser helps seniors stay safe. (Retrieved from Assisted Living Services, Inc., 2013.)

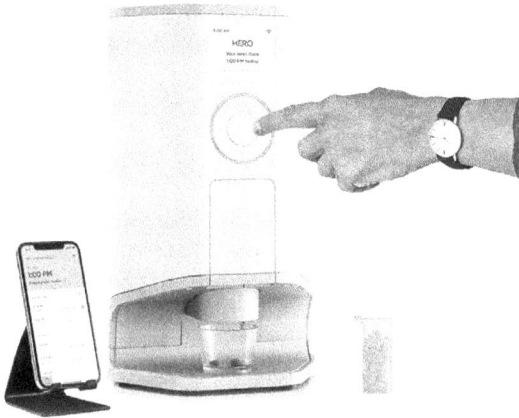

FIGURE 4.3
Managing medications has never been easier or more convenient than with the Hero platform.
(Retrieved from Hero Health, 2023.)

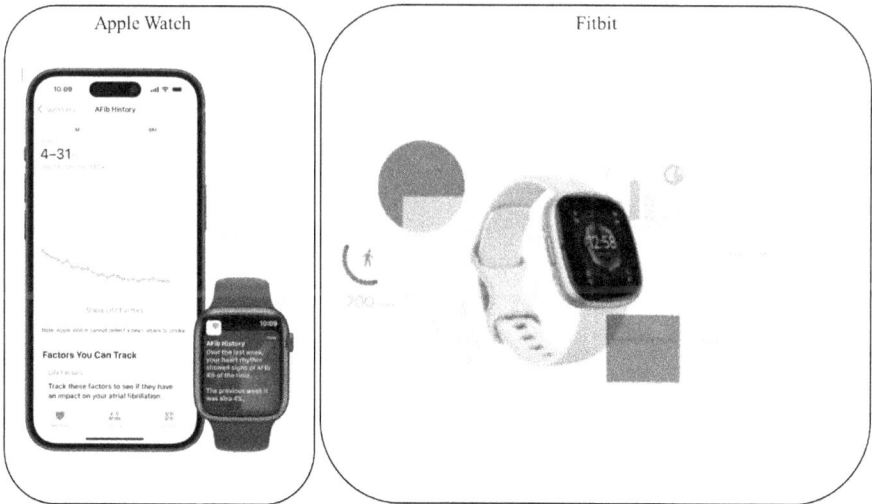

FIGURE 4.4
Left image: Apple Watch in Healthcare: Revolutionizing patient care with advanced health
monitoring and connectivity. (Adapted from Apple n.d.) Right image: Google's Device Connect
for Fitbit aims to revolutionize healthcare by integrating wearable data with clinical systems,
enhancing chronic condition management, clinical research, and overall health insights
through advanced analytics and AI. (Adapted from McCleary, 2022.)

It provides continuous health monitoring, detects early signs of health deterioration, and supports proactive healthcare management (Bächlin et al., 2010; Piwek et al., 2016).

- **Amazon Echo and Google Home**
  These smart speakers facilitate communication, provide medication reminders, and support cognitive exercises through voice-activated commands (Figure 4.5). It enhances communication, ensures medication compliance, and supports cognitive health (Chang, Chen, & Huang, 2011; Peek et al., 2014).

- **GPS Trackers (e.g., GPS-Enabled Bracelets, Shoe Inserts)**
  GPS trackers provide real-time location tracking to prevent wandering and ensure patient safety (Figure 4.6). It enhances patient safety, offers peace of mind for caregivers, and supports quick intervention in case of emergencies (Morris et al., 2013; Shoval et al., 2008).

Table 4.2 illustrates the commercial IoT tools that represent practical applications of advanced technologies in dementia care, providing comprehensive support to enhance patient safety, ensure medication compliance, and improve overall quality of life.

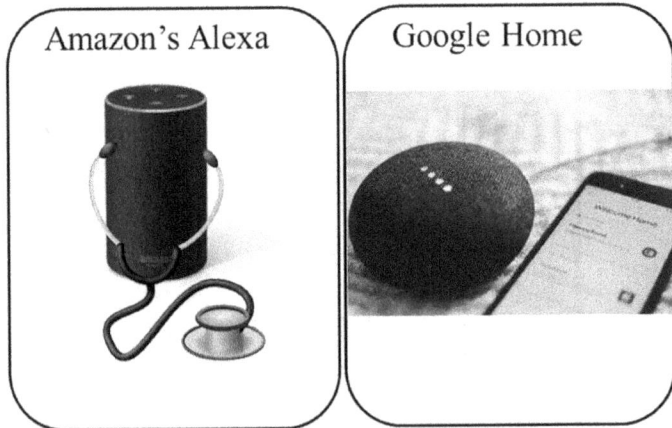

FIGURE 4.5
Left image: Amazon Alexa's health and wellness team innovates to provide advanced healthcare solutions. (Adapted from Kinsella, 2018, May 11.) Right image: Google Home serves as a crucial assistive technology for seniors with dementia, including Alzheimer's disease. This smart device aids in maintaining independence and safety by responding to voice commands for daily tasks and reminders, facilitating easier communication with caregivers, and enhancing overall daily engagement. (Adapted from Sova Healthcare, n.d.)

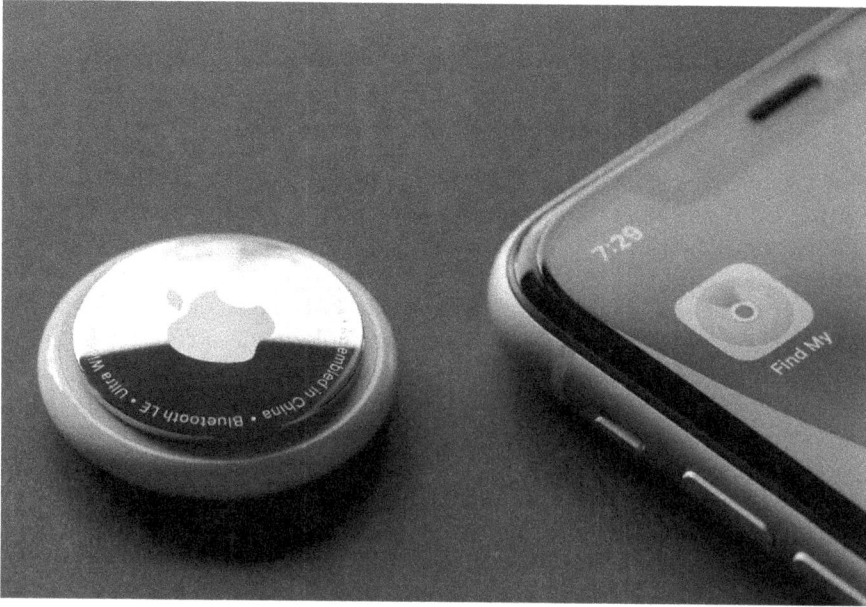

FIGURE 4.6
The GPS tracker according to the patient's lifestyle with real-time mapping. (Retrieved from Ambiq, n.d.).

TABLE 4.2

Commercial IoT Tools for Dementia Care

Tool	Description	Benefits	References
MedMinder	Smart pill dispenser with audio and visual reminders	Ensures timely medication intake, reduces errors	Gargioni, Fogli, and Baroni (2024); Mann et al. (2005); Shahani et al. (2022)
Hero Health	Automated medication management system	Improves medication adherence, integrates with mobile apps	Gargioni, Fogli, and Baroni (2024); Shahani et al. (2022)
Apple Watch and Fitbit	Wearables for tracking physiological parameters	Provides continuous health monitoring, supports proactive care	Bächlin et al. (2010); Piwek et al. (2016)
Amazon Echo and Google Home	Smart speakers for communication and reminders	Enhances communication, supports cognitive health	Chang, Chen, and Huang (2011); Peek et al. (2014)
GPS Trackers	Real-time location tracking devices	Ensures safety, prevents wandering, supports quick intervention	Shoval et al. (2008); Morris et al. (2013)

4.6 Integrative AI-Enhanced Health Monitoring Ecosystem for Elderly and Dementia Care: A Unified Approach to Real-Time Safety and Medical Response

The proposed AI-Enhanced Health Monitoring Ecosystem, illustrated in Figure 4.7, represents a cutting-edge approach to proactive healthcare for elderly populations, especially those affected by age-related conditions like dementia. Central to this ecosystem is the deployment of a network of IoT sensors and devices within residences that cater to these vulnerable groups. Key components include GPS-enabled wearable devices for tracking and safety, fall detection sensors to alert caregivers in the event of an accident, automated pill dispensers that ensure timely medication with accompanying audio prompts, and a comprehensive CCTV network. These tools are integrated into a cohesive framework that continuously feeds data to a cloud-based platform.

Here, advanced ML algorithms analyse the data to identify crucial events or potential emergencies in real-time. This system not only notifies

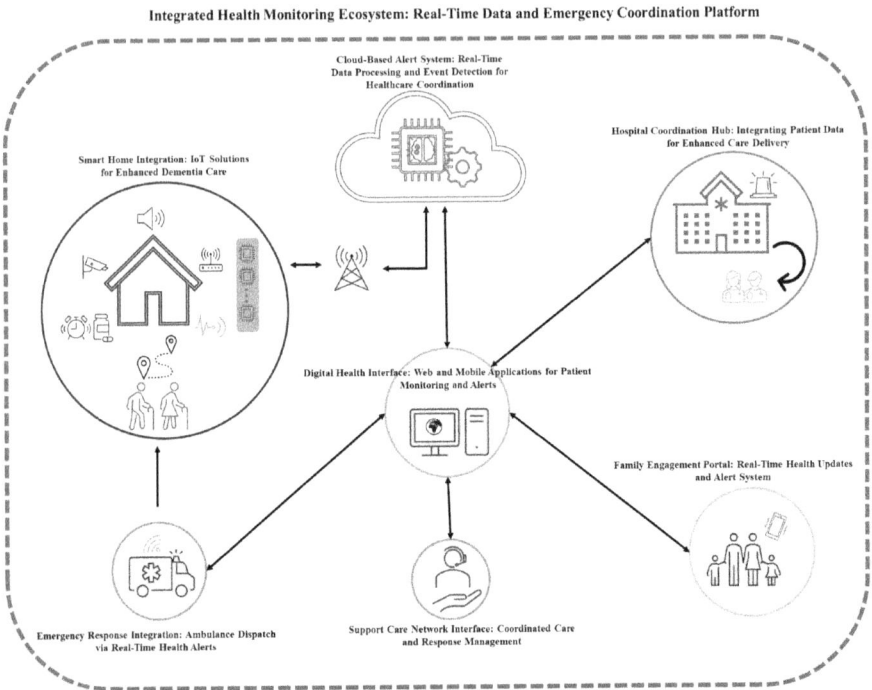

FIGURE 4.7
AI-enhanced health monitoring ecosystem: Leveraging real-time data and AI analytics for proactive emergency response and coordinated care across digital and service platforms.

healthcare providers and emergency services like ambulance crews via accessible web and mobile applications, but also enables routine monitoring by doctors and family members. To safeguard the privacy of individuals, crucial data is anonymized before it is shared, ensuring that personal information remains protected while still providing all parties with the necessary insights to deliver swift and effective care. This ecosystem offers a transformative solution to enhance the quality of life and safety for its users, promoting an integrated, technology-driven approach to age-related healthcare management.

This ecosystem addresses several critical issues faced by the elderly and their caregivers. One of the primary concerns in elderly care is the risk of falls, which can lead to serious injuries and long-term health complications. The fall detection sensors embedded in the system provide an immediate alert to caregivers and emergency services, drastically reducing the response time and potentially mitigating the severity of the injury. Moreover, GPS-enabled wearable devices ensure that elderly individuals who are prone to wandering, a common issue in dementia patients, can be quickly located and brought back to safety. This not only prevents potential accidents but also alleviates the anxiety of caregivers who constantly worry about the whereabouts of their loved ones.

Another significant aspect of the ecosystem is its ability to manage medication adherence through automated pill dispensers. Medication non-compliance is a prevalent issue among the elderly, often leading to worsening health conditions and hospitalizations. The automated dispensers ensure that medications are taken at the correct times, with audio prompts serving as reminders. This technology supports both the patient and the caregiver by reducing the burden of medication management and ensuring consistency in treatment regimens. The integration of these devices with a cloud-based platform allows healthcare providers to monitor adherence remotely, providing an additional layer of oversight and intervention when necessary.

The cloud-based platform acts as the central hub for data integration and analysis. By collecting data from various IoT devices, the platform creates a comprehensive health profile for each individual. Advanced ML algorithms then analyse this data to detect patterns and predict potential health issues before they become critical. This proactive approach to healthcare allows for timely interventions, which can prevent minor issues from escalating into major health crises. Additionally, routine monitoring and updates provided to doctors and family members ensure that everyone involved in the care process is well-informed and can make data-driven decisions.

Privacy and security are paramount in this ecosystem. The anonymization of data ensures that personal information is protected while still allowing for the necessary insights to be shared among healthcare providers and caregivers. This balance between data utility and privacy protection is crucial in gaining the trust of users and complying with regulatory standards.

4.6.1 Key Components and Benefits of the Proposed AI-Enhanced Health Monitoring Ecosystem

The key components and benefits of the proposed AI-Enhanced Health Monitoring Ecosystem highlight how each element contributes to creating a comprehensive, proactive, and integrated approach to elderly care, particularly for those with dementia.

1. **Network of IoT Sensors and Devices**
   - **GPS-Enabled Wearable Devices:** These devices track the elderly individual's location in real-time, ensuring safety, especially for those prone to wandering.
   - **Fall Detection Sensors:** Automatically detect falls and alert caregivers and emergency services, enabling rapid response to potential injuries.
   - **Automated Pill Dispensers:** Manage medication schedules with audio prompts, ensuring timely and correct dosage intake.
   - **Comprehensive CCTV Network:** Monitors the residence for unusual activities or emergencies, with real-time analysis to identify potential issues.

2. **Cloud-Based Platform**
   - **Data Integration:** Centralizes data collection from various IoT devices, ensuring seamless integration and continuous monitoring.
   - **Advanced Machine Learning Algorithms:** Analyse data to detect crucial events and potential emergencies in real time.

3. **Notification System**
   - **Healthcare Providers and Emergency Services:** Provides immediate notifications through web and mobile applications, ensuring quick and efficient dispatch of help.
   - **Routine Monitoring:** Allows doctors and family members to monitor health and well-being, receiving updates and alerts on any changes or concerns.

4. **Privacy and Security**
   - **Data Anonymization:** Ensures personal information is protected while sharing necessary insights for effective care delivery.

4.6.2 Benefits and Impact

- **Enhanced Quality of Life:** Continuous monitoring and timely interventions improve the overall well-being of elderly individuals.

- **Proactive Healthcare Management:** Advanced technologies enable a proactive approach, addressing potential issues before they escalate.
- **Peace of Mind:** Continuous monitoring provides peace of mind to caregivers and family members, reducing stress and anxiety.

Table 4.3 details the key components and features of the proposed AI-Enhanced Health Monitoring Ecosystem, illustrating how each element integrates advanced technologies to enhance elderly care, particularly for those with dementia.

This AI-Enhanced Health Monitoring Ecosystem is a transformative solution that leverages advanced technology to improve the quality of life and safety for elderly individuals, promoting a comprehensive and proactive approach to healthcare management. By integrating IoT sensors and devices with a robust cloud-based platform and advanced ML algorithms, this ecosystem ensures that elderly patients receive timely, personalized, and effective care. This not only enhances their safety and health outcomes but also supports caregivers by alleviating some of the burdens associated with elderly care.

Investing in this ecosystem represents a significant step forward in addressing the growing healthcare needs of the aging population. The combination of real-time data, advanced analytics, and seamless integration provides a holistic approach to healthcare that can adapt to the evolving needs of elderly individuals. This proactive model of care has the potential to reduce healthcare costs by preventing hospitalizations and other costly interventions, ultimately leading to a more sustainable and effective healthcare system.

TABLE 4.3

Key Components and Features of the Proposed AI-Enhanced Health Monitoring Ecosystem

Component	Features	Benefits
GPS-Enabled Wearable Devices	Real-time location tracking	Ensures safety, prevents wandering
Fall Detection Sensors	Automatic fall detection, emergency alerts	Rapid response to injuries
Automated Pill Dispensers	Scheduled medication dispensing, audio prompts	Ensures correct and timely medication intake
Comprehensive CCTV Network	Continuous monitoring, real-time analysis	Identifies unusual activities, enhances safety
Cloud-Based Platform	Data integration, machine learning algorithms	Seamless monitoring, real-time event detection
Notification System	Alerts for healthcare providers, family access	Quick help dispatch, routine health monitoring
Data Anonymization	Privacy protection	Safeguards personal information

4.7 Chapter Summary

The integration of AI and the IoT has brought about a paradigm shift in healthcare delivery, particularly in the management of Alzheimer's disease and dementia. By leveraging the capabilities of IoT devices equipped with various sensors, continuous real-time monitoring of patients' health and activity is now possible, providing caregivers and healthcare professionals with critical data for managing dementia effectively. This chapter has outlined how sensor-based IoT solutions facilitate comprehensive monitoring and seamlessly integrate with existing healthcare frameworks, enhancing the management and safety of dementia patients.

AI's role in analysing this vast amount of data is crucial, as ML algorithms can detect patterns and predict health deteriorations, enabling the dynamic customization of care plans. This shift towards proactive and preventative care models ensures that potential health issues are addressed before they escalate, significantly improving patient outcomes and quality of life.

The narrative also highlights the importance of wearable devices and smart home technologies in providing continuous health monitoring. These tools generate real-time data essential for early intervention and ongoing patient management. The ability to foresee potential health declines through ML analysis allows for timely adjustments to care plans, marking a significant move towards more personalized healthcare strategies.

Technological advancements and practical implementations of AI and IoT in dementia care are discussed, along with potential challenges such as data privacy, system interoperability, and the need for scalable solutions. Addressing these challenges is vital for the widespread adoption of these technologies, ensuring they meet the needs of an aging population.

The proposed AI-Enhanced Health Monitoring Ecosystem exemplifies a unified approach to real-time safety and medical response, integrating a network of IoT sensors and devices to continuously monitor and analyse health data. This system not only alerts healthcare providers and emergency services to potential emergencies but also enables routine monitoring by doctors and family members, ensuring comprehensive care delivery.

In summary, the integration of AI and IoT in healthcare represents a transformative solution for managing age-related conditions like dementia. By providing continuous, real-time monitoring and leveraging advanced ML algorithms, these technologies enhance patient safety, improve care quality, and promote proactive healthcare management, ultimately improving the lives of elderly individuals.

Building on the dynamic integration of AI and IoT outlined in this chapter, the subsequent discussion in "Conversational Agents in Healthcare: Leveraging Language Models and Chatbots for Patient Interaction" extends the application of AI in dementia care. This next chapter explores how conversational AI enhances the communication between patients and healthcare providers, enabling not only continuous but also interactive support tailored to the nuanced needs of dementia patients. These intelligent agents personify the next step in healthcare technology by offering responsive and adaptive interactions that foster better patient engagement and support.

Furthermore, the discussions in these chapters set the stage for the culminating insights in "Revolutionizing Dementia Care: Proposing a Comprehensive AI-Powered Global Framework for Enhanced Diagnosis and Personalized Treatment." Here, we synthesize the innovations from IoT and conversational AI to propose a visionary framework that not only addresses immediate healthcare needs but also anticipates future challenges in dementia care. This integrated approach promises a groundbreaking shift towards a more effective, efficient, and empathetic healthcare system for managing dementia on a global scale.

References

Abdulmalek, S., Nasir, A., Jabbar, W. A., Almuhaya, M. A. M., Bairagi, A. K., Khan, M. A., & Kee, S. H. (2022). IoT-based healthcare-monitoring system towards improving quality of life: A review. Healthcare (Basel), 10(10), 1993. https://doi.org/10.3390/healthcare10101993

Adibi, S., Rajabifard, A., Shojaei, D., & Wickramasinghe, N. (2024). Enhancing healthcare through sensor-enabled digital twins in smart environments: A comprehensive analysis. Sensors (Basel), 24(9), 2793. https://doi.org/10.3390/s24092793

Ahamed, F., Shahrestani, S., & Cheung, H. (2020). Internet of Things and machine learning for healthy ageing: Identifying the early signs of dementia. Sensors, 20(21), 6031. https://doi.org/10.3390/s20216031

Al-Ansi, A. M., Jaboob, M., Garad, A., & Al-Ansi, A. (2023). Analyzing augmented reality (AR) and virtual reality (VR) recent development in education. Social Sciences & Humanities Open, 8(1), 100532. https://doi.org/10.1016/j.ssaho.2023.100532

Alsharif, M. H., Kelechi, A. H., Yahya, K., & Chaudhry, S. A. (2020). Machine learning algorithms for smart data analysis in Internet of Things environment: Taxonomies and research trends. Symmetry, 12(1), 88. https://doi.org/10.3390/sym12010088

Ambiq. (n.d.). How IoT tracking devices can help people with dementia. Ambiq. Retrieved August 5, 2024, from https://ambiq.com/blog/how-iot-tracking-devices-can-help-people-with-dementia/

Assisted Living Services, Inc. (2013). MedMinder Medication Dispenser Helps Seniors Stay Safe. Assisted Living Services, Inc. Retrieved from https://www.assistedlivingct.com/medminder-medication-dispenser-helps-seniors-stay-safe/

Atzori, L., Iera, A., & Morabito, G. (2010). The Internet of Things: A survey. Computer Networks, 54(15), 2787–2805. https://doi.org/10.1016/j.comnet.2010.05.010

Botsis, T., Demiris, G., Pedersen, S., & Hartvigsen, G. (2008). Home telecare technologies for the elderly. Journal of Telemedicine and Telecare, 14(7), 333–337. https://doi.org/10.1258/jtt.2008.007002

Cahill, S. M., Begley, E., & Faulkner, J. P. (2007). "It gives me a sense of independence" – Findings from Ireland on the use and usefulness of assistive technology for people with dementia. Technology and Disability, 19(2/3), 133–142. https://doi.org/10.3233/TAD-2007-192-310

Chan, M., Estève, D., Escriba, C., & Campo, E. (2008). A review of smart homes – Present state and future challenges. Computer Methods and Programs in Biomedicine, 91(1), 55–81.

Chang, Y. J., Chen, S. F., & Huang, J. D. (2011). A Kinect-based system for physical rehabilitation: A pilot study for young adults with motor disabilities. Research in Developmental Disabilities, 32(6), 2566–2570. https://doi.org/10.1016/j.ridd.2011.07.002

Chen, M., Wan, J., & Li, F. (2012). Machine-to-machine communications: Architectures, standards, and applications. KSII Transactions on Internet and Information Systems, 6(2), 480–497.

Chimamiwa, G., Giaretta, A., Alirezaie, M., Pecora, F., & Loutfi, A. (2022). Are smart homes adequate for older adults with dementia? Sensors, 22(11), 4254. https://doi.org/10.3390/s22114254

D'Cunha, N. M., Isbel, S., McKune, A. J., Kellett, J., & Naumovski, N. (2020). Activities outside of the care setting for people with dementia: A systematic review. BMJ Open, 10(10). https://doi.org/10.1136/bmjopen-2020-040753

Dimitrov, D. V. (2016). Medical Internet of Things and big data in healthcare. Healthcare Informatics Research, 22(3), 156–163. https://doi.org/10.4258/hir.2016.22.3.156

Ding, Y., Sohn, J. H., Kawczynski, M. G., Trivedi, H., Harnish, R., Jenkins, N. W., Lituiev, D., Copeland, T. P., Aboian, M. S., Mari Aparici, C., Behr, S. C., Flavell, R. R., Huang, S. Y., Zalocusky, K. A., Nardo, L., Seo, Y., Hawkins, R. A., Hernandez Pampaloni, M., Hadley, D., & Franc, B. L. (2019). A deep learning model to predict a diagnosis of Alzheimer disease by using 18F-FDG PET of the brain. Radiology, 290(2), 456–464. https://doi.org/10.1148/radiol.2018180958

Domingos, C., Costa, P., Santos, N. C., & Pêgo, J. M. (2022). Usability, acceptability, and satisfaction of a wearable activity tracker in older adults: Observational study in a real-life context in Northern Portugal. Journal of Medical Internet Research, 24(1), e26652. https://doi.org/10.2196/26652

Doraiswamy, P. M., Narayan, V. A., & Manji, H. K. (2018). Mobile and pervasive computing technologies and the future of Alzheimer's clinical trials. npj Digital Medicine, 1, Article 1. https://doi.org/10.1038/s41746-017-0008-y

Edelstein, B., & Staats, N. (1998). Behavioral management of problem behaviors associated with dementia. In V. E. Caballo (Ed.), International Handbook of Cognitive and Behavioural Treatments for Psychological Disorders. pp. 617–648.

Ermolina, A., & Tiberius, V. (2021). Voice-controlled intelligent personal assistants in health care: International Delphi study. Journal of Medical Internet Research, 23(4), e25312. https://doi.org/10.2196/25312

Esquer, M. A., Rodríguez, L.-F., & Gutierrez-Garcia, J. O. (2023). The Internet of Things in dementia: A systematic review. Internet of Things, 22(10248), 100824. https://doi.org/10.1016/j.iot.2023.100824

Finnanger Garshol, B., Ellingsen-Dalskau, L. H., & Pedersen, I. (2020). Physical activity in people with dementia attending farm-based dementia day care – a comparative actigraphy study. BMC Geriatrics, 20(1), 219. https://doi.org/10.1186/s12877-020-01618-4

Gargioni, L., Fogli, D., & Baroni, P. (2024). A systematic review on pill and medication dispensers from a human-centered perspective. Journal of Healthcare Informatics Research, 8(2), 244–285. https://doi.org/10.1007/s41666-024-00161-w

Hallewell Haslwanter, J. D., Neureiter, K., & Garschall, M. (2020). User-centered design in AAL: Usage, knowledge of and perceived suitability of methods. Universal Access in the Information Society, 19, 57–67. Published July 23, 2018. https://link.springer.com/article/10.1007/s10209-018-0626-4

He, W., Goodkind, D., & Kowal, P. (2016). An aging world: 2015. *United States Census Bureau, International Population Reports, 95/16.*

Hero Health. (2023). Prescription Pill Dispenser, Sorter & Manager. Hero Health. Retrieved from https://herohealth.com

Holden, R. J., Campbell, N. L., Abebe, E., Clark, D. O., Ferguson, D., Bodke, K., Boustani, M. A., & Callahan, C. M. (2020). Usability and feasibility of consumer-facing technology to reduce unsafe medication use by older adults. Research in Social and Administrative Pharmacy, 16(1), 54–61. https://doi.org/10.1016/j.sapharm.2019.02.011

Holthe, T., Halvorsrud, L., & Lund, A. (2022). Digital assistive technology to support everyday living in community-dwelling older adults with mild cognitive impairment and dementia. Clinical Interventions in Aging, 17, 519–544. https://doi.org/10.2147/CIA.S357860

Islam, S. M. R., Kwak, D., Kabir, M. H., Hossain, M., & Kwak, K. S. (2015). The Internet of Things for health care: A comprehensive survey. IEEE Access, 3, 678–708.

Jeon, H. O., Chae, M.-O., & Kim, A. (2022). Effects of medication adherence interventions for older adults with chronic illnesses: A systematic review and meta-analysis. Osong Public Health and Research Perspectives, 13(5), 328–340. https://doi.org/10.24171/j.phrp.2022.0168

Jovanov, E., Milenkovic, A., Otto, C., & De Groen, P. C. (2003). A wireless body area network of intelligent motion sensors for computer assisted physical rehabilitation. Journal of NeuroEngineering and Rehabilitation, 2(1), 6.

Kinsella, B. (2018, May 11). Amazon Alexa has a health and wellness team to create healthcare solutions. Voicebot.ai. Retrieved from https://voicebot.ai/2018/05/11/amazon-alexa-has-a-health-and-wellness-team-to-create-healthcare-solutions/

Klein, D. A., Steinberg, M., Galik, E., Steele, C., Sheppard, J. M., Warren, A., Rosenblatt, A., & Lyketsos, C. G. (1999). Wandering behaviour in community-residing persons with dementia. International Journal of Geriatric Psychiatry, 14(4), 272–279. https://doi.org/10.1002/(SICI)1099-1166(199904)14:4<272::AID-GPS896>3.0.CO;2-P

Koutsouleris, N., Dwyer, D. B., Degenhardt, F., Maj, C., Urquijo-Castro, M. F., Sanfelici, R., Popovic, D., Oeztuerk, O., Haas, S. S., Weiske, J., Ruef, A., Kambeitz-Ilankovic, L., Antonucci, L. A., Neufang, S., Schmidt-Kraepelin, C., Ruhrmann, S., Penzel, N., Kambeitz, J., Haidl, T. K., Rosen, M., & … Meisenzahl, E. PRONIA Consortium (2021). Multimodal machine learning workflows for prediction of psychosis in patients with clinical high-risk syndromes and recent-onset depression. JAMA Psychiatry, 78(2), 195–209. https://doi.org/10.1001/jamapsychiatry.2020.3604

Li, C., Wang, J., Wang, S., & Zhang, Y. (2024). A review of IoT applications in healthcare. Neurocomputing, 565, 127017. https://doi.org/10.1016/j.neucom.2023.127017

Majumder, S., Aghayi, E., Noferesti, M., Memarzadeh-Tehran, H., Mondal, T., Pang, Z., & Deen, M. J. (2017). Smart homes for elderly healthcare: Recent advances and research challenges. Sensors, 17(11), 2496. https://doi.org/10.3390/s17112496

Mann, W. C., Belchior, P., Tomita, M. R., & Kemp, B. J. (2005). Computer use by middle-aged and older adults with disabilities. Technology and Disability, 17(1), 1–9. https://doi.org/10.3233/TAD-2005-17101

Mann, W. C., Ottenbacher, K. J., Fraas, L., Tomita, M., & Granger, C. V. (1999). Effectiveness of assistive technology and environmental interventions in maintaining independence and reducing home care costs for the frail elderly: A randomized controlled trial. Archives of Family Medicine, 8(3), 210–217. https://doi.org/10.1001/archfami.8.3.210

McCleary, W. (2022). Google's new plan to make Fitbit data more useful for healthcare [Image]. HealthTech Insider. Retrieved from https://healthtechinsider.com/2022/10/05/googles-new-plan-to-make-fitbit-data-more-useful-for-healthcare/

Milligan, C. (2010). Telecare and older people: Who cares where? Social Science & Medicine, 72(3), 347–354. https://doi.org/10.1016/j.socscimed.2010.08.014

Mitchell, L., & Burton, E. (2010). Designing dementia-friendly neighborhoods: Helping people with dementia to get out and about. Journal of Integrated Care, 18(6), 11–18.

Moore, K., O'Shea, E., Kenny, L., Barton, J., Tedesco, S., Sica, M., Crowe, C., Alamäki, A., Condell, J., Nordström, A., & Timmons, S. (2021). Older adults' experiences with using wearable devices: Qualitative systematic review and meta-synthesis. JMIR mHealth and uHealth, 9(6), e23832. https://doi.org/10.2196/23832

Morris, M. E., Adair, B., Miller, K., Ozanne, E., Hampson, R., Pearce, A., Santamaria, N., Viegas, L., Long, M., & Said, C. M. (2013). Smart-home technologies to assist older people to live well at home. Journal of Aging Science, 1(1), 101. https://www.researchgate.net/publication/237052835_Smart-Home_Technologies_to_Assist_Older_People_to_Live_Well_at_Home

Moyle, W., Murfield, J., & Lion, K. (2021). The effectiveness of smart home technologies to support the health outcomes of community-dwelling older adults living with dementia: A scoping review. International Journal of Medical Informatics, 153, 104513. https://doi.org/10.1016/j.ijmedinf.2021.104513

Nasir, Z., Asif, A., Nawaz, M., & Ali, M. (2023). Design of a smart medical box for automatic pill dispensing and health monitoring. Engineering Proceedings, 32(1), 7. Presented at the 2nd International Conference on Emerging Trends in Electronic and Telecommunication Engineering, Karachi, Pakistan, March 15–16, 2023. https://doi.org/10.3390/engproc2023032007

Nebeker, C., Torous, J., & Bartlett Ellis, R. J. (2019). Building the case for actionable ethics in digital health research supported by artificial intelligence. BMC Medicine, 17(1), 137.

Oskouei, R. J., MousaviLou, Z., Bakhtiari, Z., & Jalbani, K. B. (2020). IoT-based healthcare support system for Alzheimer's patients. Wireless Communications and Mobile Computing, 2020, 8822598. https://doi.org/10.1155/2020/8822598

Paul, L. C., Ahmed, S. S., Rani, T., Haque, M. A., Roy, T. K., Hossain, M. N., & Hossain, M. A. (2024). A smart medicine reminder kit with mobile phone calls and some health monitoring features for senior citizens. Heliyon, 10(4), Article e26308. https://doi.org/10.1016/j.heliyon.2024.e26308

Peek, S. T., Wouters, E. J., van Hoof, J., Luijkx, K. G., Boeije, H. R., & Vrijhoef, H. J. (2014). Factors influencing acceptance of technology for aging in place: A systematic review. International Journal of Medical Informatics, 83(4), 235–248. https://doi.org/10.1016/j.ijmedinf.2014.01.004

Piwek, L., Ellis, D. A., Andrews, S., & Joinson, A. (2016). The rise of consumer health wearables: Promises and barriers. PLoS Medicine, 13(2), e1001953. https://doi.org/10.1371/journal.pmed.1001953

Pot, A. M., Willemse, B. M., & Horjus, S. (2012). A pilot study on the use of tracking technology: Feasibility, acceptability, and benefits for people in early stages of dementia and their informal caregivers. Aging & Mental Health, 16(1), 127–134. https://doi.org/10.1080/13607863.2011.596810

Rashidi, P., & Mihailidis, A. (2013). A survey on ambient-assisted living tools for older adults. IEEE Journal of Biomedical and Health Informatics, 17(3), 579–590. https://doi.org/10.1109/JBHI.2012.2234129

Rolland, Y., Gillette-Guyonnet, S., Nourhashémi, F., Andrieu, S., Cantet, C., Payoux, P., Ousset, P. J., & Vellas, B. (2003). Déambulation et maladie de type Alzheimer. Etude descriptive. Programme de recherche REAL.FR sur la maladie d'Alzheimer et les filières de soins [Wandering and Alzheimer's type disease: Descriptive study. REAL.FR research program on Alzheimer's disease and management]. Revue de Médecine Interne, 24(Suppl 3), 333s–338s. [In French]. https://doi.org/10.1016/s0248-8663(03)80692-6

Rowe, J. W., & Kahn, R. L. (2015). Successful aging 2.0: Conceptual expansions for the 21st century. Journal of Gerontology: Series B, Psychological Sciences and Social Sciences, 70(4), 593–596. https://doi.org/10.1093/geronb/gbv025

Salvi, M., Loh, H. W., Seoni, S., Datta Barua, P., García, S., Molinari, F., & Acharya, U. R. (2024). Multi-modality approaches for medical support systems: A systematic review of the last decade. Information Fusion, 103, 102134. https://doi.org/10.1016/j.inffus.2023.102134

Savoy, A., Holden, R. J., de Groot, M., Clark, D. O., Sachs, G. A., Klonoff, D., & Weiner, M. (2024). Improving care for people living with dementia and diabetes: Applying the human-centered design process to continuous glucose monitoring. Journal of Diabetes Science and Technology, 18(1), 201–206. https://doi.org/10.1177/19322968221137907

Shahani, A., Nieva, H. R., & Czado, K., et al. (2022). An electronic pillbox intervention designed to improve medication safety during care transitions: Challenges and lessons learned regarding implementation and evaluation. BMC Health Services Research, 22, 1304. https://doi.org/10.1186/s12913-022-08702-y

Shajari, S., Kuruvinashetti, K., Komeili, A., & Sundararaj, U. (2023). The emergence of AI-based wearable sensors for digital health technology: A review. Sensors (Basel), 23(23), 9498. https://doi.org/10.3390/s23239498

Sheikhtaheri, A., & Sabermahani, F. (2022). Applications and outcomes of Internet of Things for patients with Alzheimer's disease/dementia: A scoping review. Biomed Research International, 2022, 6274185. https://doi.org/10.1155/2022/6274185

Shoval, N., Auslander, G. K., Freytag, T., Landau, R., Oswald, F., Seidl, U., … & Wahl, H. W. (2008). The use of advanced tracking technologies for the analysis of mobility in Alzheimer's disease and related cognitive diseases. BMC Geriatrics, 8(1), 7. https://doi.org/10.1186/1471-2318-8-7

Shu, S., & Woo, B. K. (2021). Use of technology and social media in dementia care: Current and future directions. World Journal of Psychiatry, 11(4), 109–123. https://doi.org/10.5498/wjp.v11.i4.109

Sokullu, R., Akkaş, M. A., & Demir, E. (2020). IoT supported smart home for the elderly. Internet of Things, 11, 100239. https://doi.org/10.1016/j.iot.2020.100239

Sova Healthcare. (n.d.). Alzheimer's assistive technology: Google Home. Retrieved from https://www.sovahealthcare.co.uk/blog/alzheimers-assistive-technology-google-home/

Teixeira, E., Fonseca, H., Diniz-Sousa, F., Veras, L., Boppre, G., Oliveira, J., Pinto, D., Alves, A. J., Barbosa, A., Mendes, R., & Marques-Aleixo, I. (2021). Wearable devices for physical activity and healthcare monitoring in elderly people: A critical review. Geriatrics (Basel), 6(2), 38. https://doi.org/10.3390/geriatrics6020038

Uddin, M. Z., Khaksar, W., & Torresen, J. (2018). Ambient sensors for elderly care and independent living: A survey. Sensors, 18(7), 2027. https://doi.org/10.3390/s18072027

Walling, A. M., Pevnick, J., Bennett, A. V., Vydiswaran, V. G. V., & Ritchie, C. S. (2023). Dementia and electronic health record phenotypes: A scoping review of available phenotypes and opportunities for future research. Journal of the American Medical Informatics Association, 30(7), 1333–1348. https://doi.org/10.1093/jamia/ocad086

World Health Organization. (2020). Dementia. Retrieved from https://www.who.int/news-room/fact-sheets/detail/dementia

Zhang, Y., Hu, Y., Jiang, N., & Yetisen, A. K. (2023). Wearable artificial intelligence biosensor networks. Biosensors and Bioelectronics, 219, 114825. https://doi.org/10.1016/j.bios.2022.114825

5

Advancing Dementia Care: AI and Machine Learning in Diagnosis and Drug Discovery

Helena Bahrami and Sasan Adibi

5.1 Introduction

Dementia refers to a range of brain disorders that impair cognitive functions such as memory, language, reasoning, and daily living skills. As a progressive condition, it often leads to a decline in the ability to process thoughts and maintain emotional control, affecting both behaviour and the ability to perform everyday activities. Although dementia is predominantly diagnosed in older individuals, it is not an exclusive part of aging.

Globally, over 55 million people are living with dementia, with an estimated 10 million new cases every year. The incidence of dementia is rising, particularly in low- and middle-income countries where over 60% of cases are now reported. This number is expected to grow substantially, with projections indicating that by 2050, around 139 million people could be living with the condition (World Health Organization (WHO), 2023; Alzheimer's Disease International (ADI), 2024).

To seamlessly transition from the foundational discussion in this chapter to subsequent explorations in "Empowering Patient Care: Leveraging Artificial Intelligence and Internet of Things for Enhanced Healthcare Delivery" and "Conversational Agents in Healthcare: Leveraging Language Models and Chatbots for Patient Interaction," we will delve deeper into how AI and IoT can be harnessed to refine care delivery methods and enhance patient interactions through conversational AI tools. These discussions will pave the way for the culminating proposal of a comprehensive AI-powered global framework, aimed at revolutionizing dementia care through enhanced diagnosis, personalized treatment, and integrated care systems.

DOI: 10.1201/9781003485681-5

5.1.1 Types of Dementia and Their Symptoms

There are over 100 different known types of dementia (Earlstein, 2016; Beller et al., 2020; Budson & Solomon, 2021; National Institute on Aging, 2023; Dementia UK, n.d.). The most common types and their characteristics are:

5.1.1.1 Alzheimer's Disease (AD)

AD is a neurodegenerative disorder characterized by progressive memory loss, cognitive decline, and behavioural changes. It is the most common form of dementia, primarily affecting older adults, and is associated with the buildup of amyloid plaques and tau tangles in the brain (Timsina et al., 2023; Gonzalez-Ortiz et al., 2024; Grigoli et al., 2024).

- **Brain Changes:** Abnormal deposits of amyloid plaques and tau tangles disrupt cell function and communication.
- **Symptoms:** Memory loss, confusion, difficulty with language and problem-solving, changes in behaviour.
- **Progression:** Gradual and progressive, with symptoms worsening over time.
- **Typical Onset:** Usually after age 65, though early-onset can occur in 30s to mid-60s.
- **Risk Factors:** Age, genetics, family history, and certain lifestyle factors.
- **Biomarkers:** The accumulation of amyloid-beta (Aβ) plaques and tau protein tangles is a well-established biomarker for AD, observed through PET scans or measured in cerebrospinal fluid (CSF). Neurofilament light (NfL) is also emerging as a biomarker for neuronal damage in Alzheimer's.
- **Genetic Factors:** The APOE ε4 allele is the most significant genetic risk factor for late-onset AD. Mutations in the PSEN1, PSEN2, and APP genes are associated with early-onset familial Alzheimer's.

5.1.1.2 Vascular Dementia (VD)

VD is a non-neurodegenerative condition caused by reduced blood flow to the brain, often following strokes or other vascular issues. It leads to cognitive impairment that can vary in severity, depending on the extent and location of the brain damage, and is the second most common type of dementia after AD (Cipollini et al., 2019; Sanders et al., 2023).

- **Brain Changes:** Result from conditions that block or reduce blood flow to various regions of the brain, depriving them of oxygen and nutrients.

- **Symptoms:** Often include problems with planning, judgement, memory, and other thought processes.
- **Progression:** Can be sudden following a stroke or slowly due to chronic conditions.
- **Typical Onset:** Can occur after age 60, especially in individuals with a history of strokes or cardiovascular issues.
- **Risk Factors:** High blood pressure, smoking, diabetes, high cholesterol, and cardiovascular diseases.
- **Biomarkers:** White matter lesions, lacunar infarcts, and microbleeds are typical indicators of vascular damage seen in VD through neuroimaging. Elevated levels of inflammatory markers like C-reactive protein and homocysteine are associated with an increased risk of VD.
- **Genetic Factors:** The APOE ε4 allele is linked to an increased risk of VD, especially post-stroke. NOTCH3 mutations are associated with CADASIL, a genetic form of VD. CLIC1 and CLU gene variants are implicated in vascular function and amyloid metabolism.

5.1.1.3 Lewy Body Dementia (LBD)

LBD is a neurodegenerative disorder characterized by the presence of abnormal protein deposits called Lewy bodies in the brain. It causes cognitive fluctuations, visual hallucinations, and Parkinsonian motor symptoms, and is closely related to both Parkinson's disease and AD (Abdelmoaty et al., 2023; Wyman-Chick et al., 2024).

- **Brain Changes:** Characterized by abnormal deposits of the protein alpha-synuclein in the brain.
- **Symptoms:** Cognitive decline, visual hallucinations, movement disorders similar to Parkinson's, and sleep disturbances.
- **Progression:** Symptoms can fluctuate daily and worsen over time.
- **Typical Onset:** Generally, begins at age 50 or older.
- **Risk Factors:** Age, male gender, and possibly genetic factors.
- **Biomarkers:** The presence of alpha-synuclein aggregates (Lewy bodies) in the brain is a defining feature of LBD. Decreased dopamine transporter uptake, visible via DaTscan, is also a biomarker used in diagnosis.
- **Genetic Factors:** Mutations in the SNCA gene, which encodes alpha-synuclein, are linked to LBD. Variants in the GBA gene, associated with Gaucher's disease, and the LRRK2 gene, often linked to Parkinson's disease, are also associated with an increased risk of LBD.

5.1.1.4 *Frontotemporal Dementia (FTD)*

FTD is a neurodegenerative condition that primarily affects the frontal and temporal lobes of the brain, leading to changes in personality, behaviour, and language. FTD typically manifests at a younger age compared to other dementias and includes a group of disorders that affect specific regions of the brain, causing a range of symptoms depending on the area involved (Katisko et al., 2022; Mravinacová et al., 2024).

- **Brain Changes:** Involves degeneration of the frontal and temporal lobes of the brain.
- **Symptoms:** Changes in personality and behaviour, language difficulties, and movement problems.
- **Progression:** Progressive and varies depending on the subtype (behavioural variant, primary progressive aphasia, etc.).
- **Typical Onset:** Often begins between the ages of 40 and 65.
- **Risk Factors:** Genetic mutations are a significant risk factor.
- **Biomarkers:** TDP-43 protein inclusions, tau protein inclusions, and decreased progranulin levels are biomarkers associated with different forms of FTD. These can be detected in brain tissue or sometimes measured in CSF or blood.
- **Genetic Factors:** Mutations in the MAPT gene (affecting tau protein), GRN gene (affecting progranulin), and repeat expansions in the C9orf72 gene are common genetic causes of FTD. TARDBP mutations are less common but also associated with FTD.

Table 5.1 offers a detailed comparison of the major types of dementia, emphasizing both shared and distinct characteristics. All types exhibit a decline in cognitive functions, manifesting common symptoms such as memory loss, confusion, and behavioural changes that significantly affect daily living and communication abilities.

Specifically, the table delineates the unique pathological brain changes associated with each type of dementia, such as the presence of different proteins and the areas of the brain they affect. These distinctions are crucial for accurately diagnosing and differentiating between types (Ahmed et al., 2014; Oldan et al., 2021; Zabihi et al., 2021; Javeed et al., 2023).

Furthermore, the table outlines the diagnostic tools commonly used across all dementia types, including brain scans and blood tests. It highlights how the presence of particular biomarkers and genetic factors can vary markedly, providing essential insights into the underlying causes and informing potential treatment approaches. Additionally, demographic factors like age, lifestyle, and medical history are noted as significant contributors to the onset and progression of each type, emphasizing the importance of personalized care strategies.

TABLE 5.1

Comparative Overview of Dementia Types: Similarities, Differences, and Diagnostic Approaches

Aspect	Alzheimer's Disease (AD)	Vascular Dementia	Lewy Body Dementia	Frontotemporal Dementia (FTD)
Similarities	Decline in cognitive function, impacts daily life	Decline in cognitive function, impacts daily life	Decline in cognitive function, impacts daily life	Decline in cognitive function, impacts daily life
Common symptoms	Memory loss, confusion, communication difficulty	Memory loss, confusion, communication difficulty	Memory loss, confusion, communication difficulty	Memory loss, confusion, communication difficulty
Differences	Tau and amyloid proteins, memory-focused symptoms	Impaired blood flow, judgement, and planning issues	Alpha-synuclein proteins, visual hallucinations	Frontal/temporal lobe degeneration, behaviour, and language symptoms
Biomarkers	Amyloid-beta (Aβ) plaques, Tau protein tangles, and Neurofilament light (NfL) in cerebrospinal fluid (CSF) or blood	White matter lesions, lacunar infarcts, microbleeds (observed via MRI or CT scans), elevated C-reactive protein, and homocysteine levels	Alpha-synuclein aggregates (Lewy bodies), decreased dopamine transporter (DAT) uptake in the brain (visible via DaTscan)	TDP-43 protein inclusions, Tau protein inclusions, Progranulin (PGRN) levels in blood/CSF
Genetic factors	APOE ε4 allele, PSEN1 and PSEN2 mutations, APP gene mutations	APOE ε4 allele, NOTCH3 mutations (associated with CADASIL), CLIC1 and CLU gene variants	Mutations in the SNCA (alpha-synuclein) gene, GBA gene, and potentially LRRK2 gene variants	Mutations in the MAPT (Microtubule-Associated Protein Tau) gene, GRN (Progranulin) gene, C9orf72 repeat expansions, and TARDBP (TAR DNA-binding protein) gene
Clinical data	Blood tests, EEG, fMRI, PET scans, neurological exams	Blood tests, EEG, fMRI, PET scans, neurological exams	Blood tests, EEG, fMRI, PET scans, neurological exams	Blood tests, EEG, fMRI, PET scans, neurological exams
Demographic factors	Older age, genetics, lifestyle	History of strokes or cardiovascular issues, older age	Older age, male gender	Middle-aged adults, genetic predisposition

5.1.2 Identifying Genetic Biomarkers across Dementia Types

Genetic biomarkers are pivotal in deciphering the complexities of various dementia types. This section delves into how these markers vary across different disorders, enhancing the precision of AI and machine learning (ML)-based diagnostics and treatment strategies. By analysing genetic indicators, we uncover vital insights into the progression and possible therapeutic interventions for these challenging conditions.

In clinical practice, the collection of genetic biomarker data is a methodical process that integrates patient history, clinical evaluations, and advanced diagnostic tools. Initially, a comprehensive medical history and neurological examination are conducted to assess cognitive functions and identify potential familial patterns of dementia. Blood samples are then collected for genetic testing, which can identify key mutations such as the APOE ε4 allele in AD or the NOTCH3 gene in VD. Advanced imaging techniques, such as MRI and PET scans, are employed to detect structural brain changes and amyloid or tau deposits, which are critical in diagnosing AD and differentiating it from other types of dementia. CSF analysis through lumbar puncture further supports the diagnosis by measuring biomarkers like Aβ and tau proteins. In addition, emerging blood tests for biomarkers such as phosphorylated tau offer non-invasive alternatives for early detection. Cognitive and neuropsychological assessments complement these findings, providing a comprehensive understanding of the patient's cognitive decline and helping to distinguish between different dementia types. This multidisciplinary approach ensures that genetic and biomarker data are integrated into a precise and personalized diagnostic process, ultimately guiding treatment decisions and improving patient outcomes (Cipollini et al., 2019; Katisko et al., 2022; Abdelmoaty et al., 2023; Sanders et al., 2023; Gonzalez-Ortiz et al., 2024; Grigoli et al., 2024; Mravinacová et al., 2024; Wyman-Chick et al., 2024).

Table 5.2 provides a clear view of the key genetic markers for each major type of dementia, highlighting the specific mutations and genetic factors that play crucial roles in the pathogenesis and diagnosis of these conditions.

TABLE 5.2

Key Genetic Biomarkers Associated with Major Types of Dementia

Type of Dementia	Genetic Biomarkers
Alzheimer's disease (AD)	Primary: APOE ε4 allele. Others: Mutations in APP, PSEN1, and PSEN2 genes associated with familial Alzheimer's.
Vascular dementia (VD)	Primary: APOE ε4 allele (associated with risk, particularly post-stroke). Others: Mutations in the NOTCH3 gene associated with CADASIL.
Lewy body dementia (LBD)	Mutations in SNCA (alpha-synuclein) and GBA genes, linked to increased risk of Parkinson's disease and Lewy body dementia.
Frontotemporal dementia (FTD)	Mutations in MAPT (tau protein), GRN (progranulin), and C9orf72 genes, leading to abnormal accumulations of tau and TDP-43 proteins.

5.1.3 Importance of Ethnicity and Geography in Diagnosis and Drug Discovery of Dementia Types

Understanding variations in dementia prevalence across different ethnicities and geographic locations is vital due to factors like genetic susceptibility, cultural and environmental influences, drug efficacy and safety, and differences in healthcare access and diagnosis. Each of these factors can significantly impact the risk, management, and treatment of dementia in diverse populations. Knowing these differences helps tailor interventions, improve drug development, and enhance healthcare strategies to better serve specific groups (Prince et al., 2013).

Table 5.3 provides a general overview of the prevalence and distribution of various types of dementia across different ethnic groups and geographic locations.

While the table provides a general overview of the prevalence of different types of dementia by ethnic group and geographic location, it is important to recognize that the patterns presented are not absolute and may vary widely. Dementia prevalence is influenced by a complex interplay of genetic, environmental, and lifestyle factors, and the representation of certain ethnic groups or regions in research may reflect disparities in healthcare access, diagnostic capabilities, and study focus rather than true differences in prevalence. For instance, AD, while frequently studied in Caucasian, Hispanic, and African American populations in North America, is a global condition affecting diverse populations worldwide. Similarly, VD is prevalent across many regions, particularly in areas with high cardiovascular disease rates, such as East Asia and the Indian subcontinent, but it is also common globally. The apparent concentration of LBD and FTD in Caucasian populations in North America and Western Europe may be more indicative of where research is concentrated rather than where these conditions are exclusively found. Consequently, the data in the table should be viewed as a reflection of current research and diagnostic trends, acknowledging the broader global impact

TABLE 5.3

Prevalence of Dementia Types by Ethnicity and Geographic Location

Dementia Type	Ethnic Group	Geographic Location
Alzheimer's disease (AD)	Primarily Caucasian, but also Hispanic and African American	North America, Western Europe, Latin America
Vascular dementia	East Asian, South Asian, Caucasian	East Asia (Japan, China), Indian subcontinent, worldwide
Lewy body dementia	Primarily Caucasian	North America, Western Europe
Frontotemporal dementia (FTD)	Primarily Caucasian	North America, Western Europe

of these dementia types. However, categorizing dementia by ethnicity and geographic location also presents risks of bias and oversimplification that can affect diagnosis and treatment. These risks include the potential for over-generalization, which might overlook individual variations within groups, and the reinforcement of stereotypes that can lead to stigma and discrimination. Additionally, uneven resource allocation may result in less represented groups being overlooked, and the limited generalizability of clinical research that does not adequately reflect diverse populations can further exacerbate disparities. Addressing these challenges requires a balanced approach that integrates personalized medicine and culturally sensitive care, ensuring that medical research and healthcare practices are free from biases and are broadly applicable. This is particularly crucial in the context of AI and ML, where biases in diagnosis and drug discovery can significantly affect the accuracy, reliability, and fairness of the outcomes (Zhang et al., 1990; Poorkaj et al., 2001; Lleó et al., 2002; Hailpern et al., 2007; Schindler & Fagan, 2015; Mayeda et al., 2016; Steenland et al., 2016; Yang et al., 2023).

The above visualization illustrates the geographical distribution of various types of dementia across the world (Figure 5.1). The left subplot highlights the prevalence of AD, FTD, and VD in different countries. The right subplot specifically focuses on the prevalence of LBD. By separating the data into two subplots, we ensure that the overlapping regions where both AD and LBD are common, such as in the United States, Canada, and the United Kingdom, are clearly represented. This dual-plot approach provides a clearer understanding of how different dementia types are distributed globally.

Figures 5.2 and 5.3 illustrate the use of PET scan and fMRI technologies, respectively, to visualize brain activity in AD alongside a normal brain. Figure 5.2 displays PET scans that highlight amyloid deposition patterns in AD. The scans demonstrate the presence or absence of amyloid plaques in the brain, with a positive result indicating plaque accumulation, a hallmark of Alzheimer's pathology. These imaging techniques represent a major advancement in the diagnosis and assessment of cognitive impairment, allowing for the visualization of changes previously detectable only through autopsy. Figure 5.3 showcases fMRI images that reveal variations in brain activity and connectivity in AD and a normal case, providing insight into the neural mechanisms affected by each condition. These imaging techniques are crucial for diagnosing and understanding the pathophysiological differences between dementia types.

5.1.4 Global Impact of COVID-19 on Dementia Research Fundings

The COVID-19 pandemic has significantly impacted vulnerable populations, especially those living with dementia. Currently, over 50 million individuals worldwide are grappling with AD and other forms of dementia. The challenges posed by the pandemic have been profound due to disruptions in critical support structures, including research funding and healthcare services.

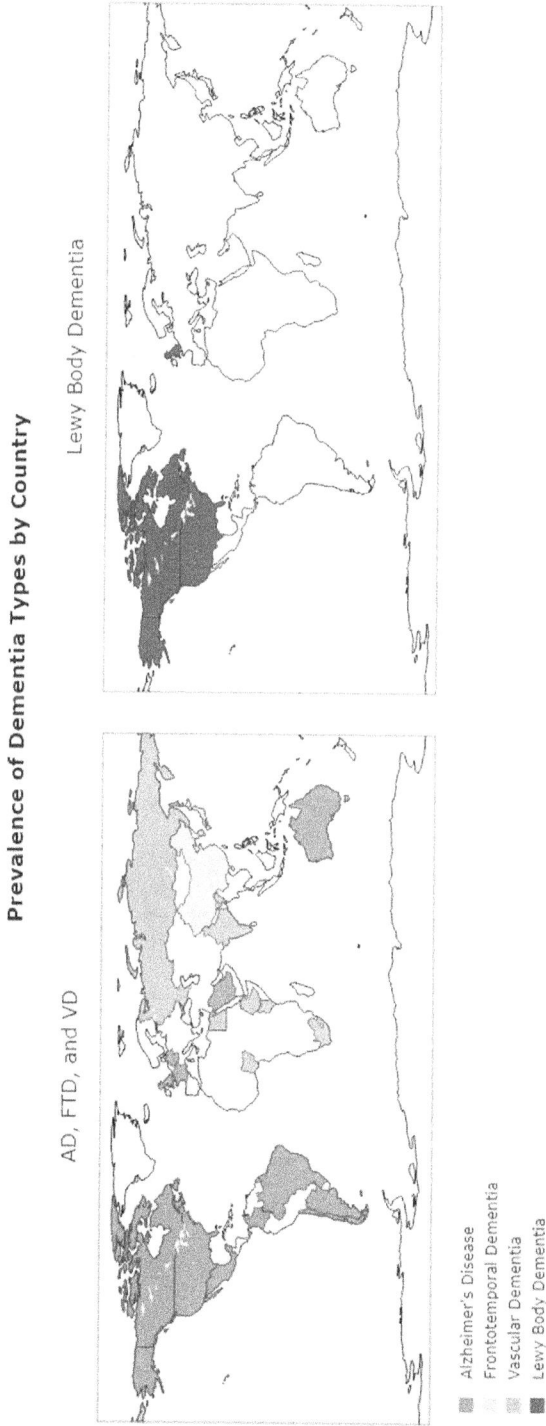

FIGURE 5.1
Global prevalence of dementia types by country.

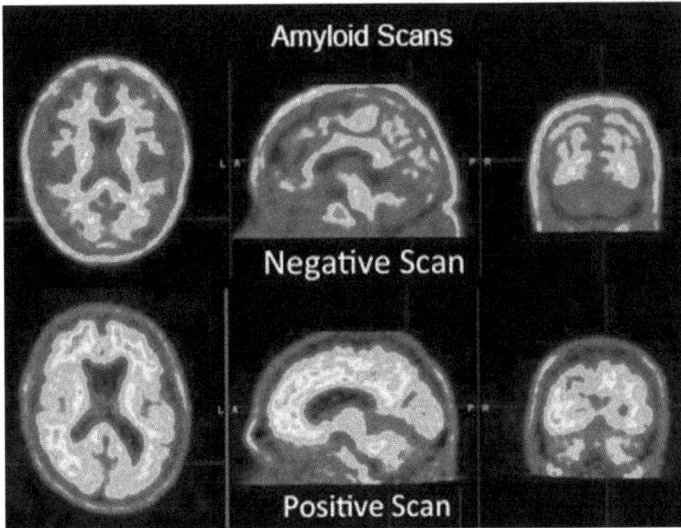

FIGURE 5.2
Examples of amyloid PET scans in Alzheimer's disease diagnosis. The upper segment shows a negative result, while the bottom segment shows a positive result, indicating the presence of amyloid plaques. Amyloid PET imaging represents a significant advancement in assessing cognitive impairment, visualizing plaques that are key in the progression of Alzheimer's disease. Previously, these plaques could only be detected post-mortem. (Retrieved from the University of California, San Francisco, Department of Radiology and Biomedical Imaging, 2024.)

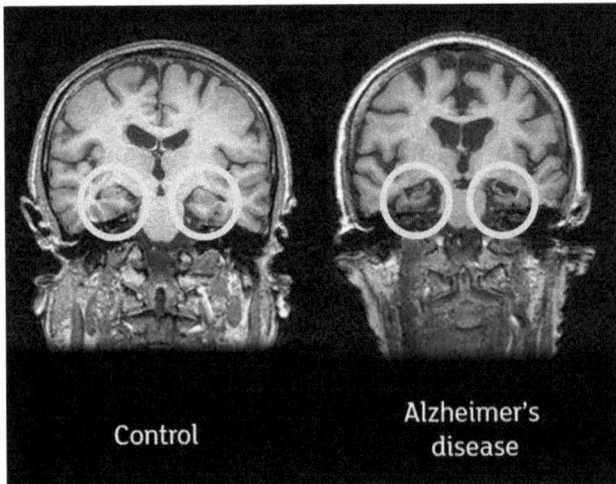

FIGURE 5.3
Functional MRI (fMRI) scans displaying neural activity in Alzheimer's disease compared to a normal brain. These images highlight the distinct patterns of brain activity that can aid in diagnosing and understanding Alzheimer's disease. (Retrieved from Alzheimer's Research UK, 2024.)

In response to these challenges, various non-profit organizations and charities dedicated to dementia research have been proactive. Since the onset of mandated lockdowns in March 2020, these entities have strived to maintain and even accelerate the momentum of AD and related dementia research. The International Alzheimer's and Related Dementia Research Funder Consortium, comprising nearly 40 funding organizations, has played a pivotal role by sharing information and coordinating efforts to ensure ongoing support for the research community.

The growing linkage between COVID-19 and increased risks or exacerbations among dementia patients highlights the ongoing need for interventions to halt or slow the disease's progression. This need is further emphasized by the decline in new dementia diagnoses and the disproportionately high number of COVID-19-related deaths within this demographic. Despite the pandemic, the dedication to supporting dementia research remains unwavering. Funding bodies have adapted by offering more flexible grant terms, extending deadlines, and providing additional financial support to retain research staff. These adaptive measures have been vital in sustaining research activities and supporting the dementia community through these challenging times. To illustrate the scale of the impact and the robust response efforts, a bar plot visualizing the estimated number of individuals living with different types of dementia worldwide highlights the extensive efforts by various organizations to adapt and bolster research during the pandemic (Meyers et al., 2022; Salcedo-Pérez-Juana et al., 2023).

As of 2024, AD remains the most prevalent form of dementia, with approximately 6.9 million Americans aged 65 and older living with the condition. This figure is part of a larger global trend, with over 55 million people worldwide affected by Alzheimer's and other dementias. VD is the second most common form, accounting for 15–20% of all dementia cases and impacting millions globally, particularly in regions with high rates of cardiovascular disease. LBD, while less recognized, affects around 1.4 million people in the United States, highlighting its significant yet underappreciated burden. FTD, though less common, particularly affects younger populations, with an estimated 60,000 cases in the United States and likely hundreds of thousands worldwide. These statistics emphasize the ongoing need for research, early diagnosis, and targeted interventions to manage and mitigate the global impact of these various dementia types (Gascón-Bayarri et al., 2007; Albrecht et al., 2019; Henríquez et al., 2022; Alzheimer's Association, 2024a, 2024b, 2024c; Liampas et al., 2024; National Institute of Neurological Disorders and Stroke, 2024).

Figure 5.4 depicts the estimated number of individuals living with different types of dementia worldwide, compared to normal cases. This visual helps to contextualize the scale of each type of dementia, highlighting the significant impact of AD relative to other forms. The plot also emphasizes the vast number of individuals considered as normal cases, useful for comparative purposes in research and public health discussions.

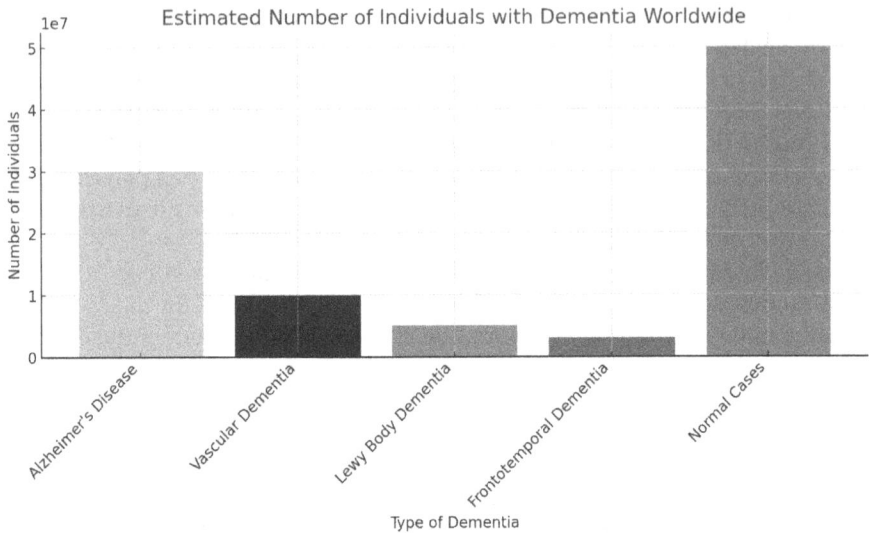

FIGURE 5.4
The estimated number of individuals living with different types of dementia worldwide.

5.1.5 Global Investment in Dementia Research: A Comparative Overview

This section details the escalating efforts by governments and institutions worldwide to enhance their investments in research and development, aimed at tackling the debilitating effects of dementia. It offers a thorough examination of the varied approaches to funding across key global regions, including the United States, Europe, and Asia-Pacific. This overview not only highlights the diversity in strategies and financial commitments but also underscores the widespread recognition of the urgent need to address this growing health challenge.

5.1.5.1 United States and Europe

In the United States, the National Institutes of Health (NIH) has bolstered Alzheimer's and dementia research funding by $100 million for the fiscal year 2024 (Alzheimer's Association, 2024a, 2024b, 2024c). Europe continues substantial investments in dementia research through the Horizon Europe program, with approximately EUR 8 billion allocated specifically to the health cluster, which includes significant funding for dementia research (Alzheimer Europe, 2024).

5.1.5.2 Asia and Pacific

In East Asia, significant investments have been made, with China investing around $500 billion in R&D in 2022, aiming to improve dementia care and early diagnosis (Liao & Brunner, 2023; CDRA, 2024; World Health Organization, 2024). South Korea and Japan have also made considerable contributions, with South Korea investing nearly $16 billion and Japan around $140 billion in R&D, fuelling advances across genetics, neuroimaging, and epidemiology (Alzheimer's Association, 2024a, 2024, 2024c). In India, the government has injected £49.9 million to create dementia trial sites, reflecting a proactive stance toward improving diagnosis and treatment within the country (India Education Diary, 2024). Australia is supporting a range of initiatives through at least $1 million to the Dementia Australia Research Foundation's Dementia Grants Program, whereas New Zealand faces challenges with adequate funding for dementia research (Australian Government Department of Health and Aged Care, 2022; Dementia Australia, 2024).

This detailed breakdown reflects a robust global effort towards enhancing dementia research infrastructure, emphasizing both national and regional strategies to combat this growing public health issue. The substantial investments in East Asia, particularly by economic powerhouses like China, Japan, and South Korea, are particularly noteworthy as they represent a significant portion of the global effort to address dementia.

5.1.5.3 Investment Figures and Projections

Significant investments in dementia research are driving advances across basic science, translational research, and clinical applications. For instance, the Alzheimer's drug market is projected to grow from $6.95 billion in 2023 to $15.08 billion by 2032. These investments reflect the growing global burden of dementia, with AD being the most prevalent form (Renub Research, 2024).

The specific allocation of funds towards the integration of AI and ML in dementia research is less distinctly defined. Despite the growing inclination to merge AI with healthcare—including in the study of dementia—distinct figures dedicated exclusively to this intersection are not typically separated from the broader scope of dementia research funding.

Table 5.4 presents the specific funding amounts designated for dementia research in 2024 by various countries. It details the substantial financial commitments from nations like the United States, China, Japan, and European Union members, among others. These investments are pivotal for driving forward research into diagnosis, treatment, and ultimately the prevention of dementia.

The accompanying bar chart in Figure 5.5 visually represents the funding data from the table, offering a clear comparative perspective of the financial efforts each country is making towards dementia research. The chart highlights the vast differences in funding scales, with countries like China and Japan making especially significant contributions compared to others. This visualization aids in understanding the global landscape of financial investment in dementia research and underscores the varied levels of commitment across the globe.

TABLE 5.4

Dementia Research Funding by Country in 2024: *This table presents the allocated funding amounts in US dollars for dementia research across various countries, illustrating the global commitment to advancing the understanding and treatment of dementia and related disorders*

Country	Funding Amount (USD)
United States	$100 million
Europe	~$8.69 billion (EUR 8 billion)
China	$500 billion (R&D overall, not dementia-specific)
South Korea	$16 billion
Japan	$140 billion
India	~$61 million (£49.9 million)
Australia	$1 million
New Zealand	Unknown

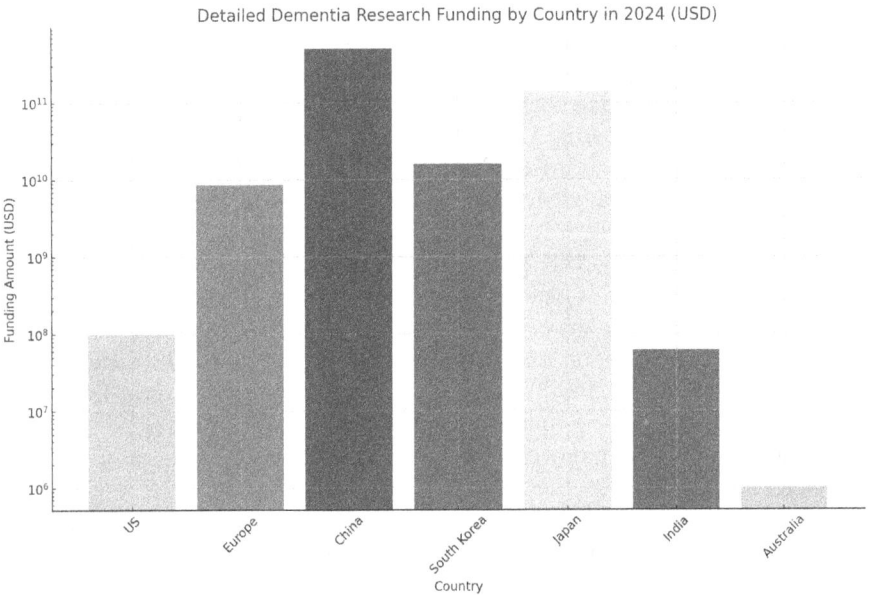

FIGURE 5.5
Bar chart of Dementia Research Funding by Country in 2024: This chart displays the comparative funding levels in US dollars dedicated to dementia research across key countries, highlighting the substantial investments made to combat the growing challenge of dementia globally.

5.2 Advancing Dementia Research: AI and Machine Learning in Data Optimization and Personalized Medicine

Building on the foundation of global funding insights, the next section will delve into the transformative potential of artificial intelligence (AI) and ML in dementia research. We will explore the innovative methods employed to preprocess—more precisely, to refine and optimize—the data. This involves a detailed review of various techniques that enhance the quality and utility of data before it is used in analytical models.

Further, we will examine the different AI models that are making significant strides in the diagnosis and drug discovery processes for dementia. Emphasis will be placed on the personalized approaches that these technologies facilitate. This personalized methodology not only promises targeted diagnosis and treatment but also introduces unique challenges, including the potential for bias within data sets. Understanding these risks is crucial for developing reliable AI tools that can offer substantial benefits in the clinical setting.

By addressing both the advantages and the inherent limitations of these AI-driven approaches, this section aims to provide a comprehensive overview of how cutting-edge technology is shaping the future of dementia research and patient care.

5.3 Leveraging Data for Diagnosis and Drug Discovery

The discovery and analysis of genetic biomarkers for various dementia types are pivotal in refining diagnostic approaches and developing targeted therapies. In AD, the presence of the APOE ε4 allele is particularly significant, alongside mutations in APP, PSEN1, and PSEN2 genes, which denote a hereditary form of the condition (Raulin et al., 2022; Quan et al., 2023). For VD, genetic predispositions such as NOTCH3 gene mutations, associated with CADASIL, are crucial for understanding its pathogenesis (Locatelli et al., 2020; Cho et al., 2021; Yuan et al., 2024). In the context of LBD, researchers have identified critical genetic markers such as mutations in the GBA and SNCA genes, which overlap with Parkinson's disease pathology (Orme et al., 2018; Abdelmoaty et al., 2023; Wyman-Chick et al., 2024). Similarly, FTD is linked with specific gene mutations in MAPT, GRN, and C9orf72, which are instrumental in the disease's protein misfolding processes (Katisko et al., 2022; Mravinacová et al., 2024). These genetic insights are essential for the development of preprocessing strategies in data analysis, setting the stage for more advanced applications of AI and ML in the realm of dementia research.

Advanced neuroimaging techniques such as fMRI, PET scans, and EEG offer critical insights into the brain's structural and functional characteristics that are affected in dementia. For instance, fMRI studies reveal disruptions in neural connectivity in AD and FTD, which are crucial for understanding cognitive decline (Chandra et al., 2019; Whitwell, 2019). PET scans provide a visual representation of amyloid and tau protein deposits in AD and show distinctive patterns of glucose metabolism across different dementia types (Márquez & Yassa, 2019; Herzog et al., 2022; Yen et al., 2023). EEG has been instrumental in showing brain activity alterations, such as the slowing of alpha rhythms in AD and the presence of sharp wave activity in LBD (Tsolaki et al., 2014; Cromarty et al., 2016; van der Zande et al., 2018). In addition to imaging, clinical tests such as blood biomarkers for Aβ and tau proteins have become fundamental in confirming the presence of AD, whereas elevated homocysteine levels might suggest VD (Cromarty et al., 2016; Lue et al., 2017; Altuna-Azkargorta & Mendioroz-Iriarte, 2021; Hosoki et al., 2021; Varesi et al., 2022). These tools collectively enhance the accuracy of differential diagnosis and help in the management of these conditions.

Demographic data, including age, genetic background, and educational attainment, play significant roles in the risk assessment and diagnosis of dementia. Epidemiological studies have shown that older age is the most significant risk factor for AD, while genetic predispositions such as the APOE ε4 allele further compound this risk (Qiu et al., 2009; Mangialasche et al., 2012; Contador et al., 2024). For VD, factors like hypertension and stroke history, linked to lifestyle and demographic data, are critical for diagnosis and treatment planning (Arvanitakis et al., 2019; Sanders et al., 2023). In FTD and LBD, family history and genetic testing for specific mutations such as those in the MAPT or GBA genes provide essential diagnostic clues (Tolea & Galvin, 2018; Carneiro et al., 2020; Rohrer et al., 2022). Understanding these demographic factors allows clinicians to better tailor treatment approaches and anticipate disease progression, enhancing patient care across dementia types.

5.3.1 Discussion on EEG, fMRI, and PET Scan Data Analysis Techniques in Dementia Research

AI and ML techniques are profoundly enhancing the preprocessing and feature extraction processes in neuroimaging, critical steps in the diagnosis and monitoring of neurological conditions like dementia.

5.3.1.1 EEG Data

EEG data preprocessing and feature extraction play critical roles in enhancing the accuracy of ML models for dementia prediction. Initially, EEG data undergoes meticulous preprocessing to remove artifacts with methods like Independent Component Analysis (ICA) and Principal Component Analysis

(PCA), and further analysis through techniques such as Fourier Transforms to dissect frequency-domain features. This precise cleaning and preparation enable more accurate diagnoses and understanding of brain activity patterns (Cassani et al., 2018; Arvanitakis et al., 2019; Ding et al., 2022; Lal et al., 2024).

In a comprehensive comparison of EEG preprocessing and feature extraction methods:

- **Finite Impulse Response (FIR):** Filtering method uses FIR filters to compute power intensity across high and low-frequency bands, effectively discriminating among AD, mild cognitive impairment (MCI), and healthy controls, achieving high accuracy in classification tasks (Alahmadi et al., 2024; Henney et al., 2024).

- Discrete Wavelet Transform (DWT) decomposes the EEG signal into wavelet coefficients, capturing both time and frequency information, crucial for identifying transient features in EEG signals associated with various dementia stages (Fiscon et al., 2018; Pirrone et al., 2022).

- Fast Fourier Transform (FFT) converts time-domain EEG signals into the frequency domain, offering a spectrum of EEG signals valuable for analysing frequency components indicative of neurological states associated with dementia (Fiscon et al., 2018; Pirrone et al., 2022).

- Feature Extraction Battery (FEB) enhances classification performance by combining several feature extraction methods, used alongside optimized support vector machines (SVMs) (Javeed et al., 2023).

- Hierarchical Modelling creates a structure of EEG-derived features, aiding efficient classification and understanding of EEG patterns related to different dementia types (Sharma et al., 2021; Smith et al., 2022).

- PCA and ICA simplify the EEG dataset and separate mixed signals into independent non-Gaussian signals, respectively, both enhancing the accuracy of dementia prediction (Javeed et al., 2023).

- Autoregressive (AR) Modelling and Classification and Regression Trees (CART) forecast future EEG behaviour based on past values and classify EEG spatial patterns, addressing complex classification challenges in EEG data related to dementia (Grajski et al., 1986; Henderson et al., 2006).

- Adaptive Synthetic Sampling (ADASYN) addresses class imbalance in ML models for dementia prediction by generating synthetic samples, enhancing classification accuracy (Ahmed et al., 2022).

These methods collectively provide a robust framework for processing and analysing EEG data, facilitating the early detection and classification of dementia, including AD and other subtypes.

5.3.1.2 fMRI and PET Scans

For fMRI and PET scans, preprocessing steps such as motion correction and spatial normalization are crucial. Motion correction adjusts for any patient movements during the scan, while spatial normalization aligns these scans with standardized brain templates, thereby enhancing the consistency and reliability of data across different studies. For feature extraction, Voxel-Based Morphometry (VBM) is employed in fMRI to analyse brain function and pathology by measuring differences in brain anatomy, and Kinetic Modelling in PET scans quantifies metabolic processes crucial for detecting disease markers (Gispert et al., 2003; Chen & Glover, 2015; Joseph & Jayaraman, 2024; Wang et al., 2024).

Similarly, MRI data preprocessing includes bias field correction and segmentation, improving the quality of the scans. Techniques like Diffusion Tensor Imaging (DTI) are then used to explore the microstructural integrity of neural pathways, providing insights into the brain's connectivity (Oldham et al., 2020; Aja-Fernández et al., 2023; Karimi, 2024).

A detailed comparison of various preprocessing and feature extraction methods used in neuroimaging for dementia prediction includes:

- **Standardization:** Normalizing PET images to a standard brain template reduces variability caused by anatomical differences (Pellegrini et al., 2018; Presotto et al., 2018; Shukla et al., 2023; Lee et al., 2024; Singh et al., 2024).

- **Smoothing:** Applying a Gaussian filter to PET scans decreases noise and enhances signal detection, aiding in feature identification for ML models (Pellegrini et al., 2018; Smith et al., 2022; Shukla et al., 2023; Singh et al., 2024).

- **Segmentation:** This step is vital for dividing the brain into anatomical or functional regions in fMRI and PET scans, helping localize brain activity and metabolic processes linked to dementia (Ahmadzadeh et al., 2023; Lee et al., 2023).

- **Feature Engineering:** Techniques that measure cortical thickness and metabolic activity help identify neurodegenerative changes indicative of dementia (Javeed et al., 2023; Lal et al., 2024).

- **Principal Component Analysis (PCA):** PCA reduces the dimensionality of imaging data, simplifying models without significant information loss (Mwangi et al., 2014; Javeed et al., 2023; O'Dell et al., 2023).

- **Independent Component Analysis (ICA):** ICA separates fMRI data into independent subcomponents, useful for identifying patterns of brain activity associated with cognitive decline (McKeown & Sejnowski, 1998; Calhoun et al., 2001; Jung et al., 2001; Guo & Pagnoni, 2008; Pellegrini et al., 2018; Shukla et al., 2023; Singh et al., 2024).

- **Voxel-Based Morphometry (VBM):** VBM assesses changes in brain anatomy, identifying structural differences between individuals with dementia and healthy controls (Bernasconi, 2005; Whitwell, 2009; Ribeiro & Busatto, 2016).

- **Time Series Analysis:** Analysing fMRI signal time series provides insights into the dynamics of brain activity, particularly valuable in the early stages of dementia (Moguilner et al., 2021; Yen et al., 2023; Rezaei et al., 2024).

- **Deep Learning (DL) Models:** CNNs and RNNs automatically extract complex patterns from neuroimaging data, enhancing the accuracy of diagnosing various stages of dementia (Ebrahimighahnavieh et al., 2020; Avberšek & Repovš, 2022; Shanmugavadivel et al., 2023; Zhao et al., 2023; Alsubaie et al., 2024).

- **Graph-Based Models:** These models analyse brain connectivity patterns, detecting subtle changes associated with dementia progression and offering insights into network dynamics (Farahani et al., 2019; García-Gutiérrez et al., 2024; Wu et al., 2024; Zhang et al., 2024).

This comprehensive examination of methods establishes a robust framework for processing and analysing neuroimaging data, which can be further enhanced by incorporating a multimodal approach. Combining data from various imaging modalities could provide a more holistic understanding and improved diagnostic accuracy in dementia research.

5.3.1.3 Multimodal Data

The integration of multimodal data—combining EEG, fMRI, PET, MRI, clinical (blood data), and demographic information—offers a comprehensive approach to diagnosing and understanding dementia. This approach not only improves the accuracy of diagnostic models but also enables the development of personalized treatment plans. By leveraging diverse data sources, AI and ML can uncover complex, multi-layered insights into how dementia evolves, highlighting the interactions between different biological markers and patient characteristics. Such an approach is instrumental in moving towards precision medicine, where treatment strategies are tailored to individual profiles, thereby optimizing therapeutic outcomes (Polikar et al., 2010; Huang et al., 2023; Alrawis et al., 2024; Malik et al., 2024; Salvi et al., 2024).

5.3.2 Integration of Clinical and Demographic Data for Comprehensive Analysis

Integrating multimodal data sources such as EEG, clinical blood data, and demographic information into the analysis of dementia using AI and ML techniques enhances diagnostic accuracy and provides a more holistic understanding of the disease's progression. For instance, EEG data processed through artifact removal and filtering techniques can capture nuanced neurophysiological changes (Jiang et al., 2019; Xu et al., 2024). Concurrently, blood biomarkers offer insights into the biochemical processes that may precede visible symptoms, thereby facilitating early diagnosis (Kandiah et al., 2022; Varesi et al., 2022; Souchet et al., 2024). Additionally, incorporating demographic variables allows for the adjustment of models based on age, genetic predispositions, and other socio-environmental factors, thus improving the predictive power and personalization of diagnostics (Mura et al., 2017; Brain et al., 2024; Chang et al., 2024).

These integrated data streams are critical in developing sophisticated ML models that can predict the onset and trajectory of dementia with greater precision. For example, the use of multimodal data in DL frameworks enhances the detection of patterns that single-mode data might miss, significantly improving the identification of early-stage dementia and tailoring interventions to individual needs. The synergy among these diverse data types not only enriches the dataset but also supports a more comprehensive approach to managing and understanding dementia, ultimately leading to improved patient outcomes and more effective use of healthcare resources.

5.4 Overview of Research Proposing AI and ML Models for Diagnosis and Drug Discovery

The integration of ML and AI in dementia research has transformed the diagnostic landscape, enhancing the ability to predict and diagnose various subtypes of dementia, including AD, FTD, VD, and Dementia with Lewy Bodies (DLB). This section outlines the significant advancements and methodologies used in leveraging ML and AI for these purposes.

5.4.1 Advancing Dementia Diagnosis: Integrating Machine Learning and Artificial Intelligence in Neurological Predictive Analytics

ML models have become increasingly vital in diagnosing and classifying dementia. These models can be categorized based on their underlying algorithms and their application in various diagnostic tasks, each offering unique strengths and challenges.

Traditional ML models, such as K-Nearest Neighbors (KNN), Random Forest (RF), and decision trees (e.g., the C4.5 algorithm), have been widely used to differentiate between dementia subtypes and healthy controls. These models are particularly effective when the data is structured and well-labelled, allowing for straightforward classification tasks. For example,

KNN and decision trees have been employed to classify patients based on extracted features from neuroimaging data, cognitive scores, and other clinical assessments. However, these models often require manual feature selection and may struggle with the complexity of multimodal data, limiting their applicability in more nuanced diagnostic scenarios (Lal et al., 2024).

DL models, particularly Convolutional Neural Networks (CNNs) and Bidirectional Long Short-Term Memory (BiLSTM) networks, have significantly advanced neuroimaging analysis. CNNs, known for their ability to capture spatial hierarchies in data, have been widely applied to MRI, PET, and EEG scans, where they automatically extract critical features for detecting Alzheimer's and Parkinson's diseases. For instance, CNNs have been integral to multimodal learning approaches that integrate brain imaging, cognitive scores, and genetic data, achieving high accuracy rates in distinguishing AD from MCI (Tajbakhsh et al., 2016; Zhao et al., 2023; Alsubaie et al., 2024).

On the other hand, BiLSTM networks are particularly well-suited for handling sequential data such as EEG signals. These networks capture temporal dependencies, making them effective in detecting subtle changes in brain activity indicative of early-stage dementia. The application of BiLSTM to EEG data analysis has resulted in state-of-the-art accuracy for MCI and AD detection, underscoring its potential as a reliable diagnostic tool (Alahmadi et al., 2024).

Multimodal learning methods, which combine various data types such as brain imaging, speech, and genetic assessments, have gained prominence due to their enhanced diagnostic capabilities. These approaches often utilize CNNs for feature extraction and latent feature representation spaces for feature fusion. By integrating different modalities, these models can accurately classify and predict disease progression, with reported accuracy rates ranging from 74.3% to 98.8% (Huang et al., 2023).

Hybrid models that combine traditional ML algorithms with DL architectures have also emerged, leveraging the strengths of both approaches. For example, models like DAD-Net, a CNN specifically designed for small datasets, combine DL with classical methods to improve AD diagnosis accuracy using MRI data (Lal et al., 2024).

The early detection of AD during the MCI stage is crucial for enabling timely intervention that could slow down disease progression. However, the success of computer-aided diagnosis (CAD) systems in this context often relies on the availability of a substantial amount of biomarker data, which is not always accessible. To address this challenge, a study introduced an instance-based transfer learning framework leveraging the Gradient Boosting Machine (GBM) algorithm, known as TrGB. This approach incorporates a weighting mechanism that adjusts the influence of source domain data based on the residual errors of base learners, enhancing the prediction accuracy of AD in target domains with limited labelled data. By transferring relevant knowledge from comprehensive datasets, such as the Alzheimer's

Disease Neuroimaging Initiative (ADNI), TrGB significantly improved classification accuracy in distinguishing between cognitively normal (CN) and MCI stages, as well as early and late MCI stages, with notable gains in accuracy and F1-scores compared to conventional methods (Shojaie et al., 2022).

The study underscores the importance of using transfer learning to overcome data scarcity in medical applications, particularly in AD diagnosis. The tailored weighting mechanism within the GBM framework effectively mitigates the risk of negative transfer, where irrelevant information from the source domain could degrade the performance of the target model. Despite its benefits, TrGB introduces increased model complexity and computational demands, suggesting future exploration of more efficient algorithms like Extreme Gradient Boosting (XGB) or Light Gradient Boosting Machine (LightGBM) to further optimize performance.

Despite the advancements in ML models, several challenges remain in their clinical application. DL models, while powerful, often require large amounts of labelled data, which are not always available in clinical settings. This limitation leads to challenges like overfitting, where models perform well on training data but poorly on new, unseen data. Additionally, the black-box nature of many DL models raises concerns about interpretability, making it difficult for clinicians to trust and adopt these models in practice (Zhao et al., 2023).

Future research needs to address these challenges by focusing on improving model robustness and reliability. This includes developing more sophisticated architectures that can generalize across diverse patient populations and integrating explainable AI (XAI) techniques to enhance model transparency. Moreover, expanding multimodal learning approaches, which combine various data types, holds promise for more comprehensive and accurate diagnostic tools that can be applied in both clinical and remote settings (Huang et al., 2023).

In addition to traditional and DL models, novel approaches like personalized predictive modelling using Spiking Neural Networks (SNNs) have emerged. This brain-inspired architecture is particularly effective for capturing the dynamic structural changes in the brain over time and space, which are crucial for predicting cognitive outcomes such as MCI and dementia. The proposed method integrates longitudinal MRI data with SNNs, enabling the model to detect intricate spatiotemporal patterns in the brain. This approach has demonstrated high accuracy in predicting cognitive decline up to two years in advance, validated using data from the Sydney Memory and Ageing Study (MAS). The added benefit of providing a 3D visualization of brain changes enhances its potential as a diagnostic tool (Doborjeh et al., 2021).

What sets this personalized approach apart is its ability to tailor predictions to individual patients by training SNN models on data from patients with similar characteristics. This personalization not only enhances prediction accuracy but also allows for the discovery of individual and group-specific biomarkers. The successful application of this methodology in the

MAS cohort underscores its potential for broader use in various clinical and neuroimaging contexts. This study highlights the importance of personalized approaches in precision medicine, especially for conditions like dementia, where early and accurate prediction is critical for effective treatment and care planning (Doborjeh et al., 2021).

Several advanced ML and AI methodologies have been instrumental in enhancing the accuracy and effectiveness of dementia diagnosis. These techniques, each with its unique capabilities, contribute to a more precise and tailored approach to patient care:

- **Support Vector Machines (SVMs):** SVMs are particularly essential for binary classification tasks, where they excel in distinguishing between different dementia subtypes by classifying imaging data and clinical variables. Their ability to create hyperplanes that best separate data points makes them a reliable choice for tasks requiring high precision, such as differentiating AD from other forms of dementia (Bougea et al., 2021).

- **DL Techniques:** DL models, including CNNs and Recurrent Neural Networks (RNNs), are pivotal in capturing complex data structures and dependencies. These models significantly improve diagnostic processes by automatically learning intricate patterns from large datasets, such as MRI and PET scans. Their application in neuroimaging allows for the extraction of critical features, facilitating early detection and accurate classification of dementia subtypes (Ebrahimighahnavieh et al., 2020; Ebrahimi & Luo, 2021; Alsubaie et al., 2024; Mohammed et al., 2024).

- **RFs:** Known for their robustness and resistance to overfitting, RFs are particularly suitable for analysing the multifactorial nature of dementia. They are capable of handling large and complex datasets, making them ideal for tasks that involve multiple variables and require high model stability. RFs' ability to aggregate results from numerous decision trees enhances their predictive accuracy in clinical diagnostics (Dimitriadis & Liparas, 2018; Velazquez & Lee, 2021).

- **Dimensionality Reduction:** Techniques such as PCA and ICA are critical in managing the extensive and high-dimensional data typical of neuroimaging studies. These methods reduce the complexity of the data while preserving the most informative features, enabling more efficient and accurate analyses. By streamlining data, PCA and ICA help in uncovering underlying patterns that are essential for accurate diagnosis (Mwangi et al., 2014; Javeed et al., 2023).

- **Clustering and Genetic Algorithms:** Clustering methods and genetic algorithms are utilized to segment patient data into meaningful subgroups. This segmentation is vital for personalized medicine approaches, where understanding specific patterns and risk factors within subgroups can lead to more individualized and effective treatment plans. These techniques contribute to the identification of distinct patient profiles, aiding in the development of tailored therapeutic strategies (Jayatilake & Ganegoda, 2021; Parikh et al., 2021).

- **Advanced Neural Networks:** Beyond basic DL architectures, advanced neural networks, including deep convolutional networks and long short-term memory (LSTM) networks, play a crucial role in discovering patterns of disease progression and identifying potential biomarkers. These networks enhance the early diagnosis and facilitate the creation of personalized treatment plans by learning from complex, longitudinal datasets (Javeed et al., 2023; Alsubaie et al., 2024; Malik et al., 2024).

Collectively, these methodologies significantly enhance the accuracy of ML models in dementia diagnosis. By leveraging these advanced techniques, healthcare professionals can better tailor treatments to individual patient profiles, ultimately improving patient outcomes and advancing the field of precision medicine.

Table 5.5 serves as a concise reference for the varied ML models employed in the ongoing battle against dementia, illustrating their specific applications and the studies that underpin their effectiveness.

5.4.2 Harnessing Machine Learning Innovations for Enhanced Drug Discovery

The integration of ML and AI in drug discovery represents a transformative shift in the pharmaceutical industry, fostering more efficient, precise, and innovative approaches. This section provides a comprehensive examination of how these technologies enhance drug discovery processes, supported by robust academic research and practical applications. ML models are increasingly central to drug discovery, offering powerful tools for predicting drug interactions, efficacy, and safety with higher accuracy and speed than traditional methods.

- **SVMs and RFs:** Traditional ML algorithms like SVMs and RFs have been foundational in developing quantitative structure-activity relationship (QSAR) models, which predict the bioactivity of chemical compounds. These models were crucial in handling structured datasets but faced limitations in managing the voluminous and complex data generated by modern high-throughput screening (HTS) techniques. SVMs are particularly effective in high-dimensional spaces, though they require careful kernel selection and may be less adaptable to unstructured data. RFs, known for their robustness against overfitting, are valuable in feature selection but can struggle with noisy or very large datasets (Chen et al., 2018; Askr et al., 2023).

TABLE 5.5

Comprehensive Overview of Machine Learning Models in Dementia Prediction

Model Type	Advantages	Disadvantages	Key Studies
LSTM networks	Captures temporal dynamics in data	High computational cost	Alahmadi et al. (2024)
Explainable AI models	Increases model transparency	May reduce model performance	Zhang et al. (2024); Zhao et al. (2023)
GBM (Gradient Boosting Machines)	Handles various data types effectively	Prone to overfitting	Shojaie et al. (2022)
Random Forests	Robust against overfitting, good for feature selection	Less effective with noisy/large data	Dimitriadis and Liparas (2018); Velazquez and Lee (2021)
SVM (Support Vector Machines)	Effective in high-dimensional spaces	Requires careful kernel selection	Bougea et al. (2021); Waghere et al. (2021)
CNNs (Convolutional Neural Networks)	Excellent in pattern recognition in imaging data	Needs extensive data for training	Alsubaie et al. (2024); Ebrahimighahnavieh et al. (2020); Tajbakhsh et al. (2016)
SNNs (Spiking Neural Networks)	Biologically plausible, efficient	Still under active development for practical applications	Doborjeh et al. (2021)
Dimensionality Reduction (PCA/ICA)	Streamlines analysis of high-dimensional data	May lose some data variance during reduction	Javeed et al. (2023); Mwangi et al. (2014)
Advanced neural networks	Discover patterns of disease progression, identify biomarkers	High computational requirements	Javeed et al. (2023); Alsubaie et al. (2024); Malik et al. (2024)
Clustering and genetic algorithms	Segments patient data into subgroups for personalized medicine	Complex implementation, computationally expensive	Parikh et al. (2021); Jayatilake and Ganegoda (2021)

- **Convolutional Neural Networks (CNNs):** CNNs have revolutionized drug discovery by processing and learning from vast amounts of unstructured data, such as molecular graphs and images. They are extensively used in predicting drug-target interactions (DTIs) and drug-drug interactions (DDIs) by analyzing structural properties of molecules. CNNs automatically extract hierarchical features, enhancing prediction accuracy and enabling the discovery of novel drug candidates (Nag et al., 2022; Kumar & Srivastava, 2024).

- **Recurrent Neural Networks (RNNs):** RNNs, especially those employing LSTM units, excel in processing sequential data, making them ideal for tasks such as generating valid SMILES strings (text-based molecular representations) and predicting protein structures. Their ability to capture temporal dependencies is crucial for modelling the progression of drug efficacy and side effects over time (Chen et al., 2018; Askr et al., 2023).

- **Variational Autoencoders (VAEs) and Generative Adversarial Networks (GANs):** VAEs and GANs are transformative in de novo molecular design, where they generate novel chemical structures with desired properties by learning continuous representations of molecules in a latent space. These generative models allow for the exploration of chemical space in an unsupervised manner, providing innovative approaches to drug discovery by enabling the creation of entirely new molecules that may possess therapeutic potential (Chen et al., 2018; Nag et al., 2022).

- **Graph Neural Networks (GNNs):** GNNs extend the capabilities of CNNs to graph-structured data, showing great promise in predicting DTIs and DDIs by leveraging the topological information of molecular graphs. These models are particularly useful in analysing interactions within biological networks, making them invaluable in understanding complex molecular interactions (Rehman et al., 2024).

- **Transfer Learning and GBMs:** In contexts where data is scarce, such as early detection of AD, transfer learning frameworks like the TrGB model, which utilizes GBMs, are essential. By leveraging large, well-annotated datasets (e.g., ADNI), these models transfer knowledge to domains with limited data, improving the prediction accuracy of drug efficacy and disease progression. The use of GBMs with tailored weighting mechanisms helps mitigate risks associated with negative transfer, making them highly effective in clinical and drug discovery applications (Shojaie et al., 2022).

- **Dimensionality Reduction Techniques:** Techniques such as PCA and ICA are crucial for managing the high-dimensional data typical in drug discovery. These methods streamline the analysis by reducing the data's complexity while retaining the most informative features, facilitating more efficient and accurate modelling in tasks like QSAR and pharmacokinetics prediction (Javeed et al., 2023).

- **Explainable AI (XAI):** XAI techniques, such as gradient-based attribution and DeepLIFT, address interpretability issues associated with DL models. In drug discovery, where understanding the model's decision-making process is crucial for regulatory approval, XAI provides transparency, helping ensure that AI-driven predictions are reliable and justifiable (Askr et al., 2023).

- **AI in Clinical Trial Optimization:** AI and ML are increasingly used to optimize clinical trials by predicting patient responses and trial outcomes. By integrating vast amounts of multi-omics data, AI models can identify and prioritize potential drug targets, refine patient cohorts, and reduce the time and cost associated with clinical trials. This application is particularly relevant in complex diseases like dementia, where patient stratification and trial design are critical challenges (Doherty et al., 2023).

- **Digital Twins and AI-Driven Simulations:** AI-driven digital twins, which simulate patient responses to drugs, represent a cutting-edge application in pharmaceutical manufacturing and clinical trial design. These digital simulations enable researchers to test the effects of drugs on virtual populations, reducing the risks and costs associated with traditional clinical trials. The use of digital twins is expected to become a standard practice in drug development, particularly in personalized medicine (Askr et al., 2023).

- **Predictive Modelling:** ML models efficiently predict DTIs and the pharmacokinetic properties of new compounds, significantly reducing the time and resources required for drug development (Wang & Zeng, 2013; D'Souza et al., 2023; Wu et al., 2023; Cheng et al., 2024; Kumar & Srivastava, 2024; Qiu & Cheng, 2024).

- **Molecular Dynamics Simulations:** ML techniques are integrated into molecular dynamics simulations to enhance the accuracy of drug-target modelling and to facilitate the discovery of lead compounds (Jiang et al., 2020).

- **Virtual Screening:** ML algorithms streamline the virtual screening process, enabling rapid and accurate identification of promising drug candidates from large chemical libraries (Doherty et al., 2023).

The integration of ML and DL techniques in drug discovery and development has significantly advanced the field, offering powerful tools for processing complex biological data, predicting drug interactions, and optimizing clinical trials. These methodologies not only enhance the efficiency and accuracy of drug discovery but also hold the potential to revolutionize the development of personalized therapies. As these technologies continue to evolve, their impact on pharmaceutical research and healthcare will likely grow, leading to more effective and safer therapeutic interventions.

Table 5.6 provides a detailed comparison of various ML models used in drug discovery, highlighting their unique advantages, potential limitations, and key studies that exemplify their application in enhancing the efficiency and effectiveness of pharmaceutical research and development.

These models demonstrate the diverse potential of ML to revolutionize drug discovery, improving not only the speed and cost-effectiveness of this process but also enhancing the precision and innovative capacity of

TABLE 5.6

Comprehensive Overview of Machine Learning Models in Dementia Drug Discovery

Model Type	Advantages	Disadvantages	Key Studies
Convolutional Neural Networks (CNNs)	High accuracy in processing molecular structures and images; automatically extracts hierarchical features	Requires large datasets; computationally intensive	Jing et al. (2018); Chen et al. (2018); Kumar and Srivastava (2024); Nag et al. (2022)
Support Vector Machines (SVMs)	Effective in high-dimensional spaces; robust classification capabilities	Sensitive to kernel choice; less adaptable to unstructured data	Zdrazil et al. (2024); Bucholc et al. (2023)
Random Forests (RFs)	Robust against overfitting; effective in feature selection and handling structured datasets	Less effective with noisy or very large datasets	Gunther et al. (2008); Guney et al. (2016); Chen et al. (2018); Askr et al. (2023)
Recurrent Neural Networks (RNNs)	Excels in processing sequential data; captures temporal dependencies	Computationally intensive; complex to train and interpret	Chen et al. (2018); Askr et al. (2023)
Generative Adversarial Networks (GANs)	Innovative in generating novel molecules and simulating interactions	Challenging to train; requires careful tuning to avoid mode collapse	Kazeminia et al. (2020); Chen et al. (2022); Nag et al. (2022)
Graph Neural Networks (GNNs)	Leverages topological information from molecular graphs; useful in drug-target and drug-drug interaction predictions	Requires graph-structured data; computationally demanding	Rehman et al. (2024); Kumar & Srivastava (2024)
Variational Autoencoders (VAEs)	Generates diverse molecular structures; efficient in exploring chemical space	Complexity in training; may require fine-tuning for specific tasks	Chen et al. (2018); Nag et al. (2022)
Gradient Boosting Machines (GBMs)	Effective in handling data scarcity; mitigates risks of negative transfer in transfer learning	Computationally intensive; potential overfitting without careful tuning	Shojaie et al. (2022)
Dimensionality Reduction Techniques (PCA, ICA)	Streamlines analysis of high-dimensional data; retains essential features for accurate modelling	May oversimplify data; interpretation can be complex	Javeed et al. (2023)
Explainable AI (XAI)	Increases model transparency; essential for regulatory approval in drug discovery	May reduce model performance if not implemented carefully	Askr et al. (2023)

TABLE 5.6 (*Continued*)

Comprehensive Overview of Machine Learning Models in Dementia Drug Discovery

Model Type	Advantages	Disadvantages	Key Studies
Predictive Modelling	Efficient in predicting drug-target interactions and pharmacokinetics; accelerates drug development	Dependent on data quality; complex model selection and tuning	Qiu and Cheng (2024); Wu et al. (2023); D'Souza et al. (2023)
Molecular dynamics simulations	Enhances accuracy in drug-target modelling; facilitates lead compound discovery	Computationally expensive; requires significant expertise	Jiang et al. (2020)
Virtual screening	Streamlines the identification of promising drug candidates; reduces time and resources	Accuracy depends on model and data quality; may generate false positives	Doherty et al. (2023)
AI in clinical trial optimization	Optimizes trial outcomes and patient stratification; reduces time and cost	Data integration and standardization challenges; complex model interpretation	Doherty et al. (2023)
Digital twins	Simulates patient responses; reduces risks and costs in drug trials	Requires high computational resources; complex to develop and validate	Askr et al. (2023)

the pharmaceutical industry. By leveraging large multi-omics datasets, AI algorithms are adept at identifying genetic targets and uncovering genetic variants linked to dementia, enhancing our understanding of the biological pathways and risk factors involved. This capacity for deep data analysis supports hypothesis-driven drug discovery by identifying high-risk mutations and potential new targets, akin to significant medical discoveries in other fields, such as PCSK9 mutations for cholesterol management.

Furthermore, AI is transforming drug design through the use of algorithms that perform virtual screenings, efficiently sorting through millions of compounds to pinpoint those with potential efficacy against dementia-related targets. This not only speeds up the drug discovery process but also facilitates the repurposing of existing drugs, offering new therapeutic opportunities for dementia treatment. Additionally, AI's predictive capabilities are crucial in clinical trials, where it analyzes extensive data from previous studies to predict the success of drug candidates, thereby optimizing trial designs and reducing the likelihood of costly failures. This comprehensive approach underscores a transformative shift towards more targeted and efficient therapeutic development in combating dementia.

5.4.3 Personalized Machine Learning in Modern Medicine: Transforming Diagnosis and Drug Discovery

The fusion of personalized ML and AI with modern medicine is profoundly reshaping both diagnostic and drug discovery processes. By tailoring medical treatments to individual patient profiles, these technologies optimize therapeutic effectiveness and significantly enhance drug development. This section explores the various personalized ML models employed in disease diagnosis and therapeutic innovation, supported by the latest research and technological advancements.

Personalized ML models are becoming central to modern diagnostics, particularly in managing complex and chronic conditions like dementia. These models are designed to analyse vast amounts of patient-specific data, including clinical, genetic, and neuroimaging information, to predict disease progression and tailor treatment strategies accordingly.

For instance, Doborjeh et al. (2021) introduced a novel approach utilizing brain-inspired SNNs to analyse longitudinal neuroimaging data, effectively classifying and predicting cognitive decline such as MCI and dementia. This personalized predictive model is highly accurate, leveraging dynamic brain patterns in MRI data to identify early markers of neurodegenerative diseases.

Ensuring the accuracy and reliability of AI-driven healthcare solutions requires rigorous validation methodologies. Algorithm validation involves comprehensive testing using diverse datasets and techniques like cross-validation, which are crucial for enhancing the generalizability and adaptability of AI systems to personalized care. Clinical validation, on the other hand, assesses the safety and efficacy of AI interventions through rigorous trials, often comparing AI-based solutions with standard treatments to evaluate their impact on patient outcomes (Maleki Varnosfaderani & Forouzanfar, 2024).

AI's application in AD research spans diagnosis, treatment, and drug discovery. In diagnosis, AI enhances the accuracy and timeliness by analysing neuroimaging and clinical data, enabling early intervention and personalized treatment plans. In drug discovery, AI accelerates the identification of new therapeutic targets and optimizes clinical trials, addressing the complexities and high failure rates in AD drug development (Angelucci et al., 2024; Cheng et al., 2024).

For example, AI-driven models integrated with multi-omics datasets can personalize treatment strategies for AD, improving clinical outcomes by targeting specific biological pathways implicated in the disease. This approach is not only more cost-effective but also increases the clinical effectiveness of new therapies.

Several advanced AI techniques are enhancing personalized medicine's scope in diagnosing and treating diseases like dementia:

- **Recurrent Neural Networks (RNNs):** RNNs, particularly LSTM networks, are pivotal in predicting cognitive outcomes following the administration of dementia medications. For instance, Liu et al.

(2022) developed an AI model that recommends dementia treatments based on patient-specific data, significantly slowing cognitive decline over time.

- **Generative Models:** VAEs and GANs are revolutionizing drug discovery by generating novel chemical structures with therapeutic potential, providing innovative approaches to creating new molecules that can be tailored to individual patient profiles (Chen et al., 2018; Nag et al., 2022).
- **GNNs:** These models extend the capabilities of traditional neural networks to graph-structured data, such as molecular graphs in DTI predictions, facilitating personalized drug discovery and development (Rehman et al., 2024).

AI and ML are increasingly critical in optimizing clinical trials, particularly for complex diseases where patient stratification and trial design pose significant challenges. AI models can predict patient responses and trial outcomes more accurately by integrating multi-omics data, ultimately reducing the time and cost associated with bringing new therapies to market (Doherty et al., 2023).

Moreover, the concept of digital twins—virtual simulations of patient responses to drugs—represents a cutting-edge application in personalized medicine. These simulations enable researchers to test the effects of therapies on virtual populations, thus reducing the risks and costs associated with traditional clinical trials (Askr et al., 2023).

While the integration of AI in personalized medicine offers tremendous potential, it also raises important ethical and societal questions, particularly regarding data privacy and bias in AI models. Ensuring the equitable application of these technologies across diverse patient populations is crucial for their successful adoption in clinical practice (Hirani et al., 2024; Javanmard, 2024).

The intersection of personalized ML and AI with modern medicine is revolutionizing how diseases are diagnosed and treated, especially in the realm of neurodegenerative conditions like AD. By harnessing advanced AI techniques, personalized medicine is becoming more precise, offering tailored therapeutic strategies that improve patient outcomes. As these technologies continue to evolve, they promise to further enhance the efficiency and accuracy of drug discovery, ultimately leading to more effective and safer therapeutic interventions.

This detailed exploration underscores the transformative impact of AI in personalized medicine, supported by cutting-edge research and clinical applications. As the field advances, continued innovation and ethical consideration will be key to fully realizing the potential of AI-driven personalized healthcare.

Table 5.7 provides a detailed comparison of various personalized ML models used in medical applications, highlighting their specific applications, key advantages, and notable studies that exemplify their effectiveness in enhancing diagnosis and drug discovery processes. RNNs are crucial in

TABLE 5.7

Overview of Personalized Machine Learning Models in Medical Applications

Model Type	Applications	Advantages	Key References
Recurrent Neural Networks (RNNs)	Longitudinal data analysis for personalized treatment adjustments	Effective in sequence prediction, crucial for predicting cognitive outcomes and adjusting treatments	Liu et al. (2022); Lavecchia (2019)
Generative Adversarial Networks (GANs)	Generating novel drug molecules tailored to individual patient profiles	Innovative in drug design, enabling the creation of personalized therapeutic agents	Kazeminia et al. (2020); Chen et al. (2022)
Graph Neural Networks (GNNs)	Modelling molecular interactions for personalized drug discovery	Accurately predicts molecular interactions, facilitating personalized drug development	Rehman et al. (2024); Patel et al. (2020)
Convolutional Neural Networks (CNNs)	Imaging data analysis for personalized disease diagnosis	High accuracy in pattern recognition, essential for identifying disease-specific biomarkers	Wang et al. (2020); Jing et al. (2018)
Transfer Learning with Gradient Boosting Machines (GBMs)	Enhancing predictive accuracy in personalized medicine	Improves accuracy in target domains with limited data, crucial for personalized drug efficacy prediction	Shojaie et al. (2022)
Variational Autoencoders (VAEs)	De novo molecular design for personalized therapies	Enables exploration of chemical space for the development of patient-specific treatments	Nag et al., (2022); Chen et al. (2018)
Digital Twins	Simulating patient-specific responses in clinical trials	Reduces risks and costs, enables personalized medicine in virtual populations	Askr et al. (2023)

personalized medicine for their ability to analyze longitudinal patient data, enabling the adjustment of treatments over time. GANs and VAEs are central to personalized drug discovery, as they facilitate the creation of new drug molecules tailored to individual needs. GNNs play a vital role in modelling complex molecular interactions, essential for understanding patient-specific drug responses. CNNs are key in diagnosing diseases through imaging, increasingly personalized through the identification of individual biomarkers. Transfer Learning with GBMs enhances predictive accuracy in settings where patient-specific data is limited, making it critical for personalized drug development. Additionally, Digital Twins are emerging as a technology that allows for the simulation of individual patient responses, supporting personalized treatment strategies in clinical trials.

Personalized ML models are pivotal in advancing modern medicine by enhancing diagnostic accuracy and accelerating drug discovery. These models not only improve clinical outcomes but also promote a shift towards more individualized, patient-centred medical care, embodying the potential to revolutionize treatments and improve quality of life.

These insights underscore the importance of continued research and adoption of personalized ML techniques in healthcare, promising significant strides in medical sciences and patient care.

5.5 Commercial AI and ML Tools in Healthcare: A Global Overview

The integration of AI and ML technologies in healthcare has led to the development of advanced commercial tools that are redefining diagnosis and drug discovery across the globe. These tools, developed by leading companies and research groups, are instrumental in enhancing the accuracy, efficiency, and personalization of healthcare services. This section provides a detailed overview of notable AI- and ML-based tools, their developers, and the countries where they are actively used.

Table 5.8 exemplifies the practical applications of AI and ML in modern healthcare, offering innovative solutions for diagnosis and drug discovery. Each tool has been developed with specific healthcare needs in mind, facilitating earlier, more accurate diagnoses, and more effective treatments. These tools, developed by diverse organizations, are being utilized across different

TABLE 5.8

Overview of Commercial AI and ML-Based Tools in Healthcare

Tool Name	Developer/Company	Country of Use	References
autoSCORE	Holberg EEG AS	USA	FDA (2024)
Butterfly iQ3	Butterfly Network, Inc.	USA	FDA (2024)
REMI AI	Epitel, Inc.	USA	FDA (2024)
TumorSight	SimBioSys, Inc.	USA	FDA (2024)
qXR-LN	Qure.ai Technologies	USA	FDA (2024)
ART-Plan	TheraPanacea	USA	FDA (2024)
MAGNETOM Sola	Siemens Medical Solutions USA, Inc.	USA	FDA (2024)
HM70 EVO	Samsung Medison Co., Ltd.	USA	FDA (2024)
PAXLOVID	Pfizer	Global	Pfizer Insights (2022)
Ultromics System	Ultromics	USA	Johnson & Johnson (2024)
Monarch Platform	Johnson & Johnson MedTech	USA	Johnson & Johnson (2024)
DASI Dimensions	DASI Simulations	USA	FDA (2024)

countries, primarily the USA, showcasing significant advancements in the integration of technology in healthcare practices globally.

5.6 Integrating Artificial Intelligence in Clinical Dementia Care: Challenges and Opportunities

The integration of AI in the diagnosis and management of dementia represents a significant leap forward in personalized medicine, enabling healthcare providers to tailor treatment strategies to the individual characteristics of each patient. AI's capacity to process and interpret vast arrays of data—from neuroimaging to genetic profiles—allows for a nuanced understanding of the disease's progression and potential therapeutic avenues. This holistic approach is crucial in dementia care, where early detection and precise intervention can substantially alter patient outcomes.

Moreover, AI extends its utility to the realm of patient care management and drug development. Predictive models harness data to forecast disease progression, facilitating early interventions that can delay the onset of severe symptoms. In drug development, AI algorithms analyse existing medical data to predict how different drugs might interact with specific biomarkers, thereby optimizing drug efficacy and minimizing adverse effects. This method of using AI for targeted therapy development is not only more efficient but also cost-effective, potentially accelerating the introduction of new treatments to the market.

However, the adoption of AI in clinical settings is not without challenges. Data privacy remains a paramount concern, as patient data used to train AI systems often contain sensitive information that must be protected against breaches. Additionally, the black-box nature of many AI models poses significant hurdles in clinical acceptability. Healthcare professionals need to understand how decisions are made by AI to trust and effectively integrate these tools into their practice.

5.6.1 Data Privacy and Security

5.6.1.1 Challenge

Patient data used in AI models often include sensitive personal information. Unauthorized access to such data can lead to significant privacy violations.

5.6.1.2 Solutions

Implementing advanced encryption methods for data storage and transmission can secure patient information. Additionally, adopting strict access controls and regular audits can help prevent unauthorized data breaches.

5.6.2 Bias and Underrepresentation

5.6.2.1 Challenge

AI systems could exhibit biases if the data used to train them are not representative of the global population. This can lead to disparities in the accuracy of diagnoses across different ethnicities, genders, and socio-economic groups.

5.6.2.2 Solutions

To combat bias, it's crucial to use diverse datasets that reflect the variability in the global population. Rigorous testing across different demographics can help identify and mitigate biases in AI models.

5.6.3 Risks from Black-Box Models

5.6.3.1 Challenge

The opaque nature of some AI models can make it difficult for clinicians to understand how decisions are made, which can hinder trust and adoption in clinical settings.

5.6.3.2 Solutions

Developing XAI models that provide insights into their decision-making processes can enhance transparency. Training clinicians on the basics of AI can also improve trust and integration.

5.6.4 Regulatory Challenges

5.6.4.1 Challenge

The regulatory environment for AI in healthcare is complex and often lagging behind technological advancements, which can slow down the adoption of AI technologies.

5.6.4.2 Solutions

Collaborative efforts between AI developers, clinicians, and regulatory bodies can expedite the creation of guidelines that ensure the safety and efficacy of AI tools. Ongoing monitoring and adaptive regulations can keep pace with technological advancements.

5.6.5 Addressing Underrepresented Data

5.6.5.1 Challenge

Data from underrepresented groups may not be sufficiently included in the datasets, leading to less effective AI solutions for these populations.

5.6.5.2 Solutions

Deliberate efforts to collect and include data from diverse populations can ensure that AI tools are effective across different demographics. Partnerships with global institutions can help gather a wide array of data.

While AI presents transformative potential for diagnosing and managing dementia, addressing these challenges through thoughtful solutions is essential to maximize benefits and minimize risks. By implementing robust data protection measures, ensuring model transparency, expanding regulatory frameworks, and enhancing data diversity, AI can be more effectively integrated into clinical practice, leading to better patient outcomes and more personalized care.

5.7 Chapter Summary

In this comprehensive chapter on the intersection of ML, AI, and dementia research, we delve into the multifaceted aspects of diagnosing and treating various types of dementia. The chapter begins by exploring the different types of dementia, including AD, FTD, VD, and DLB. Each type is distinguished by unique symptoms and progression patterns, which are critical for accurate diagnosis and management.

Following the discussion on dementia types, the chapter provides an extensive overview of the diverse datasets used in dementia research. These include genetic biomarkers, neuroimaging data such as EEG, fMRI, and PET scans, as well as clinical and demographic data. The importance of considering ethnicity and its implications on the prevalence and manifestation of dementia is also discussed, highlighting the need for diverse research approaches to understand and address the disease effectively across different populations.

The narrative then shifts to the significant investments in research and development, underscoring the funding budgets allocated globally, which underscore the critical need and commitment to advancing our understanding and treatment capabilities of dementia.

An in-depth discussion on preprocessing techniques follows, which are essential for cleaning and preparing the data for analysis. This section bridges into a detailed examination of various ML and AI models and techniques used in the diagnosis and drug discovery for dementia. It covers how these technologies have revolutionized the field by providing tools that can predict disease progression, identify new therapeutic targets, and personalize treatment plans to enhance patient outcomes.

The personalized approach to dementia treatment is highlighted as a promising area of research and application, utilizing ML models to tailor treatments based on individual patient data, thus optimizing therapeutic efficacy and minimizing adverse effects.

Lastly, the chapter reviews commercial AI and ML-based tools that have been developed and are currently used in clinical settings. This section lists specific tools, their developers, and the countries where they are in use, providing real-world examples of how AI and ML are being integrated into healthcare practices globally.

In summary, this chapter not only explores the scientific and clinical landscapes of dementia research but also emphasizes the transformative impact of ML and AI in diagnosing and treating this complex suite of diseases. The integration of these technologies into clinical and research frameworks represents a significant leap forward in our ability to understand, predict, and manage dementia, ultimately leading to improved patient care and outcomes.

To further build upon the foundational knowledge and technological advancements detailed in this chapter, the subsequent chapters will delve into more specific applications and integrations of these technologies in real-world healthcare settings. In "Empowering Patient Care: Leveraging Artificial Intelligence and Internet of Things for Enhanced Healthcare Delivery," we explore how AI and IoT devices are utilized in the continuous monitoring and management of dementia, enhancing patient safety and improving the efficacy of interventions through real-time data collection and analysis. This integration facilitates a seamless transition into "Conversational Agents in Healthcare: Leveraging Language Models and Chatbots for Patient Interaction," where the focus shifts to the use of conversational AI to further personalize patient care. Here, we examine how these agents assist in maintaining communication with patients, offering consistent support, and managing their care with unprecedented precision and adaptability. Together, these chapters illustrate a progressive and integrated approach to dementia care, highlighting a holistic system that combines diagnosis, treatment, and continuous care into a unified framework.

References

Abdelmoaty, M. M., Lu, E., Kadry, R., Foster, E. G., Bhattarai, S., Mosley, R. L., & Gendelman, H. E. (2023). Clinical biomarkers for Lewy body diseases. Cell & Bioscience, 13(1), 209. https://doi.org/10.1186/s13578-023-01152-x

Ahmadzadeh, M., Christie, G. J., Cosco, T. D., Arab, A., Mansouri, M., Wagner, K. R., DiPaola, S., & Moreno, S. (2023). Neuroimaging and machine learning for studying the pathways from mild cognitive impairment to Alzheimer's disease: A systematic review. BMC Neurology, 23(1), Article 309. https://doi.org/10.1186/s12883-023-03323-2

Ahmed, G., Er, M. J., Fareed, M. M. S., Zikria, S., Mahmood, S., He, J., Asad, M., Jilani, S. F., & Aslam, M. (2022). DAD-Net: Classification of Alzheimer's disease using ADASYN oversampling technique and optimized neural Network. Molecules, 27(20), Article 7085. https://doi.org/10.3390/molecules27207085

Ahmed, R. M., Paterson, R. W., Warren, J. D., Zetterberg, H., O'Brien, J. T., Fox, N. C., Halliday, G. M., & Schott, J. M. (2014). Biomarkers in dementia: Clinical utility and new directions. Journal of Neurology, Neurosurgery & Psychiatry, 85(12), 1426–1434. https://doi.org/10.1136/jnnp-2014-307662

Aja-Fernández, S., Martín-Martín, C., Planchuelo-Gómez, Á, Faiyaz, A., Uddin, M. N., Schifitto, G., Tiwari, A., Shigwan, S. J., Singh, R. K., Zheng, T., Cao, Z., Wu, D., Blumberg, S. B., Sen, S., Goodwin-Allcock, T., Slator, P. J., Avci, M. Y., Li, Z., Bilgic, B., Tian, Q., … & Pieciak, T. (2023). Validation of deep learning techniques for quality augmentation in diffusion MRI for clinical studies. NeuroImage: Clinical, 39, 103483. https://doi.org/10.1016/j.nicl.2023.103483

Alahmadi, T., Rahman, A. U., Alhababi, Z. A., Ali, S., & Alkahtani, H. (2024). Prediction of mild cognitive impairment using EEG signal and BiLSTM network. Machine Learning: Science and Technology, 5(2), Article ad38fe. https://doi.org/10.1088/2632-2153/ad38fe

Albrecht, J. S., Hanna, M., Randall, R. L., Kim, D., & Perfetto, E. M. (2019). An algorithm to characterize a dementia population by disease subtype. Alzheimer Disease & Associated Disorders, 33(2), 118–123. https://doi.org/10.1097/WAD.0000000000000295

Alrawis, M., Al-Ahmadi, S., & Mohammad, F. (2024). Bridging modalities: A multimodal machine learning approach for Parkinson's disease diagnosis using EEG and MRI data. Applied Sciences, 14(9), Article 3883. https://doi.org/10.3390/app14093883

Alsubaie, M. G., Luo, S., & Shaukat, K. (2024). Alzheimer's disease detection using deep learning on neuroimaging: A systematic review. Machine Learning and Knowledge Extraction, 6(1), 464–505. https://doi.org/10.3390/make6010024

Altuna-Azkargorta, M., & Mendioroz-Iriarte, M. (2021). Blood biomarkers in Alzheimer's disease. Neurología (English Edition), 36(9), 704–710. https://doi.org/10.1016/j.nrleng.2018.03.006

Alzheimer Europe. (2024). Horizon Europe research programme. Retrieved from https://www.alzheimer-europe.org/our-work/2024-work-plan

Alzheimer's Association. (2024a). Alzheimer's disease facts and figures. Alzheimer's Association. Retrieved from https://www.alz.org/media/Documents/alzheimers-facts-and-figures.pdf

Alzheimer's Association. (2024b). Congress reaches bipartisan agreement on $100 million Alzheimer's research funding increase and continued investment in Alzheimer's public health infrastructure. Retrieved from https://www.alz.org/news/2024/congress-bipartisan-funding-alzheimers-research

Alzheimer's Association. (2024c). Call for papers: Spotlight on Alzheimer's disease and related dementias research in East Asia. Alzheimer's & Dementia. Retrieved from https://alz-journals.onlinelibrary.wiley.com/hub/journal/15525279/call-for-papers

Alzheimer's Research UK. (n.d.). All you need to know about brain scans and dementia. Retrieved on June 29, 2024, from https://www.alzheimersresearchuk.org/news/all-you-need-to-know-about-brain-scans-and-dementia/#:~:text=Functional%20magnetic%20resonance%20imaging%20(fMRI)&text=fMRI%20is%20more%20commonly%20used,scan%2C%20like%20a%20thinking%20test.

Alzheimer's Research UK. (2023). Economic Value of Dementia Research. Retrieved from https://www.alzheimersresearchuk.org/wp-content/uploads/2023/07/Economic-Value-of-Dementia-Research-July-2023.pdf

Angelucci, F., Ai, A. R., Piendel, L., Cerman, J., & Hort, J. (2024). Integrating AI in fighting advancing Alzheimer: Diagnosis, prevention, treatment, monitoring, mechanisms, and clinical trials. Current Opinion in Structural Biology, 87, Article 102857. https://doi.org/10.1016/j.sbi.2024.102857

Arvanitakis, Z., Shah, R. C., & Bennett, D. A. (2019). Diagnosis and management of dementia: Review. JAMA, 322(16), 1589–1599. https://doi.org/10.1001/jama.2019.4782

Askr, H., Elgeldawi, E., Aboul Ella, H., Elshaier, Y. A. M. M., Gomaa, M. M., & Hassanien, A. E. (2023). Deep learning in drug discovery: An integrative review and future challenges. Artificial Intelligence Review, 56(7), 5975–6037. https://doi.org/10.1007/s10462-022-10306-1

Australian Government Department of Health and Aged Care. (2022). Dementia and Aged Care Services (DACS) Fund. Retrieved from https://www.health.gov.au/our-work/dementia-and-aged-care-services-dacs-fund

Avberšek, L. K., & Repovš, G. (2022). Deep learning in neuroimaging data analysis: Applications, challenges, and solutions. Frontiers in Neuroimaging, 1, Article 981642. https://doi.org/10.3389/fnimg.2022.981642

Beller, J., Beller, H., & Briggs, J. (2020). Dementia: Types, symptoms, & risk factors: Dementia guide for patients, families, caregivers, & medical professionals (11th ed.). Independently published.

Bernasconi, A. (2005). Structural analysis applied to epilepsy. In Magnetic resonance in epilepsy (2nd ed., pp. 249–269). Neuroimaging Techniques. https://doi.org/10.1016/B978-012431152-7/50012-4

Bougea, A., Efthymiopoulou, E., Spanou, I., & Zikos, P. (2021). A novel machine learning algorithm predicts dementia with Lewy bodies versus Parkinson's disease dementia based on clinical and neuropsychological scores. Journal of Geriatric Psychiatry and Neurology, 35(3). https://doi.org/10.1177/0891988721993556

Brain, J., Kafadar, A. H., Errington, L., Kirkley, R., Tang, E. Y. H., Akyea, R. K., Bains, M., Brayne, C., Figueredo, G., Greene, L., Louise, J., Morgan, C., Pakpahan, E., Reeves, D., Robinson, L., Salter, A., Siervo, M., Tully, P. J., Turnbull, D., Qureshi, N., & Stephan, B. C. M. (2024). What's new in dementia risk prediction modelling? An updated systematic review. Dementia and Geriatric Cognitive Disorders Extra, 14(1), 49–74. https://doi.org/10.1159/000539744

Bucholc, M., James, C., Al Khleifat, A., Badhwar, A., Clarke, N., Dehsarvi, A., Madan, C. R., Marzi, S. J., Shand, C., Schilder, B. M., Tamburin, S., Tantiangco, H. M., Lourida, I., Llewellyn, D. J., & Ranson, J. M. (2023). Artificial intelligence for dementia research methods optimization. Alzheimer's & Dementia, 19(12), 5934–5951. https://doi.org/10.1002/alz.13441

Budson, A. E., & Solomon, P. R. (2021). Memory loss, Alzheimer's disease, and dementia: A practical guide for clinicians (3rd ed.). Elsevier. ISBN: 978-0323795449

Calhoun, V., Adali, T., Pearlson, G., & Pekar, J. J. (2001). A method for making group inferences using independent component analysis of functional MRI data: Exploring the visual system. NeuroImage, 13(6), 88. https://doi.org/10.1016/S1053-8119(01)91431-4

Carneiro, F., Saracino, D., Huin, V., Clot, F., Delorme, C., Méneret, A., Thobois, S., Cormier, F., Corvol, J. C., Lenglet, T., Vidailhet, M., Habert, M.-O., Gabelle, A., Beaufils, É, Mondon, K., Tir, M., Andriuta, D., Brice, A., Deramecourt, V., & Le

Ber, I. (2020). Isolated parkinsonism is an atypical presentation of GRN and C9orf72 gene mutations. Parkinsonism & Related Disorders, 80, 73–81. https://doi.org/10.1016/j.parkreldis.2020.09.019

Cassani, R., Estarellas, M., San-Martin, R., Fraga, F. J., & Falk, T. H. (2018). Systematic review on resting-state EEG for Alzheimer's disease diagnosis and progression assessment. Disease Markers, 2018, Article 5174815. https://doi.org/10.1155/2018/5174815

Chandra, A., Dervenoulas, G., & Politis, M., Alzheimer's Disease Neuroimaging Initiative. (2019). Magnetic resonance imaging in Alzheimer's disease and mild cognitive impairment. Journal of Neurology, 266(6), 1293–1302. https://doi.org/10.1007/s00415-018-9016-3

Chang, T., Fu, M., Valiente-Banuet, L., Wadhwa, S., Pasaniuc, B., & Vossel, K. (2024). Improving genetic risk modeling of dementia from real-world data in under-represented populations. Research Square [Preprint]. https://doi.org/10.21203/rs.3.rs-3911508/v1

Chen, H., Engkvist, O., Wang, Y., Olivecrona, M., & Blaschke, T. (2018). The rise of deep learning in drug discovery. Drug Discovery Today, 23(6), 1241–1250. https://doi.org/10.1016/j.drudis.2018.01.039

Chen, J. E., & Glover, G. H. (2015). Functional magnetic resonance imaging methods. Neuropsychology Review, 25(3), 289–313. https://doi.org/10.1007/s11065-015-9294-9

Chen, Y., Yang, X.-H., Wei, Z., Heidari, A. A., Zheng, N., Li, Z., Chen, H., Hu, H., Zhou, Q., & Guan, Q. (2022). Generative adversarial networks in medical image augmentation: A review. Computers in Biology and Medicine, 144, 105382. https://doi.org/10.1016/j.compbiomed.2022.105382

Cheng, F., Wang, F., Tang, J., Zhou, Y., Fu, Z., Zhang, P., Haines, J. L., Leverenz, J. B., Gan, L., Hu, J., Rosen-Zvi, M., Pieper, A. A., & Cummings, J. (2024). Artificial intelligence and open science in discovery of disease-modifying medicines for Alzheimer's disease. Cell Reports Medicine, 5(2), Article 101379. https://doi.org/10.1016/j.xcrm.2023.101379

Chinese Dementia Research Association. (2024). Retrieved from https://cdra-hk.org

Cho, B. P. H., Nannoni, S., Harshfield, E. L., Tozer, D., Gräf, S., Bell, S., & Markus, H. S. (2021). NOTCH3 variants are more common than expected in the general population and associated with stroke and vascular dementia: An analysis of 200,000 participants. Journal of Neurology, Neurosurgery, and Psychiatry, 92(7).

Cipollini, V., Troili, F., & Giubilei, F. (2019). Emerging biomarkers in vascular cognitive impairment and dementia: From pathophysiological pathways to clinical application. International Journal of Molecular Sciences, 20(11), 2812. https://doi.org/10.3390/ijms20112812

Contador, I., Buch-Vicente, B., del Ser, T., Llamas-Velasco, S., Villarejo-Galende, A., Benito-León, J., & Bermejo-Pareja, F. (2024). Charting Alzheimer's disease and dementia: Epidemiological insights, risk factors, and prevention pathways. Journal of Clinical Medicine, 13(14), 4100. https://doi.org/10.3390/jcm13144100

Cromarty, P., Drummond, A., Francis, T., Watson, J., & Battersby, M. (2016). NewAccess for depression and anxiety: Adapting the UK Improving Access to Psychological Therapies Program across Australia. Australas Psychiatry, 24(5), 489–492. https://doi.org/10.1177/1039856216641310

D'Souza, S., Prema, K. V., Balaji, S., et al. (2023). Deep learning-based modeling of drug–target interaction prediction incorporating binding site information of proteins. Interdisciplinary Sciences: Computational Life Sciences, 15, 306–315. https://doi.org/10.1007/s12539-023-00557-z

Dementia Australia. (2024). About the Dementia Australia Research Foundation. Retrieved from https://www.dementia.org.au/research/

Dementia UK. (n.d.). Types of dementia. Retrieved from https://www.dementiauk. org/understanding-dementia/types-of-dementia/

Dimitriadis, S. I., & Liparas, D.; Alzheimer's Disease Neuroimaging Initiative. (2018). How random is the random forest? Random forest algorithm on the service of structural imaging biomarkers for Alzheimer's disease: From Alzheimer's disease neuroimaging initiative (ADNI) database. Neural Regeneration Research, 13(6), 962–970. https://doi.org/10.4103/1673-5374.233433

Ding, Y., Chu, Y., Liu, M., Ling, Z., Wang, S., Li, X., & Li, Y. (2022). Fully automated discrimination of Alzheimer's disease using resting-state electroencephalography signals. Quantitative Imaging in Medicine and Surgery, 12(2), 1063–1078. https://doi.org/10.21037/qims-21-430

Doborjeh, M., Doborjeh, Z., Merkin, A., Bahrami, H., Sumich, A., Krishnamurthi, R., Medvedev, O. N., Crook-Rumsey, M., Morgan, C., Kirk, I., Sachdev, P. S., Brodaty, H., Kang, K., Wen, W., Feigin, V., & Kasabov, N. (2021). Personalised predictive modelling with brain-inspired spiking neural networks of longitudinal MRI neuroimaging data and the case study of dementia. Neural Networks, 144, 522–539. https://doi.org/10.1016/j.neunet.2021.09.013

Doherty, T., Yao, Z., Al Khleifat, A., Tantiangco, H., Tamburin, S., Albertyn, C., Thakur, L., Llewellyn, D. J., Oxtoby, N. P., Lourida, I., Ranson, J. M., & Duce, J. A. (2023). Artificial intelligence for dementia drug discovery and trials optimization. Alzheimer's & Dementia. Advance online publication. https://doi.org/10.1002/alz.13428

Earlstein, F. (2016). Dementia: Types, diagnosis, symptoms, treatment, causes, neurocognitive disorders, prognosis, research, history, myths, and more! Facts & information, Nrb Publishing, Atlanta.

Ebrahimi, A., & Luo, S.; Alzheimer's Disease Neuroimaging Initiative. (2021). Convolutional neural networks for Alzheimer's disease detection on MRI images. Journal of Medical Imaging (Bellingham), 8(2), Article 024503. https://doi.org/10.1117/1.JMI.8.2.024503

Ebrahimighahnavieh, A., Luo, S., & Chiong, R. (2020). Deep learning to detect Alzheimer's disease from neuroimaging: A systematic literature review. Computer Methods and Programs in Biomedicine, 187, Article 105242. https://doi.org/10.1016/j.cmpb.2019.105242

Farahani, F. V., Karwowski, W., & Lighthall, N. R. (2019). Application of graph theory for identifying connectivity patterns in human brain networks: A systematic review. Frontiers in Neuroscience, 13, Article 585. https://doi.org/10.3389/fnins.2019.00585

FDA. (2024). FDA authorized AI/ML-enabled medical devices. Retrieved from https://www.fda.gov/medical-devices/software-medical-device-samd/artificial-intelligence-and-machine-learning-aiml-enabled-medical-devices

Fiscon, G., Weitschek, E., Cialini, A., Felici, G., Bertolazzi, P., De Salvo, S., Bramanti, A., Bramanti, P., & De Cola, M. C. (2018). Combining EEG signal processing with supervised methods for Alzheimer's patients classification. BMC Medical Informatics and Decision Making, 18(1), Article 35. https://doi.org/10.1186/s12911-018-0613-y

García-Gutiérrez, F., Hernández-Lorenzo, L., Cabrera-Martín, M. N., Matias-Guiu, J. A., & Ayala, J. L., & Alzheimer's Disease Neuroimaging Initiative. (2024). Predicting changes in brain metabolism and progression from mild cognitive impairment to dementia using multitask deep learning models and explainable AI. NeuroImage, 297, Article 120695. https://doi.org/10.1016/j.neuroimage.2024.120695

Gascón-Bayarri, J., Reñé, R., Del Barrio, J. L., De Pedro-Cuesta, J., Ramón, J. M., Manubens, J. M., Sánchez, C., Hernández, M., Estela, J., Juncadella, M., & Rubio, F. R. (2007). Prevalence of dementia subtypes in El Prat de Llobregat, Catalonia, Spain: The PratICON study. Neuroepidemiology, 28(4), 224–234. https://doi.org/10.1159/000108597

Gispert, J. D., Pascau, J., Reig, S., Martínez-Lázaro, R., Molina, V., García-Barreno, P., & Desco, M. (2003). Influence of the normalization template on the outcome of statistical parametric mapping of PET scans. NeuroImage, 19(3), 601–612. https://doi.org/10.1016/s1053-8119(03)00072-7

Gonzalez-Ortiz, F., Kirsebom, B. E., Contador, J., et al. (2024). Plasma brain-derived tau is an amyloid-associated neurodegeneration biomarker in Alzheimer's disease. Nature Communications, 15, 2908. https://doi.org/10.1038/s41467-024-47286-5

Grajski, K. A., Breiman, L., Viana Di Prisco, G., & Freeman, W. J. (1986). Classification of EEG spatial patterns with a tree-structured methodology: CART. IEEE Transactions on Biomedical Engineering, 33(12), 1076–1086. https://doi.org/10.1109/TBME.1986.325684

Grigoli, M. M., Pelegrini, L. N. C., Whelan, R., & Cominetti, M. R. (2024). Present and future of blood-based biomarkers of Alzheimer's disease: Beyond the classics. Brain Research, 1830, 148812. https://doi.org/10.1016/j.brainres.2024.148812

Guney, E., Menche, J., Vidal, M., & Barabási, A.-L. (2016). Network-based in silico drug efficacy screening. Nature Communications, 7, 10331. https://doi.org/10.1038/ncomms10331

Gunther, S., Kuhn, M., Dunkel, M., Campillos, M., Senger, C., Petsalaki, E., Ahmed, J., Urdiales, E. G., Gewiess, A., Jensen, L. J., Schneider, R., Skoblo, R., Russell, R. B., Bourne, P. E., Bork, P., & Preissner, R. (2008). SuperTarget and Matador: Resources for exploring drug-target relationships. Nucleic Acids Research, 36(Database issue), D919–D922. https://doi.org/10.1093/nar/gkm862

Guo, Y., & Pagnoni, G. (2008). A unified framework for group independent component analysis for multi-subject fMRI data. NeuroImage, 42(3), 1078–1093. https://doi.org/10.1016/j.neuroimage.2008.05.008

Hailpern, S. M., Melamed, M. L., Cohen, H. W., & Hostetter, T. H. (2007). Moderate chronic kidney disease and cognitive function in adults 20 to 59 years of age: Third National Health and Nutrition Examination Survey (NHANES III). Journal of the American Society of Nephrology, 18(7), 2205–2213. https://doi.org/10.1681/ASN.2006101165

Henderson, G., Ifeachor, E., Hudson, N., Goh, C., Outram, N., Wimalaratna, S., Del Percid, C., & Echo, F. (2006). Development and assessment of methods for detecting dementia using the human electroencephalogram. IEEE Transactions on Biomedical Engineering, 53(8), 1557–1568.

Henney, M. A., Carstensen, M., Thorning-Schmidt, M., Kubińska, M., Grønberg, M. G., Nguyen, M., Madsen, K. H., Clemmensen, L. K. H., & Petersen, P. M. (2024). Brain stimulation with 40 Hz heterochromatic flicker extended beyond red, green, and blue. Scientific Reports, 14(1), Article 2147. https://doi.org/10.1038/s41598-024-52679-z

Henríquez, F., Cabello, V., Baez, S., de Souza, L. C., Lillo, P., Martínez-Pernía, D., Olavarría, L., Torralva, T., & Slachevsky, A. (2022). Multidimensional clinical assessment in frontotemporal dementia and its spectrum in Latin America and the Caribbean: A narrative review and a glance at future challenges. Frontiers in Neurology, 12, 768591. https://doi.org/10.3389/fneur.2021.768591

Herzog, R., Rosas, F. E., Whelan, R., Fittipaldi, S., Santamaria-Garcia, H., Cruzat, J., Birba, A., Moguilner, S., Tagliazucchi, E., Prado, P., & Ibanez, A. (2022). Genuine high-order interactions in brain networks and neurodegeneration. Neurobiology of Disease, 175, 105918. https://doi.org/10.1016/j.nbd.2022.105918

Hirani, R., Noruzi, K., Khuram, H., Hussaini, A. S., Aifuwa, E. I., Ely, K. E., Lewis, J. M., Gabr, A. E., Smiley, A., Tiwari, R. K., et al. (2024). Artificial intelligence and healthcare: A journey through history, present innovations, and future possibilities. Life, 14(5), Article 557. https://doi.org/10.3390/life14050557

Hosoki, S., Tanaka, T., & Ihara, M. (2021). Diagnostic and prognostic blood biomarkers in vascular dementia: From the viewpoint of ischemic stroke. Neurochemistry International, 146, 105015. https://doi.org/10.1016/j.neuint.2021.105015

Huang, G., Li, R., Bai, Q., & Alty, J. (2023). Multimodal learning of clinically accessible tests to aid diagnosis of neurodegenerative disorders: A scoping review. Health Information Science and Systems, 11(1), Article 32. https://doi.org/10.1007/s13755-023-00231-0

India Education Diary. (2024). Major boost for dementia research: £49.9 million funding injection announced. Retrieved from https://indiaeducationdiary.in/major-boost-for-dementia-research-49-9-million-funding-injection-announced/

Javanmard, S. (2024). Revolutionizing medical practice: The impact of artificial intelligence (AI) on healthcare. Open Access Journal of Applied Science and Technology. https://doi.org/10.33140/OAJAST.02.01.07

Javeed, A., Dallora, A. L., Berglund, J. S., & Ernberg, M. (2023). Machine learning for dementia prediction: A systematic review and future research directions. Journal of Medical Systems, 47(17). https://doi.org/10.1007/s10916-023-01906-7

Javeed, A., Dallora, A. L., Berglund, J. S., Idrisoglu, A., Ali, L., Rauf, H. T., & Anderberg, P. (2023). Early prediction of dementia using feature extraction battery (FEB) and optimized support vector machine (SVM) for classification. Biomedicines, 11(2), 439. https://doi.org/10.3390/biomedicines11020439

Jayatilake, S. M. D. A. C., & Ganegoda, G. U. (2021). Involvement of machine learning tools in healthcare decision making. Journal of Healthcare Engineering, 2021, Article 6679512. https://doi.org/10.1155/2021/6679512

Jiang, X., Bian, G. B., & Tian, Z. (2019). Removal of artifacts from EEG signals: A review. Sensors (Basel), 19(5), Article 987. https://doi.org/10.3390/s19050987

Jiang, M., Li, Z., Zhang, S., Wang, S., Wang, X., Yuan, Q., & Wei, Z. (2020). Drug-target affinity prediction using graph neural network and contact maps. RSC Advances, 10(35), 20701–20712. https://pmc.ncbi.nlm.nih.gov/articles/PMC9054320/

Jing, Y., Bian, Y., Hu, Z., Wang, L., & Xie, X. Q. (2018). Deep learning for drug design: An artificial intelligence paradigm for drug discovery in the big data era. AAPS Journal, 20(3), Article 58. https://doi.org/10.1208/s12248-018-0210-0

Johnson & Johnson. (2024). How AI is revolutionizing healthcare. Retrieved from https://www.jnj.com/innovation/artificial-intelligence-in-healthcare

Joseph, A., & Jayaraman, C. (2024). Preprocessing Techniques for Neuroimaging Modalities: An In-Depth Analysis. IntechOpen. doi: 10.5772/intechopen.109803

Jung, T. P., Makeig, S., McKeown, M. J., Bell, A. J., Lee, T. W., & Sejnowski, T. J. (2001). Imaging brain dynamics using independent component analysis. Proceedings of the IEEE, 89(7), 1107–1122. https://doi.org/10.1109/5.939827

Kandiah, N., Choi, S. H., Hu, C. J., Ishii, K., Kasuga, K., & Mok, V. C. T. (2022). Current and future trends in biomarkers for the early detection of Alzheimer's disease in Asia: Expert opinion. Journal of Alzheimer's Disease Reports, 6(1), 699–710. https://doi.org/10.3233/ADR-220059

Karimi, D. (2024). Diffusion MRI with machine learning. arXiv:2402.00019v1 [eess.IV]. Retrieved from https://arxiv.org/abs/2402.00019

Katisko, K., Huber, N., Kokkola, T., Hartikainen, P., Krüger, J., Heikkinen, A. L., Paananen, V., Leinonen, V., Korhonen, V. E., Helisalmi, S., Herukka, S. K., Cantoni, V., Gadola, Y., Archetti, S., Remes, A. M., Haapasalo, A., Borroni, B., & Solje, E. (2022). Serum total TDP-43 levels are decreased in frontotemporal dementia patients with C9orf72 repeat expansion or concomitant motoneuron disease phenotype. Alzheimer's Research & Therapy, 14(1), 151. https://doi.org/10.1186/s13195-022-01091-8

Kazeminia, S., Baur, C., Kuijper, A., van Ginneken, B., Navab, N., Albarqouni, S., & Mukhopadhyay, A. (2020). GANs for medical image analysis. Artificial Intelligence in Medicine, 109, Article 101938. https://doi.org/10.1016/j.artmed.2020.101938

Kumar, N., & Srivastava, R. (2024). Deep learning in structural bioinformatics: Current applications and future perspectives. Briefings in Bioinformatics, 25(3), Article bbae042. https://doi.org/10.1093/bib/bbae042

Lal, U., Chikkankod, A. V., & Longo, L. (2024). A comparative study on feature extraction techniques for the discrimination of frontotemporal dementia and Alzheimer's disease with electroencephalography in resting-state adults. Brain Sciences, 14(4), Article 335. https://doi.org/10.3390/brainsci14040335

Lavecchia, A. (2019). Deep learning in drug discovery: Opportunities, challenges, and future prospects. Drug Discovery Today, 24(10), 2017–2032. https://doi.org/10.1016/j.drudis.2019.07.006

Lee, S. H., Lee, S., Lee, J., Lee, J. K., & Moon, N. J. (2023). Effective encoder-decoder neural network for segmentation of orbital tissue in computed tomography images of Graves' orbitopathy patients. PLoS One, 18(5), e0285488. https://doi.org/10.1371/journal.pone.0285488

Lee, W., Lee, S., Park, Y., Kim, G. E., Bae, J. B., Han, J. W., & Kim, K. W. (2024). Construction and validation of a brain magnetic resonance imaging template for normal older Koreans. BMC Neurology, 24(1), Article 222. https://doi.org/10.1186/s12883-024-03735-8

Liampas, I., Dimitriou, N., Siokas, V., Messinis, L., Nasios, G., & Dardiotis, E. (2024). Cognitive trajectories preluding the onset of different dementia entities: A descriptive longitudinal study using the NACC database. Aging Clinical and Experimental Research, 36(1), 119. https://doi.org/10.1007/s40520-024-02769-9

Liao, J., & Brunner, E. (2023). Predictions for dementia burden and policy responses in China and UK by 2050. Innovation in Aging, 7(Supplement_1), 196. https://doi.org/10.1093/geroni/igad104.0645

Liu, Q., Vaci, N., Koychev, I., et al. (2022). Personalised treatment for cognitive impairment in dementia: Development and validation of an artificial intelligence model. BMC Medicine, 20, Article 45. https://doi.org/10.1186/s12916-022-02250-2

Lleó, A., Blesa, R., Queralt, R., Ezquerra, M., Molinuevo, J. L., Peña-Casanova, J., Rojo, A., & Oliva, R. (2002). Frequency of mutations in the presenilin and amyloid precursor protein genes in early-onset Alzheimer disease in Spain. Archives of Neurology, 59(11), 1759–1763. https://doi.org/10.1001/archneur.59.11.1759

Locatelli, M., Padovani, A., & Pezzini, A. (2020). Pathophysiological mechanisms and potential therapeutic targets in cerebral autosomal dominant arteriopathy with subcortical infarcts and leukoencephalopathy (CADASIL). Frontiers in Pharmacology, 11, 321. https://doi.org/10.3389/fphar.2020.00321

Lue, L. F., Guerra, A., & Walker, D. G. (2017). Amyloid beta and tau as Alzheimer's disease blood biomarkers: Promise from new technologies. Neurology and Therapy, 6(Suppl 1), 25–36. https://doi.org/10.1007/s40120-017-0074-8

Maleki Varnosfaderani, S., & Forouzanfar, M. (2024). The role of AI in hospitals and clinics: Transforming healthcare in the 21st century. Bioengineering (Basel), 11(4), Article 337. https://doi.org/10.3390/bioengineering11040337

Malik, I., Iqbal, A., Gu, Y. H., & Al-Antari, M. A. (2024). Deep learning for Alzheimer's disease prediction: A comprehensive review. Diagnostics (Basel), 14(12), Article 1281. https://doi.org/10.3390/diagnostics14121281

Mangialasche, F., Kivipelto, M., Solomon, A., & Fratiglioni, L. (2012). Dementia prevention: Current epidemiological evidence and future perspective. Alzheimer's Research & Therapy, 4(1), 6. https://doi.org/10.1186/alzrt104

Márquez, F., & Yassa, M. A. (2019). Neuroimaging biomarkers for Alzheimer's disease. Molecular Neurodegeneration, 14, 21. https://doi.org/10.1186/s13024-019-0325-5

Mayeda, E. R., Glymour, M. M., Quesenberry, C. P., & Whitmer, R. A. (2016). Inequalities in dementia incidence between six racial and ethnic groups over 14 years. Alzheimer's & Dementia, 12(3), 216–224. https://doi.org/10.1016/j.jalz.2015.12.007

McKeown, M. J., & Sejnowski, T. J. (1998). Independent component analysis of fMRI data: Examining the assumptions. Human Brain Mapping, 6(5–6), 368–372. https://doi.org/10.1002/(SICI)1097-0193(1998)6:5/6<368::AID-HBM7>3.0.CO;2-E

Meyers, E. A., Amouyel, P., Bovenkamp, D. E., Carrillo, M. C., De Buchy, G. D., Dumont, M., Fillit, H., Friedman, L., Henderson-Begg, G., Hort, J., Murtishaw, A., Oakley, R., Panchal, M., Rossi, S. L., Sancho, R. M., Thienpont, L., Weidner, W., & Snyder, H. M. (2022). Commentary: Global Alzheimer's disease and Alzheimer's disease related dementia research funding organizations support and engage the research community throughout the COVID-19 pandemic. Alzheimer's & Dementia, 18(5), 1067–1070. https://doi.org/10.1002/alz.12472

Moguilner, S., García, A. M., Perl, Y. S., Tagliazucchi, E., Piguet, O., Kumfor, F., Reyes, P., Matallana, D., Sedeño, L., & Ibáñez, A. (2021). Dynamic brain fluctuations outperform connectivity measures and mirror pathophysiological profiles across dementia subtypes: A multicenter study. NeuroImage, 225, Article 117522. https://doi.org/10.1016/j.neuroimage.2020.117522

Mohammed, E. M., Fakhrudeen, A. M., & Alani, O. (2024). Detection of Alzheimer's disease using deep learning models: A systematic literature review. Informatics in Medicine Unlocked. Advance online publication. https://doi.org/10.1016/j.imu.2024.101551

Mravinacová, S., Alanko, V., Bergström, S., Bridel, C., Pijnenburg, Y., Hagman, G., Kivipelto, M., Teunissen, C., Nilsson, P., Matton, A., & Månberg, A. (2024). CSF protein ratios with enhanced potential to reflect Alzheimer's disease pathology and neurodegeneration. Molecular Neurodegeneration, 19(1), 15. https://doi.org/10.1186/s13024-024-00705-z

Mura, T., Baramova, M., Gabelle, A., Artero, S., Dartigues, J.-F., Amieva, H., & Berr, C. (2017). Predicting dementia using socio-demographic characteristics and the Free and cued Selective Reminding Test in the general population. Alzheimer's Research & Therapy, 9, Article 21. https://doi.org/10.1186/s13195-017-0254-x

Mwangi, B., Tian, T. S., & Soares, J. C. (2014). A review of feature reduction techniques in neuroimaging. Neuroinformatics, 12(2), 229–244. https://doi.org/10.1007/s12021-013-9204-3

Nag, S., Baidya, A. T. K., Mandal, A., Mathew, A. T., Das, B., Devi, B., & Kumar, R. (2022). Deep learning tools for advancing drug discovery and development. 3 Biotech, 12(5), Article 110. https://doi.org/10.1007/s13205-022-03165-8

National Institute of Neurological Disorders and Stroke. (2024). Focus on Alzheimer's disease and related dementias. U.S. Department of Health and Human Services. Retrieved from https://www.ninds.nih.gov/health-information/disorders/dementias

National Institute on Aging. (2023). Understanding different types of dementia. Retrieved from https://www.nia.nih.gov/health/alzheimers-and-dementia/understanding-different-types-dementia

O'Dell, R. S., Higgins-Chen, A., Gupta, D., Chen, M. K., Naganawa, M., Toyonaga, T., Lu, Y., Ni, G., Chupak, A., Zhao, W., Salardini, E., Nabulsi, N. B., Huang, Y., Arnsten, A. F. T., Carson, R. E., van Dyck, C. H., & Mecca, A. P. (2023). Principal component analysis of synaptic density measured with [11C]UCB-J PET in early Alzheimer's disease. NeuroImage: Clinical, 39, Article 103457. https://doi.org/10.1016/j.nicl.2023.103457

Oldan, J. D., Jewells, V. L., Pieper, B., & Wong, T. Z. (2021). Complete evaluation of dementia: PET and MRI correlation and diagnosis for the neuroradiologist. AJNR American Journal of Neuroradiology, 42(6), 998–1007. https://doi.org/10.3174/ajnr.A7079

Oldham, S., Arnatkevičiūtė, A., Smith, R. E., Tiego, J., Bellgrove, M. A., & Fornito, A. (2020). The efficacy of different preprocessing steps in reducing motion-related confounds in diffusion MRI connectomics. NeuroImage, 222, 117252. https://doi.org/10.1016/j.neuroimage.2020.117252

Orme, T., Guerreiro, R., & Bras, J. (2018). The genetics of dementia with Lewy bodies: Current understanding and future directions. Current Neurology and Neuroscience Reports, 18(10), 67. https://doi.org/10.1007/s11910-018-0874-y

Parikh, R. B., Linn, K. A., Yan, J., Maciejewski, M. L., Rosland, A. M., Volpp, K. G., Groeneveld, P. W., & Navathe, A. S. (2021). A machine learning approach to identify distinct subgroups of veterans at risk for hospitalization or death using administrative and electronic health record data. PLoS One, 16(2), e0247203. https://doi.org/10.1371/journal.pone.0247203

Patel, L., Shukla, T., Huang, X., Ussery, D. W., & Wang, S. (2020). Machine learning methods in drug discovery. Molecules, 25(22), 5277. https://doi.org/10.3390/molecules25225277

Pellegrini, E., Ballerini, L., Hernandez, M. D. C. V., Chappell, F. M., González-Castro, V., Anblagan, D., Danso, S., Muñoz-Maniega, S., Job, D., Pernet, C., Mair, G., MacGillivray, T. J., Trucco, E., & Wardlaw, J. M. (2018). Machine learning of neuroimaging for assisted diagnosis of cognitive impairment and dementia: A systematic review. Alzheimer's & Dementia: Diagnosis, Assessment & Disease Monitoring, 10, 519–535. https://doi.org/10.1016/j.dadm.2018.07.004

Pfizer Insights. (2022). Pfizer is using AI to discover breakthrough medicines. Retrieved from https://insights.pfizer.com/pfizer-is-using-ai-to-discover-breakthrough-medicines/

Pirrone, D., Weitschek, E., Di Paolo, P., De Salvo, S., & De Cola, M. C. (2022). EEG signal processing and supervised machine learning to early diagnose Alzheimer's disease. Applied Sciences, 12(11), 5413. https://doi.org/10.3390/app12115413

Polikar, R., Tilley, C., Hillis, B., & Clark, C. M. (2010). Multimodal EEG, MRI and PET data fusion for Alzheimer's disease diagnosis. In Proceedings of the Annual International Conference of the IEEE Engineering in Medicine and Biology Society (pp. 6058–6061). https://doi.org/10.1109/IEMBS.2010.5627621

Poorkaj, P., Grossman, M., Steinbart, E., Payami, H., Sadovnick, A., Nochlin, D., Tabira, T., Trojanowski, J. Q., Borson, S., Galasko, D., Reich, S., Quinn, B., Schellenberg, G., & Bird, T. D. (2001). Frequency of tau gene mutations in familial and sporadic cases of non-Alzheimer dementia. Archives of Neurology, 58(3), 383–387. https://doi.org/10.1001/archneur.58.3.383

Liao, J., & Brunner, E. (2023). Predictions for dementia burden in China by 2050 and long-term care insurance policy. (2023). Innovation in Aging, 7(Supplement_1), 197. https://doi.org/10.1093/geroni/igad104.0649

Presotto, L., Iaccarino, L., Sala, A., Vanoli, E. G., Muscio, C., Nigri, A., Bruzzone, M. G., Tagliavini, F., Gianolli, L., Perani, D., & Bettinardi, V. (2018). Low-dose CT for the spatial normalization of PET images: A validation procedure for amyloid-PET semi-quantification. NeuroImage: Clinical, 20, 153–160. https://doi.org/10.1016/j.nicl.2018.07.013

Prince, M., Bryce, R., Albanese, E., Wimo, A., Ribeiro, W., & Ferri, C. P. (2013). The global prevalence of dementia: A systematic review and metaanalysis. Alzheimer's & Dementia, 9(1), 63–75.e2. https://doi.org/10.1016/j.jalz.2012.11.007

Qiu, Y., & Cheng, F. (2024). Artificial intelligence for drug discovery and development in Alzheimer's disease. Current Opinion in Structural Biology, 85, 102776. https://doi.org/10.1016/j.sbi.2024.102776

Qiu, C., Kivipelto, M., & von Strauss, E. (2009). Epidemiology of Alzheimer's disease: Occurrence, determinants, and strategies toward intervention. Dialogues in Clinical Neuroscience, 11(2), 111–128. https://doi.org/10.31887/DCNS.2009.11.2/cqiu

Quan, M., Cao, S., Wang, Q., Wang, S., & Jia, J. (2023). Genetic phenotypes of Alzheimer's disease: Mechanisms and potential therapy. Phenomics, 3(4), 333–349. https://doi.org/10.1007/s43657-023-00098-x

Raulin, A. C., Doss, S. V., Trottier, Z. A., Ikezu, T. C., Bu, G., & Liu, C. C. (2022). ApoE in Alzheimer's disease: Pathophysiology and therapeutic strategies. Molecular Neurodegeneration, 17(1), Article 72. https://doi.org/10.1186/s13024-022-00574-4

Rehman, A. U., Li, M., Wu, B., Ali, Y., Rasheed, S., Shaheen, S., Liu, X., Luo, R., & Zhang, J. (2024). Role of artificial intelligence in revolutionizing drug discovery. Fundamental Research. Advance online publication. https://doi.org/10.1016/j.fmre.2024.04.021

Renub Research. (2024). Alzheimer's drugs market report by drug class (Cholinesterase inhibitors, NMDA receptor antagonist, combination drugs, and others), drug type (Galantamine, Donepezil, Memantine, Rivastigmine, and others), distribution channel (Hospital pharmacies, retail pharmacies, and online pharmacies), region and company analysis 2024–2032. Renub Research. Retrieved July 10, 2024, from https://www.renub.com/alzheimer-s-pipeline-drugs-review-alzheimer-s-disease-drug-market-and-forecast-global-analysis-131-p.php

Rezaei, A., van den Berg, M., Mirlohi, H., Verhoye, M., Amiri, M., & Keliris, G. A. (2024). Recurrence quantification analysis of rs-fMRI data: A method to detect subtle changes in the TgF344-AD rat model. Computer Methods and Programs in Biomedicine. Advance online publication. https://doi.org/10.1016/j.cmpb.2024.108378

Ribeiro, L. G., & Busatto, G. F. (2016). Voxel-based morphometry in Alzheimer's disease and mild cognitive impairment: Systematic review of studies addressing the frontal lobe. Dementia & Neuropsychologia, 10(2), 104–112. https://doi.org/10.1590/S1980-5764-2016DN1002006

Rohrer, J., Ryan, B., & Ahmed, R. (2022). MAPT-related frontotemporal dementia. In M. P. Adam, J. Feldman, G. M. Mirzaa, et al. (Eds.), GeneReviews® [Internet]. Seattle (WA): University of Washington, Seattle. Original publication date November 7, 2000; updated August 18, 2022. Retrieved from https://www.ncbi.nlm.nih.gov/books/NBK1505/

Salcedo-Pérez-Juana, M., García-Bravo, C., Jimenez-Antona, C., Martinez-Piédrola, R. M., Fernández-De-Las-Peñas, C., & Palacios-Ceña, D. (2023). Relatives' experiences during the COVID-19 pandemic: A qualitative study set in Spanish locked-down nursing homes. Japanese Journal of Nursing Science, 20(1), Article e12510. https://doi.org/10.1111/jjns.12510

Salvi, M., Loh, H. W., Seoni, S., Barua, P. D., García, S., Molinari, F., & Acharya, U. R. (2024). Multi-modality approaches for medical support systems: A systematic review of the last decade. Information Fusion, 103, Article 102134. https://doi.org/10.1016/j.inffus.2023.102134

Sanders, A. E., Schoo, C., & Kalish, V. B. (2023). Vascular dementia. In StatPearls. StatPearls Publishing. https://www.ncbi.nlm.nih.gov/books/NBK430817/

Schindler, S. E., & Fagan, A. M. (2015). Autosomal dominant Alzheimer disease: A unique resource to study CSF biomarker changes in preclinical AD. Frontiers in Neurology, 6, Article 142. https://doi.org/10.3389/fneur.2015.00142

Shanmugavadivel, K., Sathishkumar, V. E., Cho, J., & Subramanian, M. (2023). Advancements in computer-assisted diagnosis of Alzheimer's disease: A comprehensive survey of neuroimaging methods and AI techniques for early detection. Ageing Research Reviews, 91, Article 102072. https://doi.org/10.1016/j.arr.2023.102072

Sharma, N., Kolekar, M. H., & Jha, K. (2021). EEG based dementia diagnosis using multi-class support vector machine with motor speed cognitive test. Biomedical Signal Processing and Control, 63, 102102. https://doi.org/10.1016/j.bspc.2020.102102

Shojaie, M., Cabrerizo, M., DeKosky, S. T., Vaillancourt, D. E., Loewenstein, D., Duara, R., & Adjouadi, M. (2022). A transfer learning approach based on gradient boosting machine for diagnosis of Alzheimer's disease. Frontiers in Aging Neuroscience, 14, Article 966883. https://doi.org/10.3389/fnagi.2022.966883

Shukla, A., Tiwari, R., & Tiwari, S. (2023). Review on Alzheimer disease detection methods: Automatic pipelines and machine learning techniques. Sci, 5(1), 13. https://doi.org/10.3390/sci5010013

Singh, S. G., Das, D., Barman, U., & Saikia, M. J. (2024). Early Alzheimer's disease detection: A review of machine learning techniques for forecasting transition from mild cognitive impairment. Diagnostics, 14(16), 1759. https://doi.org/10.3390/diagnostics14161759

Smith, K. M., Starr, J. M., Escudero, J., Ibañez, A., & Parra, M. A. (2022). Abnormal functional hierarchies of EEG networks in familial and sporadic prodromal Alzheimer's disease during visual short-term memory binding. Frontiers in Neuroimaging, 1, Article 883968. https://doi.org/10.3389/fnimg.2022.883968

Souchet, B., Michaïl, A., Heuillet, M., et al. (2024). Multiomics blood-based biomarkers predict Alzheimer's predementia with high specificity in a multicentric cohort study. Journal of Prevention of Alzheimer's Disease, 11(5), 567–581. https://doi.org/10.14283/jpad.2024.34

Steenland, K., Goldstein, F. C., Levey, A., & Wharton, W. (2016). A meta-analysis of Alzheimer's disease incidence and prevalence comparing African-Americans and Caucasians. Journal of Alzheimer's Disease, 50(1), 71–76. https://doi.org/10.3233/JAD-150778

Tajbakhsh, N., Shin, J. Y., Gurudu, S. R., Hurst, R. T., Kendall, C. B., Gotway, M. B., & Liang, J. (2016). Convolutional neural networks for medical image analysis: Full training or fine tuning? IEEE Transactions on Medical Imaging, 35(5), 1299–1312. https://doi.org/10.1109/TMI.2016.2535302

Timsina, J., Ali, M., Do, A., Wang, L., Sung, Y. J., & Cruchaga, C. (2023). Harmonization of CSF and imaging biomarkers for Alzheimer's disease biomarkers: Need and practical applications for genetics studies and preclinical classification. bioRxiv. https://doi.org/10.1101/2023.05.24.542118

Tolea, M. I., & Galvin, J. E. (2018). The genetics of dementia with Lewy bodies. In Handbook of Clinical Neurology (Vol. 148, pp. 431–440). https://doi.org/10.1016/B978-0-444-64076-5.00028-4

Tsolaki, A., Kazis, D., Kompatsiaris, I., Kosmidou, V., & Tsolaki, M. (2014). Electroencephalogram and Alzheimer's disease: Clinical and research approaches. International Journal of Alzheimer's Disease. https://doi.org/10.1155/2014/349249

University of California, San Francisco. Department of Radiology and Biomedical Imaging. (n.d.). Amyloid PET scan for Alzheimer's disease assessment. Retrieved on June 29, 2024, from https://radiology.ucsf.edu/patient-care/services/specialty-imaging/alzheimer

van der Zande, J. J., Gouw, A. A., van Steenoven, I., Scheltens, P., Stam, C. J., & Lemstra, A. W. (2018). EEG characteristics of dementia with Lewy bodies, Alzheimer's disease, and mixed pathology. Frontiers in Aging Neuroscience, 10, 190. https://doi.org/10.3389/fnagi.2018.00190

Varesi, A., Carrara, A., Pires, V. G., Floris, V., Pierella, E., Savioli, G., Prasad, S., Esposito, C., Ricevuti, G., Chirumbolo, S., & Pascale, A. (2022). Blood-based biomarkers for Alzheimer's disease diagnosis and progression: An overview. Cells, 11(8), 1367. https://doi.org/10.3390/cells11081367

Velazquez, M., & Lee, Y.; Alzheimer's Disease Neuroimaging Initiative. (2021). Random forest model for feature-based Alzheimer's disease conversion prediction from early mild cognitive impairment subjects. PLoS One, 16(4), e0244773. https://doi.org/10.1371/journal.pone.0244773

Waghere, S., RajaRajeswari, P., & Ganesan, V. (2021). Design and implementation of a system which efficiently retrieves useful data for the detection of dementia disease. Springer Singapore. https://doi.org/10.1007/978-981-15-7961-5_144

Wang, J., Bermudez, D., Chen, W., Durgavarjhula, D., Randell, C., Uyanik, M., & McMillan, A. (2024). Motion-correction strategies for enhancing whole-body PET imaging. Frontiers in Nuclear Medicine, 4, Article 1257880. https://doi.org/10.3389/fnume.2024.1257880

Wang, H., Wang, J., Dong, C., Lian, Y., Liu, D., Yan, Z., & Chen, S. (2020). A novel approach for drug-target interactions prediction based on multimodal deep autoencoder. Frontiers in Pharmacology, 10, 1592. https://doi.org/10.3389/fphar.2019.01592

Wang, Y., & Zeng, J. (2013). Predicting drug-target interactions using restricted Boltzmann machines. Bioinformatics, 29(13), i126–i134. https://doi.org/10.1093/bioinformatics/btt234

Whitwell, J. L. (2009). Voxel-based morphometry: An automated technique for assessing structural changes in the brain. Journal of Neuroscience, 29(31), 9661–9664. https://doi.org/10.1523/JNEUROSCI.2160-09.2009

Whitwell, J. L. (2019). FTD spectrum: Neuroimaging across the FTD spectrum. Progress in Molecular Biology and Translational Science, 165, 187–223. https://doi.org/10.1016/bs.pmbts.2019.05.009

World Health Organization. (2023). Dementia. Retrieved from https://www.who.int/news-room/fact-sheets/detail/dementia

World Health Organization. (2024). China: Improving home care for dementia patients. Retrieved from https://www.who.int/news-room/feature-stories/detail/china-improving-home-care-for-dementia-patients

Wu, X., Li, Z., Chen, G., Yin, Y., & Chen, C. Y.-C. (2023). Hybrid neural network approaches to predict drug–target binding affinity for drug repurposing: Screening for potential leads for Alzheimer's disease. Frontiers in Molecular Biosciences, 10. https://doi.org/10.3389/fmolb.2023.1227371

Wu, S., Zhan, P., Wang, G., Yu, X., Liu, H., & Wang, W. (2024). Changes of brain functional network in Alzheimer's disease and frontotemporal dementia: A graph-theoretic analysis. BMC Neuroscience, 25(1), Article 30. https://doi.org/10.1186/s12868-024-00877-w

Wyman-Chick, K. A., Chaudhury, P., Bayram, E., Abdelnour, C., Matar, E., Chiu, S. Y., Ferreira, D., Hamilton, C. A., Donaghy, P. C., Rodriguez-Porcel, F., Toledo, J. B., Habich, A., Barrett, M. J., Patel, B., Jaramillo-Jimenez, A., Scott, G. D., & Kane, J. P. M. (2024). Differentiating prodromal dementia with Lewy bodies from prodromal Alzheimer's disease: A pragmatic review for clinicians. Neurology and Therapy, 13, 885–906. https://pubmed.ncbi.nlm.nih.gov/38720013/

Xu, X., Li, J., Zhu, Z., Zhao, L., Wang, H., Song, C., Chen, Y., Zhao, Q., Yang, J., & Pei, Y. (2024). A comprehensive review on synergy of multi-modal data and AI technologies in medical diagnosis. Bioengineering (Basel), 11(3), Article 219. https://doi.org/10.3390/bioengineering11030219

Yang, Y., Bagyinszky, E., & An, S. S. A. (2023). Presenilin-1 (PSEN1) mutations: Clinical phenotypes beyond Alzheimer's disease. International Journal of Molecular Sciences, 24(9), 8417. https://doi.org/10.3390/ijms24098417

Yen, C., Lin, C. L., & Chiang, M. C. (2023). Exploring the frontiers of neuroimaging: A review of recent advances in understanding brain functioning and disorders. Life (Basel), 13(7), 1472. https://doi.org/10.3390/life13071472

Yuan, L., Chen, X., Jankovic, J., & Deng, H. (2024). CADASIL: A NOTCH3-associated cerebral small vessel disease. Journal of Advanced Research. Advance online publication. https://doi.org/10.1016/j.jare.2024.01.001

Zabihi, S., Whitfield, T., & Walker, Z. (2021). SPECT/PET findings in dementia with Lewy bodies. In R. A. J. O. Dierckx, A. Otte, E. F. J. de Vries, A. van Waarde, & K. L. Leenders (Eds.), PET and SPECT in Neurology (pp. 551–561). Springer, Cham. https://doi.org/10.1007/978-3-030-53168-3_17

Zdrazil, B., Felix, E., Hunter, F., Manners, E. J., Blackshaw, J., Corbett, S., de Veij, M., Ioannidis, H., Lopez, D. M., Mosquera, J. F., Magarinos, M. P., Bosc, N., Arcila, R., Kizilören, T., Gaulton, A., Bento, A. P., Adasme, M. F., Monecke, P., Landrum, G. A., & Leach, A. R. (2024). The ChEMBL database in 2023: A drug discovery platform spanning multiple bioactivity data types and time periods. Nucleic Acids Research, 52(D1), D1180–D1192. https://doi.org/10.1093/nar/gkad1004

Zhang, M. Y., Katzman, R., Salmon, D., Jin, H., Cai, G. J., Wang, Z. Y., Qu, G. Y., Grant, I., Yu, E., Levy, P., et al. (1990). The prevalence of dementia and Alzheimer's disease in Shanghai, China: Impact of age, gender, and education. Annals of Neurology, 27(4), 428–437. https://doi.org/10.1002/ana.410270412

Zhang, L., Qu, J., Ma, H., Chen, T., Liu, T., & Zhu, D. (2024). Exploring Alzheimer's disease: A comprehensive brain connectome-based survey. Psychoradiology, 4, Article kkad033. https://doi.org/10.1093/psyrad/kkad033

Zhao, Y., Guo, Q., Zhang, Y., Zheng, J., Yang, Y., Du, X., Feng, H., & Zhang, S. (2023). Application of deep learning for prediction of Alzheimer's disease in PET/MR imaging. Bioengineering (Basel), 10(10), Article 1120. https://doi.org/10.3390/bioengineering10101120

6

Conversational Agents in Healthcare: Leveraging Language Models and Chatbots for Patient Interaction

Helena Bahrami and Sasan Adibi

6.1 Introduction

Dementia, a progressive neurological disorder, significantly impacts patients and their families, necessitating a multifaceted approach to healthcare and support. As the global population ages, the prevalence of dementia is increasing, presenting an urgent need for innovative solutions to manage its complexities. Artificial intelligence (AI) and machine learning (ML), particularly advanced language models, offer promising tools to enhance the care and support provided to dementia patients and their caregivers. By integrating these technologies, we can develop smart assistants that facilitate real-time communication and personalized care plans, tailored to the unique needs of each patient.

These AI-powered smart assistants can function as invaluable resources for healthcare professionals (HCPs), including doctors, nurses, and other providers, enabling them to deliver more effective and efficient care. By leveraging the capabilities of language models, these systems can be trained on vast datasets encompassing medical histories, treatment outcomes, and patient preferences, allowing them to offer informed suggestions and support. Furthermore, the adaptability of these models means they can be customized to different levels of knowledge and expertise, ensuring they are accessible and useful for professionals at various stages of their careers, as well as directly to patients and families needing varying degrees of information and support.

The integration of such AI-driven platforms with hospital systems and various health service providers could revolutionize the management of dementia care. These platforms can facilitate seamless communication between different care providers and centralize patient information, leading to coordinated care strategies and improved health outcomes. By providing

DOI: 10.1201/9781003485681-6

continuous learning and adaptation, these AI assistants can evolve with the advancing landscape of dementia care, ensuring up-to-date support that continuously enhances the quality of life for those affected by dementia. This convergence of technology and healthcare represents a significant stride towards a more supportive and effective care ecosystem for dementia patients and their families.

Building on the evolving landscape of dementia care, it is imperative to integrate these AI-driven tools with the latest guidelines and professional insights to effectively manage behaviors that challenge in dementia patients, focusing on non-pharmacological interventions as recommended by recent research and expert consensus.

Building on the integration of IoT and ML discussed in "Empowering Patient Care: Leveraging Artificial Intelligence and Internet of Things for Enhanced Healthcare Delivery," this chapter explores the role of conversational agents in enriching the communication and support systems for dementia care. The use of advanced language models within AI-driven conversational platforms exemplifies how technology can enhance the responsiveness and personalization of care, ensuring that interactions are tailored to the unique needs of each patient. As we progress towards concluding our series with a comprehensive proposal, these discussions will culminate in "Revolutionizing Dementia Care: Proposing a Comprehensive AI-Powered Global Framework for Enhanced Diagnosis and Personalized Treatment." This final chapter will synthesize insights from all preceding discussions, proposing a visionary framework that integrates all facets of AI-enhanced tools to transform global dementia care, setting a new standard for diagnosis, treatment, and ongoing patient support.

6.2 Establishing Standard Protocols for Patient-Centered Dementia Care

Recent studies and e-surveys among HCPs underscore a growing consensus on the critical need for guidelines to effectively manage behaviours that challenge (BtC)[1] in dementia, particularly emphasizing non-pharmacological interventions (Gray et al., 2022). The National Institute for Health and Care Excellence (NICE)[2] Guideline and a British Psychological Society—Division of Clinical Psychology briefing (BPS-DCP (2013)) highlight the shift toward interventions that minimize distress and improve quality of life without relying on antipsychotics. This shift is informed by a conceptualization of BtC as expressions of unmet needs, which, if appropriately addressed, can significantly alleviate the distress associated with dementia.

6.2.1 Implementation and Practitioner Insights

A comprehensive e-survey conducted across multidisciplinary professional dementia networks in the United Kingdom reveals that while these guidelines are deemed moderately useful, there are significant challenges in their application (Gray et al., 2022). Health professionals report a "moderate" utility in the guidelines, praising their accessibility and clarity. However, they also express concerns over the guidelines' lack of detail and specificity, particularly in outlining non-pharmacological approaches tailored to individual needs.

The survey identified several thematic challenges:

- **Lack of Detail and Clarity:** Many practitioners find the guidelines to be too generic, lacking the necessary detail to inform specific clinical practices and interventions tailored to individual patient needs.
- **Implementation Barriers:** Despite the theoretical support for non-pharmacological approaches, practical implementation remains sporadic and inconsistent, often hindered by systemic barriers within healthcare settings.
- **Medical Model Predominance:** There is a noted reliance on medical models, with insufficient emphasis on psychological and personalized approaches that consider the unique circumstances and needs of dementia patients.

Before developing AI-based language models to aid in dementia care, it is essential to address these identified challenges by establishing uniform standard protocols that are agreed upon by the community of experts and patients, ensuring that the solutions provided are both specific and universally applicable.

6.2.2 Advancing Care through Structured, Non-Pharmacological Interventions

The research findings suggest a pressing need for bespoke, setting-specific toolkits that update and refine the BPS-DCP (2013) guidelines to better meet the real-world demands of managing BtC (Gray et al., 2022). These toolkits should aim to:

- **Enhance Accessibility and Relevance:** Making the guidelines more accessible and relevant to frontline staff through comprehensive training and clear, actionable steps.
- **Promote Person-Centered Approaches:** Encouraging more personalized care strategies that focus on the patient's individual needs and conditions, moving away from a one-size-fits-all approach.

- **Strengthen Interdisciplinary Collaboration:** Facilitating better collaboration across disciplines to ensure a holistic management strategy that incorporates medical, psychological, and social interventions.

6.2.3 Integration with Conversational AI and NLP in Dementia Care

Incorporating these refined guidelines into the AI-driven platforms, such as conversational agents and chatbots, can further enhance their efficacy. By programming these tools to recognize signs of distress and respond with tailored, guideline-based interventions, AI can play a crucial role in the non-pharmacological management of BtC. This approach not only aligns with the current best practices as outlined by NICE and BPS but also leverages the continuous advancements in AI and ML to provide adaptive, sensitive, and responsive care to dementia patients.

This integration promises a dual benefit: it not only adheres to established best practices but also innovates care delivery, making it more responsive and tailored to the evolving needs of dementia patients and their caregivers. By blending structured, guideline-informed interventions with the dynamic capabilities of Natural Language Processing (NLP) and conversational AI, we can create a supportive framework that not only addresses immediate behavioral challenges but also adapts to the changing conditions and preferences of patients over time.

6.3 Introduction to NLP and Its Relevance in Healthcare

NLP is increasingly vital in healthcare for enhancing patient-provider communication, extracting insights from unstructured clinical notes, and powering conversational agents. NLP technologies enable the translation of the vast stores of textual healthcare data into actionable insights, facilitating more personalized and timely care (Salvi et al., 2023; Nazi & Peng, 2024; Woo et al., 2024). NLP tools are pivotal in improving the quality of patient-provider interactions. They assist in interpreting and responding to patient inquiries, thereby making communication more efficient and reducing the potential for miscommunication. This application is crucial in settings where clear communication can significantly impact patient outcomes (Meystre et al., 2008; Aramaki et al., 2022). One of the primary applications of NLP in healthcare is in the extraction of pertinent information from unstructured clinical notes—a task that is both time-consuming and prone to errors when performed manually. NLP systems can efficiently parse these notes, identify relevant information, and summarize findings, which supports clinical decision-making and improves patient care (Kreimeyer et al., 2017). NLP is integral to the development of intelligent conversational agents or chatbots, which are increasingly used in healthcare settings for patient triage, initial consultations, and regular follow-ups. These agents provide a scalable way to extend healthcare services, offering 24/7 availability and immediate responses to patient inquiries, which is essential for managing chronic conditions and providing continuous support (Bickmore et al., 2005, 2018).

These advancements in NLP not only enhance the efficiency and accuracy of healthcare services but also contribute significantly to a more nuanced understanding of patient needs and a more tailored healthcare experience.

6.4 Overview of Language Models and Applications in Patient Interaction

The integration of language models, particularly those based on deep learning, has significantly transformed conversational interfaces in healthcare. These models, capable of interpreting and generating human-like text, enable the development of intelligent chatbots that assist in patient triage, provide health information, and support chronic disease management (Salvi et al., 2023; Nazi & Peng, 2024; Woo et al., 2024). By leveraging NLP capabilities, deep learning technologies offer substantial advancements in patient monitoring and management, especially for chronic conditions like Alzheimer's disease (AD).

For instance, Munteanu et al. (2022) describe a prototype system that utilizes AI to monitor the daily activities of Alzheimer's patients, focusing on their eating and drinking habits. This system employs video analysis to detect and remind patients about their nutritional intake, which is crucial given the memory impairments characteristic of Alzheimer's. Such technologies not only enhance patient independence but also alleviate the burden on caregivers by automating routine monitoring tasks. Integrating these AI systems with NLP-driven tools could further personalize care delivery and improve communication channels between patients and healthcare providers, ensuring timely and contextually appropriate interventions (Munteanu et al., 2022).

Moreover, other innovative applications of language models in dementia care are emerging. For example, conversational agents designed for cognitive assessment have been developed to evaluate cognitive decline in dementia patients. El Haj et al. (2024) explored ChatGPT's potential as a diagnostic aid for AD by using detailed clinical case scenarios. The study demonstrated that ChatGPT could accurately diagnose Alzheimer's and classify patients into different stages, similar to diagnoses made by blinded specialists. However, the authors emphasize that while ChatGPT can be a valuable tool for symptom assessment, it should complement, not replace, clinical judgment due to its limitations and ethical considerations surrounding patient data privacy.

Alowais et al. (2023) highlight the transformative role of AI in clinical practice, particularly in dementia and AD care. The authors underscore how AI, especially NLP, is enhancing diagnostic accuracy, personalizing treatment plans, and improving patient outcomes. By analyzing large datasets and patient records, AI systems support clinicians in making more informed decisions, thereby elevating the standard of care for dementia and Alzheimer's patients.

Another advancement is the AI-driven communication tool developed by Qi et al. (2022), which helps dementia patients articulate their needs and emotions. This tool uses language models to predict and suggest phrases, facilitating better communication between patients and caregivers. Engagement and social interaction are also critical for dementia patients, and chatbots are proving beneficial in this area. Rodríguez-Domínguez et al. (2024) explored the use of chatbots to engage dementia patients in social conversations. Powered by deep learning language models, these chatbots help reduce loneliness and stimulate cognitive functions by initiating conversations based on the patient's interests.

Suganthi et al. (2024) presented a comprehensive methodology for implementing a medical chatbot utilizing the Retrieval-Augmented Generation (RAG) framework. The system architecture includes speech recognition for user input, a generative model leveraging Hugging Face's Transformers for enhanced response relevance and contextuality, and text-to-speech conversion for output delivery. The methodology extends to iterative model training and performance evaluation to ensure the chatbot's efficacy in providing informative, coherent responses. By integrating advanced technologies and continuous refinement, the proposed chatbot aims to support medical professionals and patients by delivering precise, accessible information and facilitating effective communication.

Ruggiano et al. (2021) explored the nascent application of chatbot technologies like ChatGPT in supporting individuals with dementia and their caregivers. They assess the growing integration of chatbots in dementia care, evaluating the quality of existing applications in terms of user interaction and content delivery. While chatbots present a promising tool for enhancing care through streamlined communication and information provision, their effectiveness is limited by drawbacks such as simplistic dialog capabilities and a lack of tailored content for dementia-specific needs. The study underscores the necessity for development grounded in rigorous evidence-based research to optimize chatbot applications for this vulnerable population, suggesting that these technologies could significantly aid in managing dementia care if developed thoughtfully and inclusively.

Moreover, the integration of chatbots with telehealth services has enhanced remote dementia care. Amjad, Kordel and Fernandes (2023) discuss the transformative impact of AI on telehealth, highlighting how AI has revolutionized remote healthcare delivery by enhancing diagnostic support, patient monitoring, and personalized patient interactions. AI's rapid data processing capabilities enable healthcare providers to make informed, real-time decisions, improving patient outcomes. AI-driven systems in telehealth offer sophisticated tools for patient communication and disease management, allowing for continuous monitoring and intervention without physical presence. This facilitates the remote management of chronic diseases and specialized care, raising the standard of patient care and optimizing healthcare resource allocation.

GECA, a chatbot specifically tailored for preventive care, is particularly beneficial for patients with dementia receiving home treatment. It provides essential information, guidance, and active monitoring to enhance patient care. Notably, GECA's bilingual capabilities and seamless integration with external healthcare resources ensure personalized and effective support. Its adaptable architecture not only accommodates dementia but can also be extended to other diseases, enhancing its versatility in preventive healthcare. GECA prioritizes patient privacy and data security, adhering to strict standards and protocols to ensure secure data handling. Demonstrating a remarkable 97% accuracy rate in response delivery, GECA is poised for further evaluation in a Portuguese hospital to assess its effectiveness and user satisfaction, underscoring its potential as a robust solution in dementia care (Maia, Vieira & Praça, 2023).

Subramanian, Yang and Khanna (2024) discussed the potential of large language models (LLMs) like GPT-4 in enhancing healthcare communication, particularly in improving the readability of patient-facing documents like discharge summaries. The study by Zaretsky et al. explored how LLMs can generate concise, patient-friendly summaries but highlighted significant concerns about safety risks, including omissions and hallucinations. While LLMs show promise in healthcare communication, the authors stress the need for strict oversight and further refinement to ensure patient safety and trust in these technologies.

Schmitz and Becker (2023) explored the development of a chatbot-mediated learning platform aimed at supporting family caregivers of people with dementia, focusing on handling agitation. Their study highlights the importance of a didactic design that considers the unique learning needs of caregivers, such as time constraints and varying prior knowledge. The platform offers tailored information through short and long learning paths, using anchored instruction to provide contextually relevant content. The chatbot enhances learning by offering feedback and encouraging reflection, though it cannot replace the role of a teacher in informal learning settings.

Additionally, Rampioni et al. (2023) conducted a thematic literature analysis on the use of embodied conversational agents (ECAs) for dementia patients.

The study identified three key themes: research frameworks used to study ECA interactions with dementia patients, the efficacy of ECAs in improving user engagement and addressing the needs of patients, and the methodological and technical challenges faced in developing ECAs. The findings underscore the potential of ECAs in dementia care but highlight the need for more sophisticated study designs and personalized solutions to improve their effectiveness.

The study by Gudala et al. (2023) explores the benefits, barriers, and needs for an AI-powered medication information voice chatbot for older adults through interviews with geriatrics experts. The experts identified key benefits, including improved usability, increased medication adherence, and enhanced overall health. Barriers include technology familiarity, cost, and privacy concerns, particularly for older adults over 75. The study emphasizes the importance of a user-friendly, affordable chatbot that connects with pharmacies, caregivers, and health providers, while addressing older adults' specific needs, like medication reminders and side effects information.

Finally, Pham, Nabizadeh and Selek (2022) discuss the growing role of AI in psychiatry, focusing on applications like chatbots, avatar therapy, and companion bots. These AI tools offer benefits such as increased accessibility, reduced stigma, and cost-effectiveness in mental healthcare. However, concerns include limited emotional nuance, legal responsibilities, and data privacy issues. The authors stress the need for large, controlled trials to assess the efficacy of AI interventions and address challenges in integrating these technologies into clinical practice.

In conclusion, these advancements in establishing standard protocols for dementia care pave the way for integrating sophisticated tools like NLP in healthcare settings. This integration not only enhances the efficiency and accuracy of services but also contributes significantly to a more nuanced understanding of patient needs, fostering the development of more tailored, user-friendly conversational interfaces in healthcare.

6.5 Designing User-Friendly Conversational Interfaces in Healthcare

Conversational interfaces, such as chatbots, are increasingly integral in healthcare settings, offering a unique avenue for patient interaction that is efficient and cost-effective. To ensure these tools are used responsibly and effectively, it is crucial to adhere to a series of strategic design principles that prioritize user-friendliness and address ethical considerations in patient communication.

6.5.1 Strategies for Building User-Friendly Chatbots in Healthcare Settings

To optimize the potential of chatbots in enhancing patient care, it is crucial to employ strategic design principles that ensure these tools are both effective and user-friendly in healthcare environments.

- **Understanding User Needs:** The first step in designing effective chatbots involves engaging with potential users—patients and healthcare providers—through surveys or interviews. This engagement helps gather insights into their needs and expectations from a healthcare chatbot. Such insights guide the functionality and design of the chatbot to ensure it meets actual user demands and fits seamlessly into the healthcare communication ecosystem (Laranjo et al., 2018).

- **Simplifying Interaction:** To enhance user experience, chatbot interactions should be designed to be simple and intuitive. Utilizing NLP effectively allows the chatbot to understand and respond to user queries in a straightforward manner, without requiring users to learn complex commands. This strategy ensures that the chatbot is accessible to users with varying levels of technical proficiency (Miner, Laranjo & Kocaballi, 2020).

- **Personalization:** Offering personalized responses based on the user's medical history or previous interactions can significantly increase engagement and satisfaction. Personalization makes the interactions feel more relevant and tailored to individual users, thereby enhancing the perceived value and effectiveness of the chatbot in managing healthcare needs (Bickmore et al., 2018).

- **Continuous Learning and Adaptation:** Implementing advanced ML algorithms enables the chatbot to learn from past interactions and continuously improve its responses. This capability allows the chatbot to adapt over time to diverse user behaviors and queries, ensuring long-term effectiveness and relevance in the dynamic environment of healthcare (Kocaballi et al., 2020).

- **Ethical Considerations:** Building ethical considerations into the design process is essential. This includes ensuring privacy, maintaining transparency about how patient data is used, and actively working to mitigate any biases in language models. Adhering to these ethical standards helps maintain trust and safety in patient communication, crucial for the successful integration of AI technologies in healthcare settings.

By focusing on these strategic and ethical elements, healthcare providers can develop chatbots that not only support patient needs effectively but also contribute positively to the healthcare outcomes without compromising patient trust or safety. This comprehensive approach ensures that conversational AI tools remain beneficial and ethical components of modern healthcare systems.

6.6 Patient Engagement and Support

Davies et al. (2020) highlight the critical role of online support for older family carers of people with dementia, especially towards the end of life. Family carers often face unique challenges and may feel isolated; digital platforms can provide essential resources and a sense of community that are accessible from home. The study emphasizes the need for online resources that are easy to navigate and can provide both informational and emotional support tailored to the late stages of dementia care. Carers value platforms that help them feel prepared and equipped, maintain connections with others, balance their needs with those of their loved ones, and coordinate care effectively (Davies et al., 2020). While many carers appreciate the flexibility and accessibility of online support, the study also notes a preference for a blend of digital and face-to-face interactions, underscoring the importance of personalized and multifaceted support approaches.

6.7 Integrating AI and ML in Dementia Care: Towards a Comprehensive Support Ecosystem

The integration of AI and ML into dementia care heralds a new era of technological advancement, poised to revolutionize the management of this complex condition. As the global population ages, the prevalence of dementia increases, creating an urgent need for more effective, scalable, and personalized care solutions. AI and ML technologies offer promising avenues for addressing these challenges, facilitating the development of tools that can analyze vast amounts of data to predict outcomes, personalize treatments, and enhance the daily management of dementia. This approach not only aims to improve the quality of life for patients and ease the burden on caregivers but also optimizes healthcare resources, making comprehensive, high-quality care more accessible to all affected.

6.7.1 Patient-Centered Digital Support for Dementia Caregivers

Recent research by Davies et al. (2020) highlights the critical role of online support platforms for family carers of people with dementia, particularly in the later stages of care. These platforms offer essential resources and a sense of community, crucial for carers who may feel isolated. Digital resources that are easily navigable and tailored to the complex needs of late-stage dementia are highly valued for their ability to provide both informational and emotional support. This need underscores the importance of developing AI-enhanced platforms that offer comprehensive, personalized support. In their systematic review, Kruse et al. (2015) explore the characteristics of patient portals that garner positive feedback from both patients and providers and identify areas necessitating improvement. This study synthesizes findings from various studies to assess how patient portals aid in managing chronic diseases. Notably, patient-provider communication is a significant positive attribute, with enhanced interaction facilitated by these portals. However, issues like security concerns and user-friendliness persist, posing challenges for less tech-savvy users and deterring some providers due to the high costs of implementation and maintenance. The review suggests that a standardized design for patient portals could foster broader adoption by making these tools more accessible and effectively supporting patients in managing their chronic conditions, ultimately enhancing the quality of healthcare service delivery.

6.7.2 Enhancing Patient Engagement through AI-Driven Conversational Interfaces

The implementation of AI-driven conversational interfaces can revolutionize the way patient input is collected, enhancing the personalization of care. Chatbots are instrumental in delivering timely information and resources, significantly improving patient engagement and satisfaction. These interfaces serve not only to gather critical patient data but also to facilitate more nuanced interactions that can adapt to individual patient needs (Nazi & Peng, 2024; Woo et al., 2024).

6.7.3 Optimizing Healthcare Connectivity with AI

The connectivity between patients and HCPs is vital for effective care delivery. This section delves into strategies that improve patient-HCP interactions through the use of digital tools and interdisciplinary teams. Effective communication techniques like motivational interviewing and shared decision-making are pivotal in enhancing engagement and care quality. Digital platforms such as telemedicine, patient portals, and mobile health apps extend the reach and efficiency of healthcare services, ensuring that care is both accessible and comprehensive.

6.7.4 AI-Enhanced Tools for Remote Consultations and Referrals

Conversational agents are increasingly used to streamline remote consultations, acting as intermediaries that facilitate scheduling, preliminary data collection, and follow-up instructions. Additionally, sophisticated referral systems within chatbots, as noted by Salvi et al. (2023), optimize healthcare workflows by automating patient triage and directing them to appropriate services based on their symptoms and medical history. These innovations are crucial in creating a seamless, efficient healthcare experience.

6.7.5 Advancing Care through Structured, Non-Pharmacological Interventions

The evolving landscape of dementia care emphasizes the need for structured, non-pharmacological interventions that address the unique needs of patients. Updated guidelines and toolkits, tailored to real-world demands, are essential for managing challenging behaviors associated with dementia. By integrating AI tools, these guidelines can be dynamically adapted to enhance both accessibility and relevance, promoting a personalized approach to care.

6.7.6 Innovative Approaches to Shared Decision-Making in Dementia Care

The EMBED-Care Framework, introduced by Aworinde et al. (2024), exemplifies innovative shared decision-making in dementia care. This framework supports holistic assessments linked with decision-support tools, fostering an environment where care decisions are aligned with the individual preferences and needs of dementia patients. This personalized approach is crucial for effectively managing a condition as complex as dementia.

6.7.7 Leveraging Language Models for Enhanced Dementia Care

A study by Shawaqfeh et al. (2024) illustrates how language models can enhance the understanding of carer experiences with anticholinergic medications in dementia care. By integrating these models, healthcare providers can develop tools that offer personalized prescribing practices and communication strategies, ensuring that care is informed by a comprehensive understanding of both the benefits and risks associated with treatment options.

6.8 Ethical Considerations in AI-Powered Healthcare Interventions

As the integration of AI into healthcare continues to expand, ethical considerations become paramount to ensure that these technological interventions are conducted responsibly. This section explores the critical ethical issues surrounding the use of AI in healthcare, particularly focusing on maintaining patient privacy, ensuring data security, avoiding biases in AI algorithms, and upholding transparency in AI decision-making processes. It is essential to address these challenges proactively to build trust and ensure the equitable delivery of healthcare services through AI-powered interventions.

6.8.1 General Ethical Principles in AI Deployment

Ethical considerations in deploying NLP and AI in healthcare underscore the importance of ensuring privacy, maintaining transparency about how patient data is used, and avoiding biases in language models. It is crucial that these systems are continuously monitored and updated to align with ethical standards in patient care (Salvi et al., 2023). This includes navigating the delicate balance between the potential benefits and ethical risks of using AI to predict health outcomes, especially for chronic diseases like Alzheimer's (Ursin, Timmermann & Steger, 2021).

6.8.2 Specific Challenges in Predictive Health Analytics

Using AI to predict Alzheimer's in asymptomatic individuals presents ethical challenges, such as ensuring informed consent, preserving patient autonomy, and managing the potential psychological impact of predictive information in the absence of effective treatments. The principles of beneficence and non-maleficence are critical here, demanding that AI deployments do more good than harm. This involves managing rights like the right to know versus the right not to know and handling incidental findings that predictive algorithms may uncover well before symptoms manifest.

6.8.3 Impact on Patient-Physician Dynamics

The accuracy and explicability of AI predictions are paramount in ensuring that patients and their families can make informed decisions. As AI systems can predict disease risk with significant accuracy, they notably influence how healthcare providers communicate diagnoses and manage patient expectations and planning. This necessitates a new level of transparency in healthcare interactions, requiring that patients be adequately informed about how AI tools contribute to their healthcare outcomes and the limitations of these technologies.

6.8.4 Ethical Use of Language Models in Patient Communication

As conversational AI and predictive analytics become more integrated into healthcare, ethical considerations must guide their deployment to ensure patient trust and safety. Challenges include ensuring strict adherence to regulations such as HIPAA or General Data Protection Regulation (GDPR) for data security, maintaining high standards of chatbot accuracy to prevent misinformation, being transparent about chatbot capabilities, and actively mitigating biases in language models (Luxton, 2014; Dignum, 2019; Grote & Berens, 2020; Sun & Zhou, 2023; Singh, Sillerud & Singh, 2023; Li, 2023). By focusing on user-friendly design, personalization, and continuous learning, healthcare providers can develop chatbots that effectively support patient needs while adhering to ethical standards.

6.8.5 The Need for a Global Ethical Regulatory Organization

The diverse and complex ethical challenges posed by AI and language models in healthcare underscore the need for a global ethical regulatory organization. This entity would be responsible for setting universal standards and guidelines specifically tailored to healthcare applications, including those related to privacy, data security, accuracy, transparency, and bias mitigation. For areas such as dementia care, standardized ethical regulations would ensure that technologies are used responsibly and effectively, supporting global cooperation and enhancing the quality of care delivered worldwide.

6.9 Commercial AI Chatbots and Tools Enhancing Dementia Care

Advancements in AI have paved the way for the development of chatbots and tools specifically designed to support individuals with dementia. These innovations not only offer companionship but also assist in daily tasks and caregiver management, ultimately aiming to improve the quality of life for dementia patients.

One notable example is **Memory Lane**, a voice-enabled chatbot that engages users through storytelling. This tool is particularly beneficial in stimulating cognitive functions and providing a comforting presence in the home environment (Memory Lane, n.d.).

Another impactful technology is **ElliQ**, an AI companion robot that supports elderly users, including those with dementia. ElliQ helps users remain active and engaged by providing reminders for important tasks and medications, along with delivering news and entertainment (ElliQ by Intuition Robotics, n.d.).

Additionally, **SafelyYou** utilizes AI-powered video analysis to prevent falls, a common issue among dementia patients. By detecting falls and alerting caregivers promptly, SafelyYou significantly enhances safety within dementia care settings (SafelyYou, n.d.).

These technologies represent a significant stride towards integrating AI in healthcare, particularly in managing age-related conditions such as dementia. They not only demonstrate the potential of AI in medical applications but also underscore the importance of innovative approaches in enhancing patient care.

6.10 Revolutionizing Dementia Care: Proposing A Comprehensive AI-Powered Global Framework for Enhanced Diagnosis and Personalized Treatment

Building on the foundational principles discussed in the previous chapters, "Advancing Diagnosis and Drug Discovery: AI and Machine Learning Models for Dementia and Alzheimer's Disease" and "Empowering Patient Care: Leveraging Artificial Intelligence and Internet of Things for Enhanced Healthcare Delivery," this section proposes a revolutionary framework titled "Pioneering the Future of Dementia Care: A Global Collaboration of AI Experts and Physicians Working Together to Transform Data into Solutions for Diagnosis, Treatment, and Support."

This framework embodies a holistic and integrative approach to dementia care, leveraging multimodal data—including EEG, clinical and demographic information, PET and fMRI scans, and genomic profiles—housed within a centralized cloud platform. This global network facilitates a seamless collaboration among a diverse cadre of physicians and ML experts. Together, they harness advanced AI and clustering techniques to develop diagnostic tools that are both inclusive and sensitive to variations in ethnicity, age, and gender, thus minimizing biases and enhancing diagnostic accuracy.

In alignment with the innovative strategies explored in earlier chapters, this framework significantly enhances the capabilities for personalized drug discovery and treatment planning. It builds on established AI and IoT frameworks, integrating these with a sophisticated medical expert chatbot designed to interact and provide tailored assistance across various levels of medical expertise and patient interaction. This chatbot, trained on extensive medical texts, acts as a conduit for effective communication, offering insights and support tailored to the needs of medical professionals, patients, and their families.

As a nexus for global data sharing and analysis, this framework not only streamlines the process from diagnosis to treatment but also enriches the collective understanding of dementia management. By strategically mitigating data biases and focusing on precision in treatment and care, it promises to elevate the standard of dementia care globally. This ambitious framework aims to reshape the landscape of healthcare for dementia and AD, providing a scalable and sustainable model that anticipates the evolving needs of the global population. This comprehensive ecosystem, as detailed in the chapters, epitomizes the potential of AI and technology in transforming healthcare delivery and patient management in profound and impactful ways.

The necessity for such an advanced framework in dementia care cannot be understated. As dementia and AD continue to impact a growing segment of the global population, the demand for more effective and efficient diagnostic and treatment methodologies becomes critical. This framework not only facilitates the development of targeted treatments but also promises significant reductions in the long-term healthcare costs associated with chronic dementia care. By enabling early diagnosis and personalized treatment plans, it reduces the need for more intensive medical interventions later, which are often more costly and less effective.

To realize the full potential of this visionary framework, a broad coalition of stakeholders must come together. Governments, research institutes, healthcare providers, and technology companies must collaborate closely to provide the necessary expertise, resources, and regulatory support. Such collaborations can harness the strengths of each sector, ensuring that the framework is robust, secure, and adaptable to the needs of diverse populations. Government agencies can play a pivotal role by funding initial research and development efforts, while private tech companies can contribute cutting-edge technologies and scalability solutions.

Additionally, international health organizations and non-governmental organizations (NGOs) specializing in health innovation could be instrumental in bridging gaps between different stakeholders, especially in lower-resource settings. This wide-reaching collaboration will not only accelerate the development and deployment of the framework but also ensure that it is accessible and affordable to all, thereby democratizing the benefits of advanced AI and IoT in healthcare.

Long-term funding for this project could be sourced from a combination of government health departments, international grants, and private investments. Leveraging such funding not only fosters innovation but also aligns with broader public health goals of improving healthcare outcomes and reducing costs through enhanced preventative care and management of chronic diseases. By investing in such transformative projects, stakeholders can expect substantial returns in terms of reduced healthcare burdens, improved patient outcomes, and overall enhancement of healthcare efficiency across the globe.

The implementation of this comprehensive framework signifies a paradigm shift in how dementia care is approached and delivered. It embodies a future where technology and healthcare converge to create a system that is not only more effective but also more humane and equitable.

6.11 Essential Technological Tools for Developing an AI-Integrated Global Dementia Care Framework

As articulated in the vision for "Pioneering the Future of Dementia Care," the realization of this comprehensive AI-powered framework hinges on the deployment of state-of-the-art technological tools that enable the seamless integration of data, ML, and healthcare delivery across global platforms. This section elaborates on the detailed technological requirements that are essential for building and maintaining the proposed unified AI-driven framework in dementia care, ensuring that the architecture supports both current needs and future expansions.

6.11.1 Data Acquisition and Management

To facilitate a robust and reliable foundation for global dementia research and care, standardized data collection protocols must be implemented across global hospitals and research institutes. Secure APIs will enable safe and efficient data transfers, maintaining patient confidentiality while fostering a collaborative research environment. The use of distributed databases such as Apache Cassandra and MongoDB, coupled with cloud storage solutions like AWS S3, Azure Blob Storage, and Google Cloud Storage, will ensure data scalability and accessibility. These platforms will integrate sophisticated data management tools like AWS Redshift, Azure Synapse Analytics, and Google BigQuery to handle large-scale data warehousing and analytics, allowing researchers and clinicians to derive meaningful insights rapidly and efficiently.

6.11.2 Data Preprocessing and Integration

To ensure that the data used is of high quality and devoid of biases, comprehensive data cleaning libraries like Pandas and scikit-learn will be utilized for preprocessing. Tools such as the ARX Data Anonymization Tool will protect patient identities and comply with global privacy standards. The integration of data across multiple sources and formats will be managed by platforms like Talend and Informatica, with support from ETL tools such as Apache NiFi and StreamSets, ensuring that the data landscape within the dementia care framework is both integrated and versatile.

6.11.3 Machine Learning Models and Inference

The framework will employ a wide range of ML models to support various aspects of dementia care—from basic statistical models like linear and logistic regression to more complex classifiers and clustering algorithms. Advanced techniques will involve LLMs and deep learning frameworks such as CNNs implemented using TensorFlow and PyTorch. Feature extraction techniques like PCA, Fourier Transform, and Wavelet Transform will further enhance the model's ability to interpret complex neurological data effectively. Cloud-based platforms like AWS SageMaker, Azure Machine Learning, and Google AI Platform will facilitate the development, training, and deployment of these models at scale, ensuring that the framework remains at the forefront of technological advancements.

6.11.4 User Interface and Security Measures

The user interface, crucial for the accessibility of the framework, will be developed using modern web frameworks such as React, Angular, and Vue.js. Tools like Tableau and Power BI will enhance data visualization, making complex data more accessible to healthcare providers and researchers. Security is paramount; therefore, measures like AES and SSL/TLS encryption will protect data at rest and in transit. Regular security audits and adherence to standards such as HIPAA and GDPR will ensure that the framework not only protects patient information but also aligns with global regulatory requirements.

By leveraging these technological tools, the proposed framework will create a synergistic ecosystem where technology and expertise converge to transform dementia care. This holistic approach ensures that from data acquisition to delivery of care, every element is seamlessly integrated, promoting a future where dementia care is more predictive, personalized, and accessible across the globe. These technological underpinnings are crucial in realizing the ambitious goals set forth in previous chapters, establishing a scalable and sustainable model that evolves with the advancing landscape of global healthcare needs.

The proposed Figure 6.1 and accompanying Table 6.1 delineate a comprehensive AI-driven framework designed for the global management of

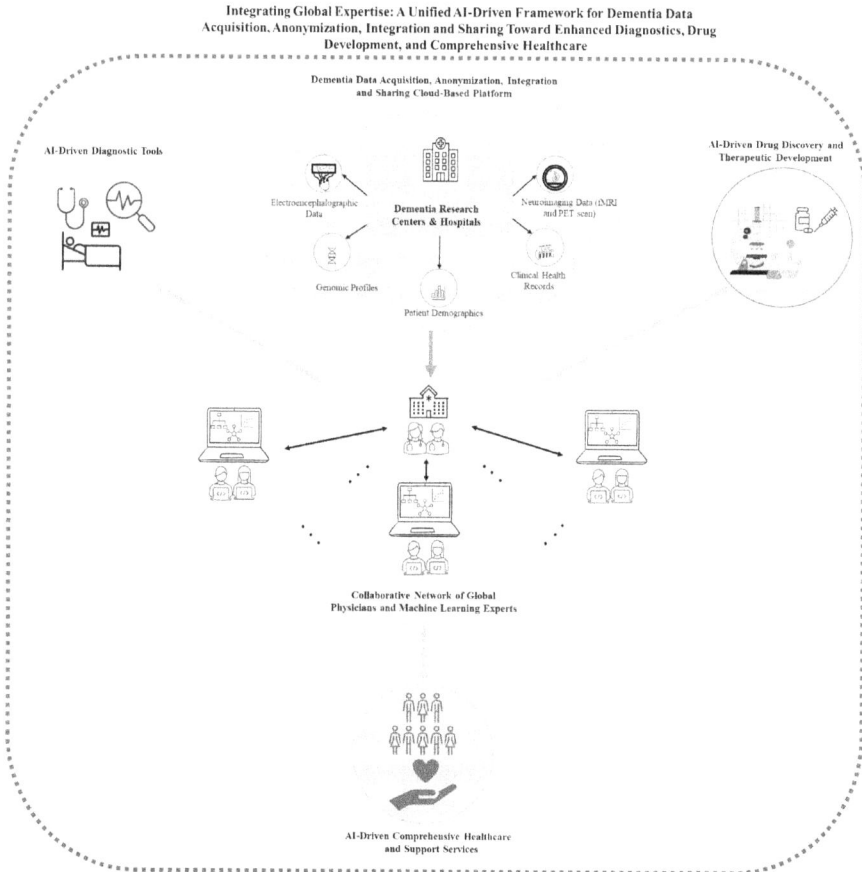

FIGURE 6.1
Pioneering the future of dementia care: a global collaboration of AI experts and physicians working together to transform data into solutions for diagnosis, treatment, and support.

TABLE 6.1

Detailed Technological Requirements for a Unified AI-Driven Framework in Dementia Care

Category	Technologies/Tools
Data Acquisition	Standardized data collection protocols across global hospitals and research institutes Secure APIs for data transfer
Data Storage and Management	Distributed databases (e.g., Apache Cassandra, MongoDB) Cloud storage solutions (AWS S3, Azure Blob Storage, Google Cloud Storage) Sophisticated data management tools integrated within cloud platforms: • **AWS**: Utilizing services like AWS Redshift for data warehousing • **Azure**: Leveraging Azure Synapse Analytics for big data and analytics solutions • **Google Cloud**: Implementing BigQuery for serverless, highly scalable data analysis • **Databricks**: Using Databricks for data engineering, machine learning, and analytics on a unified platform
Data Preprocessing	Data cleaning libraries (e.g., Pandas, scikit-learn) Anonymization tools (e.g., ARX Data Anonymization Tool)
Data Integration	Data integration platforms (e.g., Talend, Informatica) ETL (Extract, Transform, Load) tools (e.g., Apache NiFi, StreamSets)
Machine Learning Models	• **Basic Statistical Models**: Linear regression, logistic regression • **Classifiers**: Decision Trees, Support Vector Machines, Random Forests • **Clustering Algorithms**: K-means, hierarchical clustering, DBSCAN • **Advanced Techniques**: Large Language Models (LLMs), Deep Learning Models (e.g., CNNs using TensorFlow, PyTorch), LSTMs • **Feature Extraction Techniques**: PCA, Fourier Transform, Wavelet Transform
Model Training & Inference	Cloud-based machine learning platforms explicitly utilizing: • **AWS SageMaker**: For building, training, and deploying machine learning models at scale • **Azure Machine Learning**: For enterprise-grade machine learning service to build and deploy models • **Google AI Platform**: Comprehensive machine learning service with pre-trained models and a service to generate your own tailored models
User Interface	• Web-based interfaces (using frameworks like React, Angular, Vue. js) • Dashboard development tools (e.g., Tableau, Power BI for data visualization) • Secure user authentication (OAuth, SAML)
Security Measures	• Data encryption both at rest and in transit (e.g., AES, SSL/TLS) • Role-based access control systems • Regular security audits and compliance checks with standards such as HIPAA and GDPR

dementia data, from acquisition through to therapeutic insights. This framework leverages a unified, sophisticated approach utilizing state-of-the-art technologies and platforms across a spectrum of disciplines. The figure illustrates the collaborative network involving global physicians and ML experts who utilize this framework to enhance diagnostic precision, accelerate drug discovery, and optimize therapeutic strategies. Concurrently, the table categorizes and details the essential technological components that constitute this framework: from data acquisition standards and secure transfer protocols, through advanced data storage and management solutions provided by leading cloud services such as AWS, Azure, Google Cloud, and Databricks, to a diverse array of ML models including basic statistical methods, advanced neural networks, and feature extraction techniques. These elements ensure robust, scalable processing and analysis of sensitive medical data, maintaining high standards of security and compliance. Together, the figure and table encapsulate a synergistic system where technology and global expertise converge to push the boundaries of dementia care, embodying a holistic approach from data to delivery.

6.12 Comprehensive Validation and Verification Framework for AI-Driven Diagnostic, Drug Discovery, and Patient Care Solutions

The validation and verification of AI models in healthcare are critical to ensuring that these models provide accurate, reliable, and interpretable results. This section is divided into two parts: Validation by AI and ML experts and Verification by physicians, doctors, and medical scientists. The validation section includes metrics for different types of models, while the verification section focuses on the processes used by HCPs to confirm the results.

6.12.1 Validation of the Models by AI and Machine Learning Experts

Validation by AI and ML experts is an essential process to ensure the accuracy, reliability, and robustness of models employed in diagnostics, drug discovery, and patient care. AI and ML models can be broadly categorized into classifiers (prediction models), clustering models, regression models, and LLMs or NLP models. Each category requires a distinct set of validation metrics tailored to its specific application, reflecting the unique challenges and objectives of the healthcare domain (Zheng, 2015; Varoquaux & Colliot, 2023; Guo et al., 2023; Alammar & Grootendorst, 2024).

6.12.1.1 Classification Models

Validation of classification models in AI-driven diagnostics and drug discovery involves a range of metrics to ensure accuracy and reliability. Here are some common metrics:

- **Accuracy:** The proportion of correct predictions made by the model. It's a basic measure but can be misleading in imbalanced datasets.
- **Precision:** The proportion of true positives among all predicted positives. Critical in scenarios like drug discovery, where false positives can be costly.
- **Recall (Sensitivity):** The proportion of true positives among all actual positives, essential in diagnosis to minimize false negatives.
- **F1-Score:** The harmonic mean of precision and recall, balancing the two metrics and useful when the class distribution is uneven.
- **Area Under the Receiver Operating Characteristic Curve (AUC-ROC):** Measures the trade-off between true positive rate and false positive rate, providing insight into the model's discriminative ability.
- **Matthews Correlation Coefficient (MCC):** Considers true and false positives and negatives, offering a balanced measure even with imbalanced classes.

6.12.1.2 Clustering Models

Clustering models in healthcare are evaluated using several metrics to ensure meaningful subgrouping. Here are some common metrics:

- **Silhouette Score:** Measures how similar an object is to its own cluster compared to other clusters. Ranges from −1 to 1, with higher values indicating better-defined clusters.
- **Davies-Bouldin Index:** Evaluates the average similarity ratio of each cluster with its most similar cluster, where lower values signify better clustering.
- **Adjusted Rand Index (ARI):** Measures the similarity between two data clustering's accounting for chance, with a focus on healthcare applications where patient subgrouping is essential.
- **Normalized Mutual Information (NMI):** Evaluates the mutual dependence between the predicted and true cluster assignments, ensuring that clusters are meaningful.

6.12.1.3 Regression Models

Regression models in AI for healthcare rely on the following metrics to assess predictive performance. Here are some common metrics:

- **Mean Absolute Error (MAE):** The average of the absolute differences between the predicted and actual values, offering a straightforward interpretation.
- **Mean Squared Error (MSE):** The average of squared differences between the predicted and actual values, penalizing larger errors more than MAE.
- **R-squared (Coefficient of Determination):** Represents the proportion of the variance in the dependent variable that is predictable from the independent variables, crucial in modelling relationships like dosage-response in drug discovery.
- **Root Mean Squared Error (RMSE):** The square root of MSE, providing error estimates in the same units as the output variable.
- **Concordance Correlation Coefficient (CCC):** Evaluates the agreement between the predicted and observed values, emphasizing both precision and accuracy.

6.12.1.4 Validation Metrics for LLMs and NLP Models

Validation of LLMs and NLP models, particularly in healthcare applications, involves several key metrics. Here are some common metrics (Guo et al., 2023; Alammar & Grootendorst, 2024):

- **Perplexity:** Measures the model's uncertainty in predicting the next word in a sequence, with lower values indicating better performance.
- **BLEU (Bilingual Evaluation Understudy) Score:** Commonly used to evaluate the quality of text generated by models, especially in translating or summarizing medical texts.
- **ROUGE (Recall-Oriented Understudy for Gisting Evaluation) Score:** Measures the overlap between the predicted and reference summaries, particularly important in generating concise medical reports.
- **Factual Accuracy:** Ensures the generated content by LLMs is factually correct, which is paramount in the healthcare domain.
- **Entity-Level Precision and Recall:** Used in Named Entity Recognition (NER) tasks to identify medical terms and entities, critical for information extraction from medical texts.

6.12.2 Verification by Physicians, Doctors, and Medical Scientists

Verification by physicians, doctors, and medical scientists is a critical phase in the deployment of AI models in healthcare, ensuring that model predictions are rigorously evaluated and validated against real-world clinical data, current medical practices, and expert consensus.

- **Clinical Validation Studies:** Models must undergo rigorous clinical trials where predictions are tested against real-world data, with outcomes reviewed by medical experts.
- **Expert Consensus and Review Panels:** A panel of medical professionals reviews the AI model's predictions to ensure they align with current clinical practices and guidelines.
- **Cross-Disciplinary Collaboration:** Involving data scientists, clinicians, and domain experts in an iterative review process to verify model outputs and refine them based on expert feedback.
- **Real-World Evidence (RWE) Integration:** Utilizing observational data collected outside of randomized clinical trials to validate the model in diverse patient populations.
- **Continuous Monitoring and Post-Deployment Audits:** Ongoing verification of the model's performance in clinical settings, ensuring that predictions remain accurate and relevant as new data is encountered.

6.12.3 Responsible and Explainable AI (XAI)

Responsible and Explainable AI (XAI) is essential in healthcare to ensure that AI models are not only accurate but also transparent, fair, and ethically sound, thereby fostering trust among clinicians and aligning with regulatory and ethical standards (Siala & Wang, 2022; Sivarajah et al., 2023).

- **Interpretability:** Models must be interpretable to ensure that clinicians understand the reasoning behind predictions. Techniques such as SHAP (Shapley Additive Explanations) and LIME (Local Interpretable Model-agnostic Explanations) are used to provide transparency.
- **Bias and Fairness Assessments:** Regular assessments to detect and mitigate biases in the model's predictions, ensuring equitable outcomes across different patient groups.
- **Ethical AI Frameworks:** Adhering to ethical guidelines such as the AI4People framework to ensure that AI models respect patient autonomy, justice, and beneficence.
- **Model Documentation and Communication:** Detailed documentation of the model's development, validation, and verification processes, ensuring that all stakeholders understand its limitations and scope.
- **Regulatory Compliance:** Ensuring the AI models meet regulatory standards set by bodies like the FDA, EMA, or MHRA, which govern the use of AI in medical devices and healthcare.

To ensure AI and ML models in healthcare are accurate, reliable, and aligned with the highest standards of patient care, a multidisciplinary approach that integrates technical validation with clinical expertise is essential. This comprehensive strategy not only guarantees model accuracy and reliability but also ensures interpretability, ethical compliance, and clinical relevance. By combining robust validation metrics with thorough verification processes, these models can be effectively integrated into clinical practice, significantly enhancing the quality of healthcare delivery. The next section will address the critical concerns surrounding data privacy in AI applications within healthcare.

6.13 Data Privacy and Security in AI Applications for Healthcare

The integration of AI in healthcare, particularly in the use of medical data, presents significant challenges related to data privacy and security. Protecting patient information is paramount, given the sensitive nature of healthcare data and the potential risks associated with its misuse. This section addresses the key concerns and best practices for ensuring data privacy and security in AI-driven healthcare applications (Gu et al., 2023; Moon & Lee, 2023; Wang et al., 2023; Pati et al., 2024).

6.13.1 Ethical and Legal Considerations

Healthcare data is subject to stringent ethical and legal requirements, such as the Health Insurance Portability and Accountability Act (HIPAA) in the United States, the GDPR in the European Union, and other regional regulations. AI applications must comply with these regulations to protect patient privacy and avoid legal liabilities. This includes obtaining informed consent, ensuring data anonymization, and maintaining transparency in how patient data is used (Bradford, Aboy & Liddell, 2020).

6.13.2 Data Anonymization and De-Identification

To safeguard patient privacy, AI applications should employ robust anonymization and de-identification techniques. These techniques strip identifiable information from datasets, reducing the risk of re-identification. However, maintaining the balance between data utility and privacy is crucial; overly aggressive anonymization may degrade the quality of data, impacting the performance of AI models (Lee et al., 2022).

6.13.3 Secure Data Storage and Transmission

AI systems must incorporate strong encryption protocols to protect data both at rest and in transit. This includes the use of advanced encryption standards (AES) for data storage and secure socket layer (SSL) or transport layer security (TLS) for data transmission. Additionally, secure data storage solutions should include multi-factor authentication (MFA) and role-based access control (RBAC) to limit access to sensitive data (Jaime et al., 2023).

6.13.4 Data Access Controls and Audit Trails

Implementing strict data access controls is essential to prevent unauthorized access to sensitive healthcare data. Role-based access control (RBAC) mechanisms ensure that only authorized personnel have access to specific data based on their role within the organization. Furthermore, maintaining audit trails of data access and usage is critical for monitoring and tracking any potential breaches, thereby enabling prompt responses to security incidents (de Carvalho Junior & Bandiera-Paiva, 2018).

6.13.5 Risks of Data Breaches and Mitigation Strategies

Data breaches in healthcare can have severe consequences, including financial penalties, loss of trust, and harm to patients. AI applications must include robust security measures to detect, prevent, and respond to data breaches. This includes regular security assessments, vulnerability testing, and the implementation of incident response plans. Additionally, continuous monitoring of AI systems for potential security threats is essential to protect patient data proactively.

6.13.6 Ensuring Compliance with Regulatory Standards

AI developers and healthcare providers must ensure that their AI applications comply with relevant regulatory standards and industry best practices. This includes adhering to guidelines for data privacy and security, such as those provided by the International Organization for Standardization (ISO) and the National Institute of Standards and Technology (NIST). Regular compliance audits and updates to security protocols are necessary to keep pace with evolving threats and regulatory requirements (Díaz-Rodríguez et al., 2023).

6.13.7 Patient Empowerment and Data Control

Patients should be empowered to control how their data is used in AI applications. This involves providing clear and accessible information about data usage, obtaining explicit consent, and offering options for patients to opt out of data sharing. Transparency in data practices not only enhances trust but also aligns with ethical standards for patient autonomy.

Given the significant risks associated with data breaches, data privacy and security are critical components of AI applications in healthcare. By adhering to stringent ethical, legal, and technical standards, AI developers and healthcare providers can protect sensitive patient data while harnessing the power of AI to improve healthcare outcomes. Robust data privacy and security measures ensure that AI technologies are both effective and trustworthy, paving the way for their widespread adoption in the healthcare industry.

6.14 Chapter Summary

This chapter provides a detailed exploration of how NLP and AI-driven conversational agents are reshaping the landscape of dementia and AD care. By developing user-friendly interfaces that enhance patient engagement, improve communication, and support effective therapeutic interventions, these technologies play a pivotal role in facilitating social interaction, supporting mental health, and alleviating caregiver burdens through sustained engagement and interactive dialogue.

Building on the integration of AI and IoT discussed in "Empowering Patient Care: Leveraging Artificial Intelligence and Internet of Things for Enhanced Healthcare Delivery," this chapter further highlights the critical role of AI in facilitating real-time communication and personalized care planning through smart assistants. These tools are invaluable for HCPs, allowing them to deliver efficient and effective care by leveraging extensive datasets to provide informed care suggestions and support tailored to individual patient needs.

The narrative progresses to address how conversational AI and NLP enhance the non-pharmacological management of challenging behaviors in dementia, adhering to and dynamically incorporating the latest care guidelines. This integration showcases a seamless progression from the monitoring capabilities introduced in the previous chapters to active patient engagement and intervention.

Furthermore, the chapter explores the ethical dimensions of deploying AI in healthcare. It emphasizes the importance of maintaining patient privacy, autonomy, and the ethical use of AI and NLP technologies. A comprehensive framework is introduced, integrating conversational AI with diagnostic and treatment data to facilitate personalized, continuous care that respects and enhances patient autonomy and well-being.

In conclusion, the chapter underscores the transformative potential of these sophisticated tools in managing chronic neurological conditions, highlighting significant improvements in therapeutic interventions and the quality of life for those affected by dementia and AD. It connects the discussions from previous chapters on AI and IoT integration and sets the stage for a comprehensive examination of current research, commercial implementations, and academic advancements in the field. This offers a forward-looking perspective on how AI and NLP can revolutionize support systems for patients and their families, effectively tying together the advancements discussed in prior chapters to envision a future where technology profoundly enhances dementia care.

Notes

1 BtC can be defined as an expression of distress by the person living with dementia (or others in the environment) that arises from unmet health or psychosocial need(s).
2 The National Institute for Health and Care Excellence is an executive non-departmental public body of the Department of Health in the United Kingdom. NICE provides national guidance and advice to improve health and social care services, including publishing guidelines on health technologies, clinical practices, and the appropriate treatment and care of people with specific diseases and conditions.

References

Alammar, J., & Grootendorst, M. (2024). Hands-on large language models. O'Reilly Media, Inc.

Alowais, S. A., Alghamdi, S. S., Alsuhebany, N., Alqahtani, T., Alshaya, A. I., Almohareb, S. N., Aldairem, A., Alrashed, M., Bin Saleh, K., Badreldin, H. A., Al Yami, M. S., Al Harbi, S., & Albekairy, A. M. (2023). Revolutionizing healthcare: The role of artificial intelligence in clinical practice. BMC Medical Education, 23(1), 689. https://doi.org/10.1186/s12909-023-04698-z

Amjad, A., Kordel, P., & Fernandes, G. (2023). A review on innovation in healthcare sector (telehealth) through artificial intelligence. Sustainability, 15(8), 6655. https://doi.org/10.3390/su15086655

Aramaki, E., Wakamiya, S., Yada, S., & Nakamura, Y. (2022). Natural language processing: From bedside to everywhere. Yearbook of Medical Informatics, 31(1), 243–253. https://doi.org/10.1055/s-0042-1742510

Aworinde, J., Evans, C. J., Gillam, J., Ramsenthaler, C., Davies, N., Ellis-Smith, C., & EMBED-Care Programme. (2024). Co-design of the EMBED-care framework as an intervention to enhance shared decision-making for people affected by dementia and practitioners, comprising holistic assessment, linked with clinical decision support tools: A qualitative study. Health Expectations, 27(1), e13987. https://doi.org/10.1111/hex.13987

Bickmore, T. W., Caruso, L., Clough-Gorr, K., & Heeren, T. (2005). 'It's just like you talk to a friend'relational agents for older adults. Interacting with Computers, 17(6), 711–735.

Bickmore, T. W., Trinh, H., Olafsson, S., O'Leary, T. K., Asadi, R., Rickles, N. M., & Paasche-Orlow, M. K. (2018). Patient and consumer safety risks when using conversational assistants for medical information: An observational study of Siri, Alexa, and Google Assistant. *Journal of Medical Internet Research*, 20(9), e11510. https://doi.org/10.2196/11510

Bradford, L., Aboy, M., & Liddell, K. (2020). International transfers of health data between the EU and USA: A sector-specific approach for the USA to ensure an "adequate" level of protection. *Journal of Law and the Biosciences*, 7(1), Article lsaa055. https://doi.org/10.1093/jlb/lsaa055

Davies, N., Iliffe, S., Hopwood, J., Walker, N., Ross, J., Rait, G., & Walters, K. (2020). The key aspects of online support that older family carers of people with dementia want at the end of life: A qualitative study. *Aging & Mental Health*, 24(10), 1654–1661. https://doi.org/10.1080/13607863.2019.1642299

de Carvalho Junior, M. A., & Bandiera-Paiva, P. (2018). Health information system role-based access control: Current security trends and challenges. *Journal of Healthcare Engineering*, 2018, Article 6510249. https://doi.org/10.1155/2018/6510249

Díaz-Rodríguez, N., Del Ser, J., Coeckelbergh, M., López de Prado, M., Herrera-Viedma, E., & Herrera, F. (2023). Connecting the dots in trustworthy artificial intelligence: From AI principles, ethics, and key requirements to responsible AI systems and regulation. *Information Fusion*, 99, Article 101896. https://doi.org/10.1016/j.inffus.2023.101896

Dignum, V. (2019). *Responsible artificial intelligence: How to develop and use AI in a responsible way*. Springer Nature.

El Haj, M., Boutoleau-Bretonnière, C., Gallouj, K., Wagemann, N., Antoine, P., Kapogiannis, D., & Chapelet, G. (2024). ChatGPT as a diagnostic aid in Alzheimer's disease: An exploratory study. *Journal of Alzheimer's Disease Reports*, 8(1), 495–500. https://doi.org/10.3233/ADR-230191

ElliQ by Intuition Robotics. (n.d.). *New Companion: AI Companion for Aging Adults*. Retrieved 12/8/2024, from https://elliq.com/

Gray, K. L., Moniz-Cook, E., Reichelt, K., Duffy, F., & James, I. A. (2022). Professional perspectives on applying the NICE and British Psychological Society Guidelines for the management of Behaviours that Challenge in dementia care: An e-survey. *British Journal of Clinical Psychology*, 61(1), 112–131. https://doi.org/10.1111/bjc.12316

Grote, T., & Berens, P. (2020). On the ethics of algorithmic decision-making in healthcare. *Journal of Medical Ethics*, 46(3), 205–211. https://doi.org/10.1136/medethics-2019-105586

Gu, X., Sabrina, F., Fan, Z., & Sohail, S. (2023). A review of privacy enhancement methods for federated learning in healthcare systems. *International Journal of Environmental Research and Public Health*, 20(15), 6539. https://doi.org/10.3390/ijerph20156539

Guo, Z., Jin, R., Liu, C., Huang, Y., Shi, D., SupryadiYu, L., Liu, Y., Li, J., Xiong, B., & Xiong, D. (2023). *Evaluating large language models: A comprehensive survey* [Version 3]. arXiv. https://arxiv.org/abs/2310.19736

Jaime, F. J., Muñoz, A., Rodríguez-Gómez, F., & Jerez-Calero, A. (2023). Strengthening privacy and data security in biomedical microelectromechanical systems by IoT communication security and protection in smart healthcare. *Sensors*, 23(21), 8944. https://doi.org/10.3390/s23218944

Kocaballi, A. B., Quiroz, J. C., Rezazadegan, D., Berkovsky, S., Magrabi, F., Coiera, E., & Laranjo, L. (2020). Responses of conversational agents to health and lifestyle prompts: Investigation of appropriateness and presentation structures. Journal of Medical Internet Research, 22(2), e15823. https://doi.org/10.2196/15823

Kreimeyer, K., Foster, M., Pandey, A., Arya, N., Halford, G., Jones, S. F., Forshee, R., Walderhaug, M., & Botsis, T. (2017). Natural language processing systems for capturing and standardizing unstructured clinical information: A systematic review. Journal of Biomedical Informatics, 73, 14–29. https://doi.org/10.1016/j.jbi.2017.07.012

Kruse, C. S., Argueta, D. A., Lopez, L., & Nair, A. (2015). Patient and provider attitudes toward the use of patient portals for the management of chronic disease: A systematic review. Journal of Medical Internet Research, 17(2), e40. https://doi.org/10.2196/jmir.3703

Laranjo, L., Dunn, A. G., Tong, H. L., Kocaballi, A. B., Chen, J., Bashir, R., Surian, D., Gallego, B., Magrabi, F., Lau, A. Y. S., & Coiera, E. (2018). Conversational agents in healthcare: A systematic review. Journal of the American Medical Informatics Association, 25(9), 1248–1258. https://doi.org/10.1093/jamia/ocy072

Lee, J., Jeong, J., Jung, S., Moon, J., & Rho, S. (2022). Verification of de-identification techniques for personal information using tree-based methods with Shapley values. Journal of Personalized Medicine, 12(2), 190. https://doi.org/10.3390/jpm12020190

Li, J. (2023). Security implications of AI chatbots in health care. Journal of Medical Internet Research, 25, e47551. https://doi.org/10.2196/47551

Luxton, D. D. (2014). Artificial intelligence in psychological practice: Current and future applications and implications. Professional Psychology: Research and Practice, 45(5), 332. https://doi.org/10.1037/a0034559

Maia, E., Vieira, P., & Praça, I. (2023). Empowering preventive care with GECA chatbot. Healthcare (Basel), 11(18), 2532. https://doi.org/10.3390/healthcare11182532

Memory Lane. (n.d.). Digital Care Giver for Your Parents. Retrieved 12/8/2024, from https://www.memory-lane.ai/

Meystre, S. M., Savova, G. K., Kipper-Schuler, K. C., & Hurdle, J. F. (2008). Extracting information from textual documents in the electronic health record: A review of recent research. Yearbook of Medical Informatics, 2008(1), 128–144. PMID: 18660887.

Miner, A. S., Laranjo, L., & Kocaballi, A. B. (2020). Chatbots in the fight against the COVID-19 pandemic. npj Digital Medicine, 3, 65.

Moon, S., & Lee, W. H. (2023). Privacy-preserving federated learning in healthcare. In 2023 International Conference on Electronics, Information, and Communication (ICEIC). IEEE. https://doi.org/10.1109/ICEIC57457.2023.10049966

Munteanu, D., Bejan, C., Munteanu, N., Zamfir, C., Vasić, M., Petrea, S.-M., & Cristea, D. (2022). Deep-learning-based system for assisting people with Alzheimer's disease. Electronics, 11(19), 3229. https://doi.org/10.3390/electronics11193229

Nazi, Z. A., & Peng, W. (2024). Large language models in healthcare and medical domain: A review. arXiv preprint arXiv:2401.06775v2 [cs.CL]. https://doi.org/10.48550/arXiv.2401.06775

Pati, S., Kumar, S., Varma, A., Edwards, B., Lu, C., Qu, L., Wang, J. J., Lakshminarayanan, A., Wang, S., Sheller, M. J., Chang, K., Singh, P., Rubin, D. L., Kalpathy-Cramer, J., & Bakas, S. (2024). Privacy preservation for federated learning in health care. Patterns, 5(7), Article 100974. https://doi.org/10.1016/j.patter.2024.100974

Pham, K. T., Nabizadeh, A., & Selek, S. (2022). Artificial intelligence and chatbots in psychiatry. Psychiatric Quarterly, 93(1), 249–253. https://doi.org/10.1007/s11126-022-09973-8

Qi, J., Wu, C., Yang, L., Ni, C., & Liu, Y. (2022). Artificial intelligence (AI) for home support interventions in dementia: A scoping review protocol. BMJ Open, 12(9), Article e062604. https://doi.org/10.1136/bmjopen-2022-062604

Rodríguez-Domínguez, M. T., Bazago-Dómine, M. I., Jiménez-Palomares, M., Pérez-González, G., Núñez, P., Santano-Mogena, E., & Garrido-Ardila, E. M. (2024). Interaction assessment of a social-care robot in day center patients with mild to moderate cognitive impairment: A pilot study. International Journal of Social Robotics, 16, 513–528. https://doi.org/10.1007/s12369-024-01106-4

Ruggiano, N., Brown, E., Roberts, L., Framil Suarez, C., Luo, Y., Hao, Z., & Hristidis, V. (2021). Chatbots to support people with dementia and their caregivers: Systematic review of functions and quality. Journal of Medical Internet Research, 23(6), e25006. https://doi.org/10.2196/25006

SafelyYou. (n.d.). Revolutionizing Your Approach to Falls Management. Retrieved 12/8/2024, from https://www.safely-you.com/

Salvi, M., Loh, H. W., Seoni, S., Barua, P. D., García, S., Molinari, F., & Acharya, U. R. (2023). Multi-modality approaches for medical support systems: A systematic review of the last decade. Information Fusion, 102134. https://doi.org/10.1016/j.inffus.2023.102134

Schmitz, D., & Becker, B. (2024). Chatbot-mediated learning for caregiving relatives of people with dementia: Empirical findings and didactical implications for multiprofessional health care. Journal of Multidisciplinary Healthcare, 17, 219–228. https://doi.org/10.2147/JMDH.S424790

Shawaqfeh, B., Hughes, C. M., McGuinness, B., & Barry, H. E. (2024). Carers' experiences and perspectives of the use of anticholinergic medications in people living with dementia: Analysis of an online discussion forum. Health Expectations, 27, e13972. https://doi.org/10.1111/hex.13972

Siala, H., & Wang, Y. (2022). SHIFTing artificial intelligence to be responsible in healthcare: A systematic review. Social Science & Medicine, 296, Article 114782. https://doi.org/10.1016/j.socscimed.2022.114782

Singh, J., Sillerud, B., & Singh, A. (2023). Artificial intelligence, chatbots and ChatGPT in healthcare—narrative review of historical evolution, current application, and change management approach to increase adoption. Journal of Medical Artificial Intelligence, 6(0). https://jmai.amegroups.org/article/view/8271

Sivarajah, U., Wang, Y., Olya, H., & Mathew, S. (2023). Responsible Artificial Intelligence (AI) for digital health and medical analytics. Information Systems Frontiers, 1–6. https://doi.org/10.1007/s10796-023-10412-7

Subramanian, R. C., Yang, D. A., & Khanna, R. (2024). Enhancing health care communication with large language models—the role, challenges, and future directions. JAMA Network Open, 7(3), e240347. https://doi.org/10.1001/jamanetworkopen.2024.0347

Suganthi, S., Kumar, N. R., Logeswaran, S. R., Kumar, R. M., & Hariprasad, V. (2024). AI Chaperone: Awareness chatbot for Alzheimer's disease. International Research Journal of Engineering and Management (IRJAEM), 2(05), 1245–1249. https://doi.org/10.47392/IRJAEM.2024.0168

Sun, G., & Zhou, Y. H. (2023). AI in healthcare: Navigating opportunities and challenges in digital communication. Frontiers in Digital Health, 5, 1291132. https://doi.org/10.3389/fdgth.2023.1291132

Ursin, F., Timmermann, C., & Steger, F. (2021). Ethical implications of Alzheimer's disease prediction in asymptomatic individuals through artificial intelligence. Diagnostics, 11(3), 440. https://doi.org/10.3390/diagnostics11030440

Varoquaux, G., & Colliot, O. (2023). Evaluating machine learning models and their diagnostic value. In G. Varoquaux & O. Colliot (Eds.), Machine learning for brain disorders (pp. 601–630). Neuromethods, Volume 197. Springer.

Wang, W., Li, X., Qiu, X., Zhang, X., Brusic, V., & Zhao, J. (2023). A privacy-preserving framework for federated learning in smart healthcare systems. Information Processing & Management, 60(1), Article 103167. https://doi.org/10.1016/j.ipm.2022.103167

Woo, B., Huynh, T., Tang, A., Bui, N., Nguyen, G., & Tam, W. (2024). Transforming nursing with large language models: From concept to practice. European Journal of Cardiovascular Nursing, 23(5), 549–552. https://doi.org/10.1093/eurjcn/zvad120

Zheng, A. (2015). Evaluating machine learning models. O'Reilly Media, Inc.

7

Artificial Intelligence for Dementia

Olalekan Balongun and Sasan Adibi

7.1 Introduction

A significant number of people living with dementia remain undiagnosed, and healthcare professionals experience challenges in navigating this complicated and variable condition, which currently has no cure (Schwertner et al., 2022). Currently, more than 55 million individuals are diagnosed with dementia worldwide, with over 60% of them living in low- and middle-income countries (LMICs). The impact of dementia on individuals varies significantly, which is most dependent on underlying causes, other health conditions, and the cognitive functioning of the person preceding the manifestation of the illness. The illness gets worse with time. It predominantly impacts the elderly population; however, not every individual will experience it as they age (WHO, 2023). Recent studies have shown that approximately 90% of individuals diagnosed with dementia will suffer from additional psychological or behavioural symptoms and that these symptoms are important factors that impacts and increase the burden on caregivers (Schwertner et al., 2022).

Dementia is not a single disease; rather, it is a collective term to describe several cognitive disorders (Javeed et al., 2023) that arise from variety of diseases and injuries traumas that affect cerebral function. Alzheimer's disease (AD) is the predominant form of dementia, estimated to represent 60–70% of the identified cases (WHO, 2023). According to Lennon et al. (2022), AD ranks as the sixth leading cause of death in the United States and the fifth leading cause of death among individuals 65 years and older. It is estimated that the global financial burden of dementia will rise in the next 5 years tto US$2.8 trillion compared to US$1.3 trillion in 2019 (Shin, 2022). Individuals suffering from dementia may display a lack of recognition of family members or friends, may have difficulties moving around, experience difficulties eating and drinking, and loss of regulation over their bladder and bowel functions. At present, dementia ranks as the seventh leading cause of death and constitutes one of the principal factors contributing to disability and dependence among the elderly population worldwide (WHO, 2023).

DOI: 10.1201/9781003485681-7

While an absolute cure for dementia is yet to be discovered, several approaches can be initiated to facilitate support for individuals living with this illness and their respective caregivers (WHO, 2023). Most clinical symptoms are likely to progressively worsen over time, while others might disappear or be more apparent during the later stages of dementia. As the disease progresses, the requirement for support in personal care increases (Joling et al., 2020).

7.1.1 What Is Dementia?

Dementia is a syndrome marked by the progressive decline of cognitive function of an individual beyond normal, which is associated with the biological process of aging. It is characterized by a disruption of multiple higher cortical functions including learning and memory, complex attention, executive function, language, motor perception, and social cognition, and impacts an individual's ability to perform their everyday tasks without assistance. According to the World Health Organization (WHO), "the current number of the people with dementia across the globe is approximately 55 million, with projection of the numbers expected to rise to approximately 78 million by 2030 and 139 million by 2050." The most common clinical presentation of AD is a slow onset and gradually progressive loss of memory, which is common with the inability to learn new information, especially autobiographical information, such as recent events in the life of the patient (Arvanitakis et al., 2019).

7.1.2 Types of Dementia?

7.1.2.1 Alzheimer's Disease

AD is the main cause of dementia and one of the great healthcare challenges of the 21st century (Scheltens et al., 2016). AD is assumed to develop when abnormal amounts of amyloid beta (A) build up in the brain, either extracellularly as amyloid plaques, tau proteins, or intracellularly as neurofibrillary tangles, affecting neuronal function, connectivity, resulting in a gradual decline in cognitive functions. Usually, the reduced ability to remove proteins with ageing is controlled by brain cholesterol and is related to other neurodegenerative illnesses. Apart from 1% to 2% of cases where deterministic genetic anomalies have been detected, the aetiology of most individuals diagnosed with AD remains unexplained (Javeed et al., 2023).

7.1.2.2 Vascular Dementia

Vascular dementia (VaD) is a subtype of dementia characterized by a complicated mix of cerebrovascular illnesses, caused by problems with the brain's blood flow, that result in structural changes in the brain, owing to strokes and lesions, thus leading to a gradual decline of cognitive abilities (Javeed et al., 2023). Studies of VaD show it is the second most common cause of dementia after AD, causing around 15% of cases, and unlike AD, there are no licensed treatments for VaD (O'Brien & Thomas, 2015).

7.1.2.3 Lewy Body Dementia

Lewy body dementia (LBD) is the second most common cause of neuro-degenerative dementia, and it comprises both dementia with Lewy bodies and Parkinson's disease (Taylor et al., 2020). LBD is a subtype of dementia which is characterized by an abnormal deposit of the protein called alpha-synuclein in the brain. These deposits are called Lewy bodies, and they affect the brain chemistry, leading to problems with thinking, movement, behaviour, and mood. Individuals with LBD usually experience progressive loss of cognitive functions, visual hallucinations, as well as changes in alertness and concentration. They exhibit signs and symptoms of Parkinson's disease, which include tight muscles, delayed movement, difficulty walking, and tremors. LBD might be difficult to identify because its symptoms can be mistaken for other brain diseases or mental disorders (Javeed et al., 2023).

7.1.2.4 Frontotemporal Dementia

Frontotemporal dementia (FTD) is a subtype of dementia characterized by nerve cell loss in the frontal and temporal lobes of the brain, thus resulting in lobes contraction. FTD is common in both men and women, and it usually impacts the behaviour, attitude, and movement of patients diagnosed with it. FTD primarily affects individuals between the ages of 40 and 65 years; nonetheless, it can affect younger adults and the elderly (Javeed et al., 2023).

7.1.2.5 Mixed Dementia

Mixed dementia is a subtype of dementia characterized when more than one kind of dementia coexists in a patient, and it is believed to affect approximately 10% of all cases of dementia. AD and VaD are the two predominant subtypes that are most common in mixed dementia (MD). This condition is often linked with factors such as old age, high blood pressure, and brain blood vessel damage, and results in early symptoms. It is important to note that MD can be difficult to identify because one dementia subtype is often dominant, and owing to this, individuals affected by MD are rarely treated and miss out on potentially life-changing medicines. MD can cause symptoms to begin earlier than the actual diagnosis of the disease, and spread rapidly to affect the most areas of the brain (Javeed et al., 2023).

7.1.3 How Is Dementia Diagnosed at Present?

Dementia is typically diagnosed by a specialist physician who conducts a series of clinical assessments which involves acquiring an individual's personal and informant history pertaining to cognitive symptoms, a physical examination, pen and paper cognitive assessments, blood tests to eliminate other conditions that may exhibit similar features to dementia mimics of dementia (e.g., low vitamin B12 levels), and also brain scans to assess for localized brain atrophy. The entire diagnostic process is time consuming, expensive, and somewhat subjective – and solely relies on the interpretation of the clinician (Li et al., 2022).

The diagnosis of AD requires that patients exhibit both cognitive and functional deterioration. Most findings reveal that the onset of the symptoms of AD is notably subtle that both the patient and relatives are unable to pinpoint exact date of occurrence (Cipriani et al., 2020).

7.1.4 Why Detect Dementia Earlier?

Dementia embodies a complex and diverse process that is always related to cognitive decline and impaired functioning. As the disease progresses, individuals suffering from dementia experience faces alongside declined cognitive functions, a gradual dysfunction and loss of individual autonomies. In addition to the decline in memory and/or other cognitive areas, the diagnosis criteria for dementia require loss of functional reserve and deterioration in functional status (Cipriani et al., 2020).

Dementia is characterized by a lengthy preclinical period during which individuals display no noticeable cognitive impairments; however, neurogenerative changes are taking place. As a result, it is essential to identify those individuals at high risk of dementia at an earlier stage to avert the potential development of the disease in the later stages of life (Revathi et al., 2022).

Nevertheless, dementia remains significantly underdiagnosed, especially in LMICs. Actually, some research studies have shown that only 3% of individuals suffering from dementia are diagnosed by their primary caregivers during the later stages of their life.

7.2 Understanding Artificial Intelligence (AI) and Machine Learning (ML)

7.2.1 Artificial Intelligence and Machine Learning Defined

AI is a general term used to describe a concept of imitating intelligent human behaviour with minimal human intervention. Research into AI applications commenced shortly after the formal designation of the term "artificial intelligence" during a meeting held at Dartmouth College in the year 1956 (Tsoi et al., 2022).

ML is a subfield of AI which focuses on examining and learning patterns of input datasets to build models for classification, regression, and clustering. Deep learning, reinforcement learning, and transfer learning are more specific subsets of ML (Tsoi et al., 2022).

Machine learning algorithms, a subset of AI, are designed to automatically learn from data without being explicitly programmed. They could analyze complex patterns, identify correlations, and make predictions or recommendations based on historical data. In the context of business intelligence, machine learning algorithms can serve the purpose of uncovering hidden patterns in data, perform advanced data analysis, and provide great insights for informed decision-making (Sarker, 2021).

7.2.1.1 Types of Real-World Data

Structured Data: This is a kind of data with well-defined structure that conforms to a data model which follows a standard order, and is highly organized and easily accessed, and can be used by an entity or a computer program. Examples of structured data include names, dates, addresses, credit card numbers, stock information, geolocation, etc., and are stored in tabular format for well-defined schemes, such as relational database (Sarker, 2021).

Unstructured Data: In unstructured data, there is no pre-defined format or organization and that makes it much more difficult to capture, process, and analyze. They usually consist mainly of text and multimedia material. Examples of unstructured data include sensor data, emails, blog entries, wikis, word processing documents, PDF files, audio files, videos, images, presentations, web pages, etc. (Sarker, 2021).

Semi-structured: With semi-structured data, they are not stored in a relational database like the structured data mentioned above; nonetheless, it has certain organizational attributes that make it easier to analyze. Examples of semi-structured data include HTML, XML, JSON documents, NoSQL databases, etc. (Sarker, 2021).

Metadata: They are not the conventional form of data; rather, it represents data about a data. This form of data describes the relevant information and giving it more meaning for data users. Examples of document metadata can be the author, file size, date generated by the document, keywords used to define the document, etc. (Sarker, 2021).

7.2.2 Types of Machine Learning Techniques

7.2.2.1 Supervised Learning

Supervised learning is a ML technique that requires learning a function that maps an input to an output based on sample input-output pairs. Supervised learning is carried out when specific goals are identified to be attained from a certain set of inputs (i.e., a task driven approach.) The most common supervised tasks are classification and regression. Classification separates the data, while regression fits the data. Example of supervised learning is text classification. For instance, it is the case of predicting the class label or sentiment of a piece of text, like a product review (Sarker, 2021). In supervised learning, the task of training a model efficiently is easier as the dataset is composed of organized data itself (Shah et al., 2022).

7.2.2.2 Unsupervised Learning

In unsupervised learning, unlabelled dataset analyses sets are analyzed without needing any form of interference from humans (i.e., a data-driven process). This form of learning is widely used for extracting generative features, identifying meaningful trends and structures, groupings in results, and for exploratory purposes. The most common tasks in unsupervised learning include clustering, density estimation, feature learning, dimensionality reduction, finding association rules, anomaly detection, etc. (Sarker, 2021). Analysis of raw datasets is easily facilitated in unsupervised ML, thereby helping in generating analytic insights from unlabelled data (Usama et al., 2019).

7.2.2.3 Semi-Supervised Learning

Semi-supervised learning involves combining supervised and unsupervised learning by using both labelled and unlabelled data. Consequently, it falls between learning "without supervision" and learning "with supervision." The main goal of a semi-supervised learning model is to provide a better outcome for prediction than that produced using the labelled data alone from the model. Semi-supervised learning is used in machine translation, fraud detection, labelling data, and text classification (Sarker, 2021). It is important to know that in practice, semi-supervised learning methods have also been used where no significant lack of labelled data exists: if the unlabelled data points provide additional information relevant for prediction, they can potentially be used to obtain an improved classification performance.

7.2.2.4 Reinforcement Learning

Reinforcement learning is a type of ML method that enables software agents and machines to automatically evaluate the best behaviour in a particular context or environment to improve their efficiency (i.e., an environment-driven approach). This type of learning is based on reward or penalty, and its main goal is to use insights obtained from environmental activists to take action to increase the reward or minimize the risk. This is a useful tool for training AI models, which can help increase automation or optimize the operational efficiency of complex systems such as robotics, autonomous driving tasks, manufacturing, supply chain logistics, etc. (Sarker, 2021).

7.3 Application of AI in Dementia Care and Treatment

7.3.1 Socially Assistive Robots

Considering how complex dementia care is, along with the ever-growing population of aged people across the globe, researchers have been exploring ways to use advanced robotic technology to assist the elderly. One such invention was the design of an interactive pet robot called PARO, it looks like a baby harp seal, and it provides companionship and emotional interaction with its users (Tsoi et al., 2022). PARO is still being used as a robotic pet in dementia care studies. Other socially interactive robots provide support in daily engagement for those who have MCI or are at the early stage of dementia. Another socially interactive robot for people diagnosed with early stage of dementia or MCI is the CompanionAble, which provide support in their daily engagement by connecting to a smart home environment. CompanionAble focuses on cognitive and social support, such as cognitive training, video calls, suggesting activities, daily activity reminders, and this was tested with five (5) couples in their various homes over a span of two (2) days, and it was confirmed to reduce the burden for caregivers. RobuLAB10 is another special robot designed to monitor emotions, it can make calls, provide cognitive training, and offer other support for daily activities, and during health emergencies. It is important to know that research was done on the social robots with minimal participants during a short period of time, but they are not widely adopted yet in the real world (Tsoi et al., 2022).

7.3.2 Drug Discovery

Discovering a new drug usually takes a long process, it goes through the preclinical processes and clinical trials. Usually, the preclinical process in vitro tests include target identification and validation, compound screening, and lead discovery, but with the introduction of AI techniques, it could be applied in every aspect of this process to accelerate new drug development. In one case, a researcher applied Naïve Bayesian and recursive partitioning algorithms to predict active compounds bound to as many targets as possible (e.g., the Amyloid Precursor Protein) with great success. The methods were evaluated with internally fivefold cross-validation and an external test dataset with an average AUC of 0.965. The researcher and his team also proposed a network-based AI framework to identify potential drug targets by integrating multiomics data, human protein–protein networks, and other related data (Tsoi et al., 2022). Another important application of AI in drug discovery is the identification of the effect of drug-to-drug interactions when they are combined for the same or different diseases for a patient, resulting in altered effects or adverse reactions (Blanco-González et al., 2023).

7.4 Application of AI in Dementia Diagnosis and Prognosis

7.4.1 Genetics

Research shows that there can be changes in genes for patients with both early-onset and late-onset AD. Some studies have confirmed that they are inheritable. With the evolution of genomics, high-dimensional genetic-related data can be generated, which can be used for the analysis of genes of patients diagnosed with dementia. Several AI methods, such as Support Vector Machine (SVM), have shown excellent performance on gene identification and pathway analysis. Also, Random Forest (RF) is well suited for microarray data, and a group of researchers applied the SVM model to predict AD by using protein sequence, and the accuracy rate was 85.7%, where RF, Naïve Bayes, AdaBoost, and Bayes network were also applied and compared with the result of SVM to check for variation. Another group of researchers integrated genetic data, multimodal neuroimaging, cerebrospinal fluid (CSF) biomarkers, genetic factors, and measures of cognitive resilience data to develop an SVM model that could predict the progress of MCI to AD within three years, and generated an accuracy rate of up to 93%. It is also important to note that ML methods can also be used in detecting significant genetic variants, gene expression, and gene–gene interaction (Tsoi et al., 2022).

7.4.2 Speech and Language

It is known that speech and language abilities are usually impaired early in several types of dementia, with symptoms such as aphasia, pauses, reduced vocabulary, and other language impairments (Li et al., 2022). Recent research has revealed that language dysfunction is one of the earliest signs of cognitive decline and a potential biomarker for the early detection of dementia. Speech and language have long been used as important clinical information in the diagnosis of dementia, an example is the Boston naming test, which has been studied and reported since 1986. This information can be obtained through content-based (specific tasks) or content-free approaches (spontaneous conversation). Methods for checking the dysfunction include word retrieval difficulties (e.g., verbal naming, accurate meaning communication, and pulsation) and the ability to repeat words or sentences. To extract prosodic, acoustic and other features in dementia analysis, the concept of Natural Language Processing plays a major role in speech and text data analysis, and deep learning can be used during the process to quickly acquire to effective characteristics from training data, and Convolutional Neural Network (CNN) and Recurrent Neural Networks (RNN) are two popular models that could be used (Tsoi et al., 2022). A great deal of results has been yielded from research on automatic processing of speech and language with AI and ML methods, which includes computational linguistics, computational paralinguistics, signal processing, etc. (De la Fuente Garcia et al., 2020).

7.4.3 Neuroimaging

A very prominent change in people diagnosed with dementia is the obvious change in their brain structure. Changes in the brain structure and other metabolite responses in the brain can be evaluated using modern techniques like positron emission tomography (PET) and magnetic resonance imaging. ML can be used to detect numerous diseases through neuroimaging, utilizing improved medical imaging and greater accessibility of neuroimaging data (Tsoi et al., 2022). Neuroimaging generates large, complex data which are beyond interpretation for humans or traditional statistical approaches, but are appropriate to AI methods for understanding disease mechanisms and assisting in clinical diagnosis (Ranson et al., 2023).

7.4.4 CSF and Blood Biomarkers

The measure of Amyloid-Beta, total tau (T-tau), and hyperphosphorylated tau (p-tau) in CSF proteins has shown a remarkable degree of accuracy in diagnosing AD. Although these biomarkers are expensive and relatively invasive. With the recent emergence of highly sensitive and specific immune and mass spectrometry-based assays, CSF biomarkers can also be detected through blood. Other blood biomarkers exist, which are N-methyl-D-aspartate receptor-mediated biomarkers and metabolite biomarkers. A glutamate-based study was published in 2021, and it demonstrated how ML models were applied to detect both MCI and AD in healthy people. The predictive model was designed using machine learning algorithms (SVM, LR, RF, and Naïve Bayes), a total of 133 AD patients, 21 MCI patients, and 31 healthy controls were recruited to distinguish MCI or AD patients from healthy controls, with sex, age, and d-glutamate as predictors. Both the Naïve model and the RF model showed the best performance with an area under the curve (AUC) of 0.82 and 0.79. Other researchers have also applied deep learning, extreme gradient boosting, and RF on plasma metabolites data to help distinguish healthy people from patients diagnosed with AD. They also showed better AUC than the results from amyloid, p-tau, and t-tau (Tsoi et al., 2022).

7.4.5 Electroencephalogram (EEG) and Retinal Imaging (RI)

EEG is a medical test used to measure the electrical activity of the brain or to detect abnormalities in brain waves. They have been used to diagnose a number of conditions that have to do with the brain, such as brain tumours, epilepsy, sleep disorders, etc. In the recent decade, researchers have focused their investigation on the diagnosis and progression of AD using EEG. In view of the complexity of EEG data, feature extraction is a crucial step, which includes time-domain and frequency-domain features, nonlinear features, entropies, spatiotemporal features, and complex networks. Each of the features contains a series of indices and has been explored by many studies. SVM is widely used for binary classification. In a research conducted in 2021 using a multiclass SVM, 12 EEG features were initially extracted, and then 5 of them were selected through analysis of variance, and the result confirms a diagnostic accuracy of 87.6%. The use of deep learning methods, such as RNN and ANN, is rapidly increasing in EEG studies. Another researcher also proposed a multimodal ML that integrated multilayer perceptron, LR, and SVM to classify MCI and dementia using EEG data (Tsoi et al., 2022).

RI is a cost-effective replacement for neuroimaging. Changes in retinal can reveal pathology in the brain. The quantitative analysis of vessel calibres, tortuosity, and network complexity in RI data provides diagnostic value for dementia. A researcher proposed a multistage pipeline that involved SVM and CNN and achieved an average diagnostic accuracy of 82.4% for AD (Tsoi et al., 2022).

7.5 Issues in Dementia Research

7.5.1 Interpretability of Machine Learning Models

The interpretability of machine learning algorithms plays a critical role in many applications, particularly in fields like healthcare and dementia research, especially when they are involved in making decisions that can significantly impact people's lives. This is particularly important in dementia research and healthcare, where these decisions can have significant consequences. For both clinicians and patients to trust the outcomes of an algorithm, it's important to understand how its predictions are made. Without transparency, it becomes difficult to move from research to practical use in a clinical setting. The interpretability of an algorithm can be classified into two types: global and local. On the one hand, global interpretability involves understanding how the various components of an algorithm, such as features and weights, combine to make decisions. On the other hand, local interpretability focuses on individual cases, explaining how a decision was made for a specific sample or patient. Achieving global interpretability is often challenging due to the complexity of many algorithms. It is possible to examine algorithms at a detailed level to understand how changes in one feature or weight affect the decisions being made. In dementia research, a commonly used method for interpreting algorithmic decisions is permutation feature importance, which shows how much each feature influences the outcomes. Algorithms frequently used in dementia research, such as decision trees, SVMs, and Bayesian networks, are naturally interpretable, as they learn a set of rules or relationships between variables that can be explored by the user. However, the best-performing algorithm varies depending on the data, the specific application, and how success is measured (Bucholc et al., 2023).

7.5.2 Reproducibility and Replicability

As new computational models are being created to better understand dementia, issues of reproducibility and replicability become increasing significant. Reproducibility means achieving the same results with the same model and data, while replicability refers to applying the model to different datasets to assess the consistency of the findings. Reproducibility has long been a challenge in scientific research, especially in experimental medicine, where outcomes can vary due to both controllable factors, such as following the identical protocols, and uncontrollable factors, like system stochasticity. Using computational models greatly improves reproducibility, as a trained algorithm will always produce the same results when used with the same data. However, for research to be fully reproducible, both the data and the code must be accessible (Bucholc et al., 2023).

Advanced methods like transfer learning and multitask learning have the potential to enhance the replicability and generalizability of research findings. Transfer learning involves using a shared representation in a sequential manner, while multitask learning develops a shared representation across different tasks at the same time. For instance, transfer learning can be applied to train an algorithm using data from different studies, provided that some variables are the same across datasets, by finding a mapping between the data domains. This approach can enhance the generalizability of findings and minimize overfitting to the cohort used for training, thus increasing the chance of replicability in further cohorts. Researchers have already demonstrated successful use of transfer learning in dementia research. So far, only a few studies have applied the multitask learning approach in dementia research. One example involves using a deep feedforward neural network (DFNN) based on multitask learning, which employs multiple loss functions to detect AD and assess its progression stage simultaneously. This proposed model can effectively classify and predict AD and its stages, using both binary and multiclass classifications (with three or four class labels) over periods of five and ten years (Bucholc et al., 2023).

7.5.3 Clinical Applicability Issues

Using speech analysis to detect dementia is an emerging area of research, but most research has been centred on English speakers, which limits its applicability to other languages. Recent findings suggest that using multilingual datasets for training improves performance, with an F-score of 0.85, compared to an F-score of 0.80 when using only English data. Also, technical challenges such as difficulties in extracting patient data in a standardized, machine-readable format; a lack of clarity about how model predictions work; differences between clinical environments (such as variations in equipment, coding standards, and electronic health record systems); and differences in local clinical practices add further complexity to the adoption of ML solutions in dementia care (Bucholc et al., 2023).

7.6 Limitations and Future Directions

Access to large, diverse, and high-quality datasets remains a challenge. Many current studies focus on data from a limited demographic or geographic region, particularly English-speaking populations, which limits the generalizability of the findings. Future research should focus on developing models that work across languages and cultures, increasing the generalizability of dementia detection and progression prediction. Many of the advanced methods used in dementia research, such as deep learning models, lack transparency, making it difficult for clinicians to understand how decisions are made, which can hinder trust and clinical adoption. Advancements in explainable models are needed to increase transparency and make these tools more accessible to clinicians. Methods that offer insights into how specific features contribute to predictions can enhance trust in these systems. More research is needed to assess the long-term accuracy of models in predicting dementia progression. Longitudinal data from multiple sources could provide a better understanding of how dementia develops over time and improve the accuracy of predictions. By addressing these limitations and focusing on these future directions, the potential of AI to transform dementia research and care can be fully realized.

7.7 Recommendations and Conclusions

To foster trust and adoption in clinical settings, AI models must be more transparent and interpretable. Developing explainable AI methods that clinicians and caregivers can understand will help bridge the gap between research and real-world use. Also, efforts should be made to bridge the gap between AI research and its application in clinical practice. This includes improving the integration of AI tools with electronic health record systems and ensuring that clinicians are trained in using these technologies.

AI holds significant promise in transforming dementia research and care by improving early diagnosis, tracking disease progression, and personalizing treatment. However, several challenges must be addressed to fully realize this potential. Enhancing data access and diversity, improving model interpretability, establishing ethical guidelines, and fostering collaboration between various fields are key steps. By focusing on these areas, AI can be more effectively integrated into clinical practice, leading to better outcomes for dementia patients and their families. As the field evolves, a balanced approach that considers both technological advancements and ethical considerations will be crucial in ensuring AI's responsible and impactful use in dementia care.

Acknowledgement

All authors have checked the revised manuscript and agreed to the resubmission. We look forward to your favourable consideration for publication in Future Generation Computer Systems Journal.

References

Arvanitakis, Z., Shah, R.C. and Bennett, D.A., 2019. Diagnosis and management of dementia. *Jama*, 322(16), pp. 1589–1599.

Blanco-González, A., Cabezon, A., Seco-Gonzalez, A., Conde-Torres, D., Antelo-Riveiro, P., Pineiro, A. and Garcia-Fandino, R., 2023. The role of AI in drug discovery: challenges, opportunities, and strategies. *Pharmaceuticals*, 16(6), p. 891.

Bucholc, M. et al., 2023. Artificial intelligence for dementia research methods optimization. *Alzheimer's & Dementia*, 19(12), pp. 5934–5951. doi:10.1002/alz.13441.

Cipriani, G., Danti, S., Picchi, L., Nuti, A. and Fiorino, M.D., 2020. Daily functioning and dementia. *Dementia & Neuropsychologia*, 14(2), pp. 93–102.

De la Fuente Garcia, S., Ritchie, C.W. and Luz, S., 2020. Artificial intelligence, speech, and language processing approaches to monitoring Alzheimer's disease: a systematic review. *Journal of Alzheimer's Disease*, 78(4), pp. 1547–1574.

Javeed, A., Dallora, A.L., Berglund, J.S., Ali, A., Ali, L. and Anderberg, P., 2023. Machine learning for dementia prediction: a systematic review and future research directions. *Journal of Medical Systems*, 47(1), p. 17.

Joling, K.J., Janssen, O., Francke, A.L., Verheij, R.A., Lissenberg-Witte, B.I., Visser, P.J. and van Hout, H.P., 2020. Time from diagnosis to institutionalization and death in people with dementia. *Alzheimer's & Dementia*, 16(4), pp. 662–671.

Li, R., Wang, X., Lawler, K., Garg, S., Bai, Q. and Alty, J., 2022. Applications of artificial intelligence to aid early detection of dementia: a scoping review on current capabilities and future directions. *Journal of Biomedical Informatics, 127*, p. 104030.

O'Brien, J.T. and Thomas, A., 2015. Vascular dementia. *The Lancet, 386*(10004), pp. 1698–1706.

Ranson, J.M., Bucholc, M., Lyall, D., Newby, D., Winchester, L., Oxtoby, N.P., Veldsman, M., Rittman, T., Marzi, S., Skene, N. and Al Khleifat, A., 2023. Harnessing the potential of machine learning and artificial intelligence for dementia research. *Brain Informatics, 10*(1), p. 6.

Revathi, A., Kaladevi, R., Ramana, K., Jhaveri, R.H., Rudra Kumar, M. and Sankara Prasanna Kumar, M., 2022. Early detection of cognitive decline using machine learning algorithm and cognitive ability test. *Security and Communication Networks, 2022*(1), p. 4190023.

Sarker, I.H., 2021. Machine learning: algorithms, real-world applications and research directions. *SN Computer Science, 2*(3), p. 160.

Scheltens, P., Blennow, K., Breteler, M.M., De Strooper, B., Frisoni, G.B., Salloway, S. and Van der Flier, W.M., 2016. Alzheimer's disease. *The Lancet, 388*(10043), pp. 505–517.

Schwertner, E., Pereira, J.B., Xu, H., Secnik, J., Winblad, B., Eriksdotter, M., Nägga, K. and Religa, D., 2022. Behavioral and psychological symptoms of dementia in different dementia disorders: a large-scale study of 10,000 individuals. *Journal of Alzheimer's Disease, 87*(3), pp. 1307–1318.

Shah, D., Singh, A. and Prasad, S.S., 2022, November. Sentimental analysis using supervised learning algorithms. In *2022 3rd International Conference on Computation, Automation and Knowledge Management (ICCAKM)* (pp. 1–6). IEEE.

Shin, J.H., 2022. Dementia epidemiology fact sheet 2022. *Annals of Rehabilitation Medicine, 46*(2), pp. 53–59.

Taylor, J.P., McKeith, I.G., Burn, D.J., Boeve, B.F., Weintraub, D., Bamford, C., Allan, L.M., Thomas, A.J. and O'Brien, J.T., 2020. New evidence on the management of Lewy body dementia. *The Lancet Neurology, 19*(2), pp. 157–169.

Tsoi, K.K., Jia, P., Dowling, N.M., Titiner, J.R., Wagner, M., Capuano, A.W. and Donohue, M.C., 2022. Applications of artificial intelligence in dementia research. *Cambridge Prisms: Precision Medicine, 1*, p. e9.

Usama, M., Qadir, J., Raza, A., Arif, H., Yau, K.L.A., Elkhatib, Y., Hussain, A. and Al-Fuqaha, A., 2019. Unsupervised machine learning for networking: techniques, applications and research challenges. *IEEE Access, 7*, pp. 65579–65615.

WHO, 2023. https://desapublications.un.org/publications/world-social-report-2023-leaving-no-one-behind-ageing-world

8

Mobile and Platforms, Sensors, and IoT (Internet of Things): Smart Dementia Networks (SDNs) Devising on Real-Time Wearable IoT Platforms

---

Gurdeep Singh

8.1 Introduction

Dementia is considered a brain disease rather than just ageing conspiracy or conceptual understanding, it can affect mood, memory, thinking, and behaviour (MMTB), and it can peak with older age or over 65. However, it can happen at any age and to anyone.[1] Dementia is one of the primary causes impacting many population numbers suffering during different stages of the lifecycle, it also means imperatively to different age groups from young to elderly human beings. Dementia can also lead to more complex subsidiary health disorders, with some similar physical and psychological changes in the body, also reflecting similar underlying physiological features or parameters related to the core bodily measurements associated with heart rate beats per minute (HR-BPM), body temperature, activity recognition which can include repetitive tasks in a **Specified Area**, e.g., if it is self-health or under observation of family member or carer. Some other scenarios for dementia health monitoring can be at **Home-based care,** which is referred to as an **Internal Environment with further classification of Indoor Settings** and **Open-range areas,** where patients or individuals are walking activities, even hiking, or undertaking other activities to stay fit or calm or to refresh the mind, expecting release of good chemicals, which might endorse better memory functions. However, smart gadgets or devices like smartwatches, pendants, rings, or any other wearable smart sensor devices enable continuous context-aware computing mechanisms to collect real-time data from different parts of the body to depict onset and study the dementia episode behaviour through artificial intelligence (AI) and underlying machine learning methodologies. Most of the wired and non-wired networks have already been experimented with or are prevalent as Body Area Networks (BANs),

DOI: 10.1201/9781003485681-8

and in combination with wireless sensor networks (WSNs), are applied to many disorders. However, the combination and integration of BANs and WSNs can enhance solutions or implementation on small scale or distributed systems leading to SDNs, entirely to study dementia traits, among different age groups with customised architectures to application environments.

Context-aware IoT framework [1] is related to the widespread adoption and development of assisted living technologies from health monitoring to emergency response are well adopted in the healthcare industry, from standalone, dual, or multiple feature applications and solutions to predict and respond in adverse situations for various stakeholders involved in the observation, provision, and deliverance of healthcare services. It includes economic options or solutions for assisted living vulnerable groups of people. These healthcare solutions adopted among an extensive section of the society for self-health monitoring can enhance or be used for the observation, onset, and culmination of dementia episodes to care and management. We highlight the effective utilisation and implementation of SDNs to figure out any important underlying information related to physiological parameters. It can be useful for vital observations for cardiac functionality during the onset of a dementia episode, various other smart wearable sensors can be utilised to collect real-time data to formulate machine learning models to ascertain better healthcare management and emergency response during dementia or Alzheimer's or other related short-term memory loss episodes.

Some questions require answers or in-depth analysis for dementia management via adopting logical features to build machine learning models on classification and regression, it can further be integrated to build neural networks and deep learning models to manage dementia in various age groups and multiple underlying health conditions, those can impact the variability of physiological features to build real-time robust solutions with concrete thresholds and evident implementation for accurate dementia analysis, predictive solutions like web applications and customised Dementia Health Management System (DHMS) associating different stakeholders from healthcare teams e.g., general practitioners, specialist physicians, nurses, etc. and other stakeholders with encryption and customised permission or access controls with teams stakeholders, involved in healthcare management of specific manageable disorders with a technological implementation like dementia care.

8.2 Some Questions to Answer Are

a. How physiological parameters can define dementia observation and early management procedures with design protocols and an understanding of policy development?

b. How elevation and decline in real-time heart-rate patterns can insti-gate in-depth observation for dementia episodes, onset or intervals (intermediate), and at end stages?

c. How integrated smartwatch onboard sensors, data generation, and threshold observation can enhance predictive solutions towards dementia management?

8.3 Objective

This chapter aims to develop a generalised SDN, generic architecture or framework approach, including different wearable devices as integral com-ponents, in combination or prevalent BANs and WSNs, along with flow diagram steps supporting the development of the system for dementia diag-nosis and management strategies for different age groups. A more specific and generalised approach for comprehensive implementation of assisted living solutions to deliver semantic, historical prediction, and real-time solutions for wider healthcare stakeholders. There are many reasons for the origin and implementation of this research, particularly during the pan-demic dementia patients suffered the most while restrictions were in place in metropolitan cities, so many vulnerable impacted groups suffered the most and felt the aftereffects. However, in this chapter, we provide guid-ance towards dementia networks utilising wearables or Internet of Things (IoT) components to effectively serve the framework or ecosystem among distributed implementation or approach, as well as service or design to deliver for real-time healthcare needs specifically cognitive and demen-tia functions. In addition, we also present an entire wearable sensor and high-level IoT network or service design model to present applications, solu-tions, and systems for any need and technological requirements for future dementia networks, IoT, and AI with underlying machine learning meth-odologies and automated features development for healthcare provision, management, and problem identification with thresholds for cognitive to cardiac functions.

8.3.1 Numeral Proportions

In the USA ageing population numbers by 2030 projection stands at 70.3 million and 18.6 million people over the age of 65 to 80, respectively. Americans over 65 and older are projected to jump from 58 million in 2022 to 82 million by 2050, which is a 47% increase, and the 65-and-older age group's proportion of the total population is estimated to rise from 17% to 23%.[2]

8.3.2 Dementia Figures

In 2024 projection about Victoria in Australia more than 107,600 people live with all forms of dementia. This figure will incline to 216,400 by 2054. Australia – dementia among younger people is estimated at almost 29,000 people living with younger onset dementia. This figure is projected to increase to almost 41,000 by 2054 with an increased proportion of 41% increase, which is almost 50% approximately on a general basis, which is very alarming.[3]

8.3.3 Dementia Data around the World

Around 55 million people suffer from dementia worldwide, with an increase of 10 million cases every year. Moreover, most people are affected by Alzheimer's, which is the most common form of dementia among the suffering population. On facts in 2019, dementia cost dearly to the economies of the world, cost comes to 1.3 trillion dollars. However, this repeated failure of excessive costs spent on dementia around the world is quite serious and shameful, especially for the countries and governments by not allocate healthcare budget for the elimination and cure of diseases like dementia. Among genders, Women are extremely affected by dementia, in any case, both directly and indirectly. Their experience leads to higher disability and higher mortality rates.[4] Some underlying risk factors of dementia include age (more common in those 65 or older), hypertension, diabetes, smoking, alcohol or drinking, and depression.

Figure 8.1 represents graphical data of people suffering from dementia in all forms by age up to 2018.[5] These are estimates gathered by the

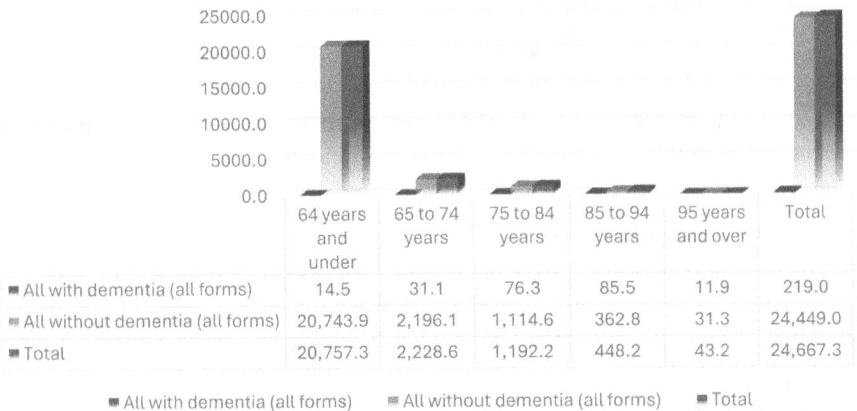

ALL PERSONS WITH DEMENTIA (ALL FORMS), BY AGE – 2018, ESTIMATES (COMMONWEALTH OF AUSTRALIA)

	64 years and under	65 to 74 years	75 to 84 years	85 to 94 years	95 years and over	Total
■ All with dementia (all forms)	14.5	31.1	76.3	85.5	11.9	219.0
■ All without dementia (all forms)	20,743.9	2,196.1	1,114.6	362.8	31.3	24,449.0
■ Total	20,757.3	2,228.6	1,192.2	448.2	43.2	24,667.3

■ All with dementia (all forms)   ■ All without dementia (all forms)   ■ Total

FIGURE 8.1
Graphical data of people suffering from dementia.

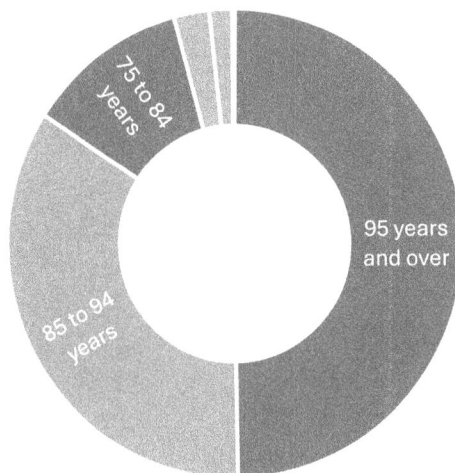

FIGURE 8.2
Worldly numeral proportions.[6]

Commonwealth of Australia. So, in total 64 years and under statistically stand at 20,757.3, However, other categories of age from 65–74, 75–84, 85 to 94 and lastly 95 and over, just add 4000 cases approximately, which shows us that, with the onset of dementia the numbers are massive, however middle and post management period during rising age group exhibits quite a substantial improvement in the post numbers in comparison to the age group of 64 and under. This data depicts a lot to learn and examine factual strategies to control dementia.

These solutions or systems should integrate with other health systems to care for the elderly, which the chart shows predominantly 75 years old and above (Figure 8.2).

Figure 8.3 presents the top ten causes of death according to United Nations (UN) data, where dementia or Alzheimer's ranked seventh in 2021. However, in the 2000s, it was not anywhere closer in the charts, we can imagine the impact of these disorders on mortality, especially in older populations or populations anywhere after 65 years old, regardless of other age groups that are impacted or don't have a diagnosis of Alzheimer's.

8.3.4 Economic Viability

Customised solutions covering specific needs to observe dementia behaviour or underlying conditions with monitoring specific features can be easily developed and implemented as minimal or extensive changes in certain physiological features in terms of standalone or multiple feature applications, utilising certain sensors or economic gadgets like smart devices or

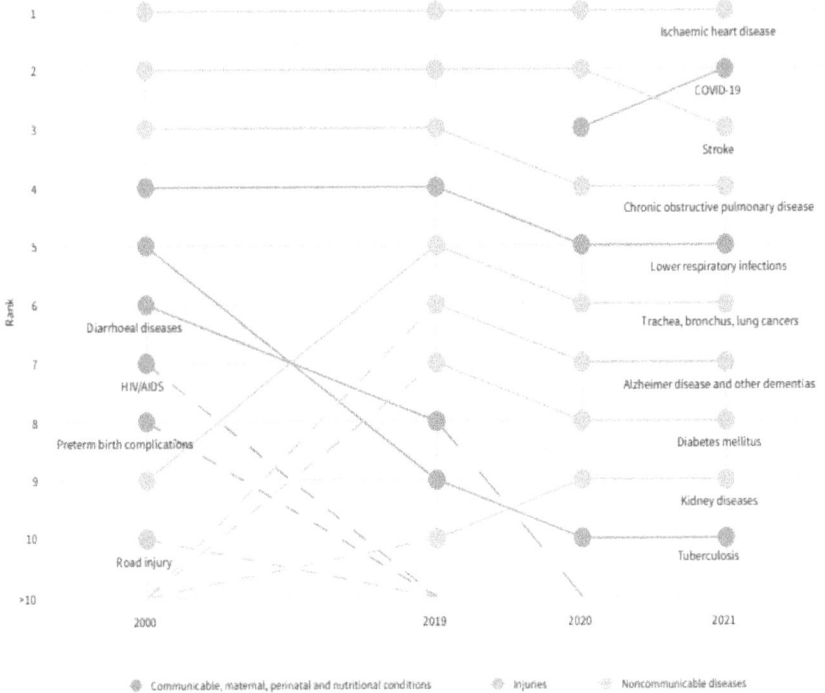

Note: Solid lines represent movement within the top 10 causes of death. Dashed lines represent movement in or out of the top 10 causes of death.

FIGURE 8.3
(Examples, Facts, Proportions, Examples, impacted individual's + or – deserving population).[7]

context-aware pervasive gadgets. Low-cost single or multiple feature solutions, some standalone or off-the-shelf experimental sensor equipment or solutions, those can specifically monitor bodily or single health features, on health needs, especially wearable, exhibit low economic cost or approach among wider population to monitor their physiological parameters.

8.4 Background

Some dementia solutions in wearable, wireless, sensor and BANs include technologically integrated solutions in smart homes, generalised or standalone solutions, whereas standalone solutions, which we define as SDNs, include sensor-based capabilities to collect data, amend, and transcend real-time data for solutions in real-time, historical data for predictive analytics. Some examples of the different networks are as follows:

8.4.1 Body Area Networks

8.4.1.1 This Solution with Context-Aware Dementia Helmet for Enhanced Safety and Navigation

The proposed context-aware dementia helmet is a wearable device designed to improve the quality of life and safety for individuals with dementia or blindness. By integrating various sensors and haptic feedback mechanisms, this helmet can provide real-time information about the wearer's environment, helping them navigate their surroundings with greater confidence. The device utilises a combination of infrared sensors and mobile phone vibrator motors to detect and alert the user to nearby obstacles. The helmet's design incorporates a comfortable and easily wearable headband, ensuring optimal comfort for extended use. The helmet's obstacle detection system provides timely alerts, reducing the risk of accidents and injuries. **Mobility:** By providing real-time environmental information, the helmet empowers individuals with dementia or blindness to navigate their surroundings more confidently and **enhanced quality of life** helmet can significantly improve the overall quality of life for individuals with cognitive impairments by providing a sense of security and independence. **Customisable:** The helmet can be tailored to meet the specific needs of individual users, allowing for adjustments to sensitivity, vibration intensity, and other settings. The context-aware dementia helmet represents a promising solution for addressing the challenges faced by individuals with dementia or blindness. By combining advanced technology with a user-friendly design, this device has the potential to revolutionise the way these individuals interact with their environment and improve their overall well-being.

8.4.2 Wearable or Wireless Sensor Networks (WSNs)

This research proposes a WSN solution for **real-time health monitoring**. The **system utilises a cloud-based architecture** to enable remote monitoring of vital signs, including heartbeat, body temperature, and blood pressure. **Data collected from wearable sensors is transmitted directly to the cloud platform,** allowing for real-time analysis and visualisation. Additionally, an on-device LCD screen provides an alternative for immediate access to health data. The proposed solution aligns with the broader framework of the IoT for healthcare, where a sensing layer is employed to continuously observe and track user health status. This WSN solution enables real-time health monitoring through an IoT-enabled system. The cloud-based platform supports continuous tracking of vital signs like heartbeat, body temperature, and blood pressure using various wearable sensors. Collected data is transmitted directly to the cloud for analysis and can also be displayed in real time on an LCD screen. This solution aligns with the general IoT architecture for healthcare, **featuring a sensing layer dedicated to observing user health status.**

8.4.3 Smart Networks, Smart Homes

This includes scenarios or use cases involving home-based care or scenario, smart spaces or environments within (SEoT) smart environment of things or integrated AI-featured smart homes [2], literally covering more detailed and distributed applications, e.g., a household with four family members, using wearable devices like smartwatch or smart gadgets like smart pendant, smart emergency response gadgets with integrated or enhanced functionality, smartphones and smart appliance, as an example. So overall smart homes with distributed pervasive or smart devices can be one use case towards distributed architecture applications or adoption, and secondly, a healthcare environment scenario or use case, where multiple stakeholders or staff utilise or interact with smart objects to accomplish daily tasks. For example, doctors, nurses, allied health, mobile health, or paramedics can wear smartwatches, smart alarm systems, or pendants for on-call or emergency procedures, and all health and daily use smart appliances or objects in use. So, this can be another distributed architectural implementation or use-case towards the smart environments to manage dementia patients in the day as more tiringly at night by providing continuous digital alarms and instructions in high volume to divert the course of dementia patients in an organised way or track to accomplish the task and reporting back at the starting point or bed, for example.

8.5 Extend on Smart Homes, Multiple Features or Sensors to Control and Observe Movements

Smart solutions on a personal or user basis, as every individual differs in disease symptoms, management, and cure. So personalised solutions can be worked out for small settings or self-health on mobile and web networks, which can be economical, add more value, real-time predictive solutions, fewer wait times or physician directions, personalised responses and predictions for various parameters.

8.6 Frameworks and Design

8.6.1 Context-Aware Design [1]

Context-aware computing systems operate diverse data sources [3] to gather, process, and keep circumstantial data in real-time [4, 5], thereby providing services according to user needs, interaction with the environment, entity, and their localisation [3]. Context-aware systems are considered a crucial part of ubiquitous or pervasive computing technologies [6]. Mostly, the smart technologies or gadgets or devices form a part of it, however they should intact, define and exhibit features of ubiquitous or pervasive computing solving real-world problems in the modern world with exceptions to the off the shelf technology and product design, hardware and other components in an experimental stage.

8.6.2 Context-Aware Pervasive Technology Holds Significant Promise in Enhancing Dementia

care by providing tailored support and improving the quality of life for individuals with cognitive impairments. These technologies, which leverage sensors, wearable devices, and ambient intelligence, are designed to adapt to the needs and behaviours of dementia patients in real-time. For example, smart home systems can monitor daily activities and detect deviations from established routines, thereby alerting caregivers or healthcare providers about potential issues such as wandering or changes in physical health [1]. The integration of context-aware technology into dementia care has been shown to facilitate timely interventions, reduce the burden on caregivers, and enhance patient safety [2].

8.6.3 Context-Aware Pervasive Technology Offers Substantial Potential to Revolutionise Dementia Care by Providing Personalised Assistance and Elevating the Quality of Life for Those with Even Cognitive Impairments

These technologies, which utilise sensors, wearable devices, and ambient intelligence, are designed to dynamically adapt to the specific needs and behaviours of dementia patients. These technologies can also highlight different or unique behaviours of dementia patients in real time. For instance, smart home systems can track daily activities and identify deviations from normal routines, enabling caregivers or healthcare professionals to be alerted during potential concerns such as wandering or changes in physical well-being [7]. Which of those can be integrated with **Home Health Systems** [8]: Connecting the smartwatch to home health monitoring systems can provide a more comprehensive view of a patient's health.

Recent studies highlight the effectiveness of these technologies in various aspects of dementia management. For instance, research by Kluge et al. [9] demonstrated that a context-aware system could significantly improve the detection of falls and emergencies in dementia patients, leading to quicker responses and reduced injury rates [3]. Similarly, a review by Gagnon et al. [10] underscores the potential of wearable devices and smart home technologies in providing continuous monitoring and personalised feedback, which can help in managing behavioural symptoms and ensuring medication

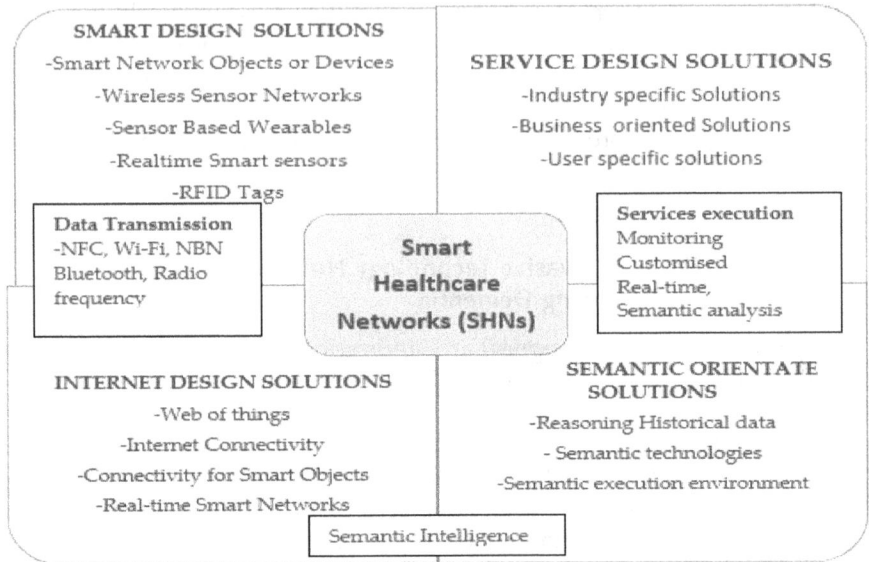

FIGURE 8.4
Smart healthcare networks.

adherence [4]. The continued advancement and integration of these pervasive technologies offer a promising avenue for enhancing dementia care as well as creating safer and more supportive environments for patients and their families.

Figure 8.4 shows general frameworks for the design of smart applications, solutions, machine learning and deep learning systems by the use of different data sources, which include continuous, tabular and non-tabular for predictive modelling to deal with defined physiological parameters including e.g., from PPG(), EEG, cognitive analysis or waves, activity range or acceleration or de-acceleration or fatigue, inclination capability, only if consented, speech recognition, urination, confusion with forgetfulness of talking or thoughts, etc. are some features to establish with an underlying time of the day, e.g., morning, afternoon, evening. Also, impact on different features after the use of medication or use of stimulants during morning and evening. So, overall, when the study of these features is important for daily routine checkups, it becomes important and precious to collect, analyse, study and draw real-time, predictive or classification machine learning results of different algorithms to study, rectify and manage dementia through SDNs [11, 12].

Some general frameworks utilised with extensive data patterns or design will be studied and presented for the development and study of Dementia Management, which include Flask on lightweight and Django on heavy or complex Python solutions, and tkinter software solutions. Similarly, Amazon, Hitoe Sensor Frameworks, Google, and Microsoft.

8.6.4 Mobile, Smart Devices, Wearables

Other smart sensor-embedded watches can lead to the development of different applications, solutions, and systems based on machine and deep learning methodologies. Prevalent frameworks like web frameworks, data handling, Python-based Django or Flask frameworks for solution implementation and features can certainly change the adoption and monitoring of smart devices in different environments, and for many treatments or reminders, optimal tracking and activities of the subject in any environment and any age bracket. Some essential data collection sources through JSON-type frameworks or database schemas on tabular, non-tabular, and real-time sensor data can make predictive models to help individuals or patients suffering from dementia. Many new and existent features should be combined to feel the impact of the onset of the dementia episodes, certain behaviours portrayed during the episode, timeline of the episode, occurrence of the episode with time or hours or day of the week. SDN networks on single wearable features on continuous data or integrated WSNs and BANs integrated data sources and features can easily help deter or notify the onset along with other underlying stages of dementia to counter them effectively by the nursing or aged care staff at healthcare or aged care settings, similarly by the carers in self-health dwellings and for patients sharing accommodation among other colleagues. These technology features or enhanced complete set of integrated multiple-feature services can transform the living quality of the individuals or patients, along with increased efficiency, to deal with counter-effective procedures for aged care workers, nurses, and carers daily. These criteria can be used alternatively to help improve and manage the condition of dementia sufferers quite appropriately. Moreover, among different management stakeholders, regardless of the frontline multiple, customised or encrypted services on a smartphone and other smart device frameworks can be universally adopted, to counter dementia management from commencement to the end of the entire experience or episode. Some other stakeholders can include family members, shift workers or irregular carers, friends, colleagues, or charity volunteers for professional and personal use to take effective care before, during and after end or cessation of the Dementia episodes by monitoring behaviour daily and using predictive machine learning modelling on semantic data, purposing with historical and real-time data coverage for affective detailed data coverage for different activities, behaviour, features, physiological parameters, metabolism or movement among older adults before and after the food, etc. These are some of the data governance features, which can be applied to the work or social environment immediately to provide specific medications or therapies to help the patient.

Some basic big data web to implementation frameworks will be described or defined for the use of continuous real-time, batch processing, tabular, or non-tabular data to present an understanding of the predictive use or purposeful utilisation procedures that can be used for healthcare stakeholders, emergency response stakeholders, and relevant management teams.

8.6.5 Smart Dementia Networks (SDNs)

For monitoring, observation, or for the onset of dementia episodes, machine learning modelling and sustainable AI systems enables superior dementia healthcare diagnosis and management. (The diagram below represents smart devices with multiple features and various stages involved in the delivery of specific AI systems or Generalised Smart Network Architectures.)

Figure 8.5 shows general context-aware SDNs Architecture with additional wearable, BANs, and WSNs devices or their capabilities with user acceptance on various modes of graphical user interfaces. The context-aware frameworks can constantly work in real-time and according to changes within the sensor measurements, and surroundings environments with use of physiological parameters equipment for adopting the measurements of the required features for constant and real-time observation and changes

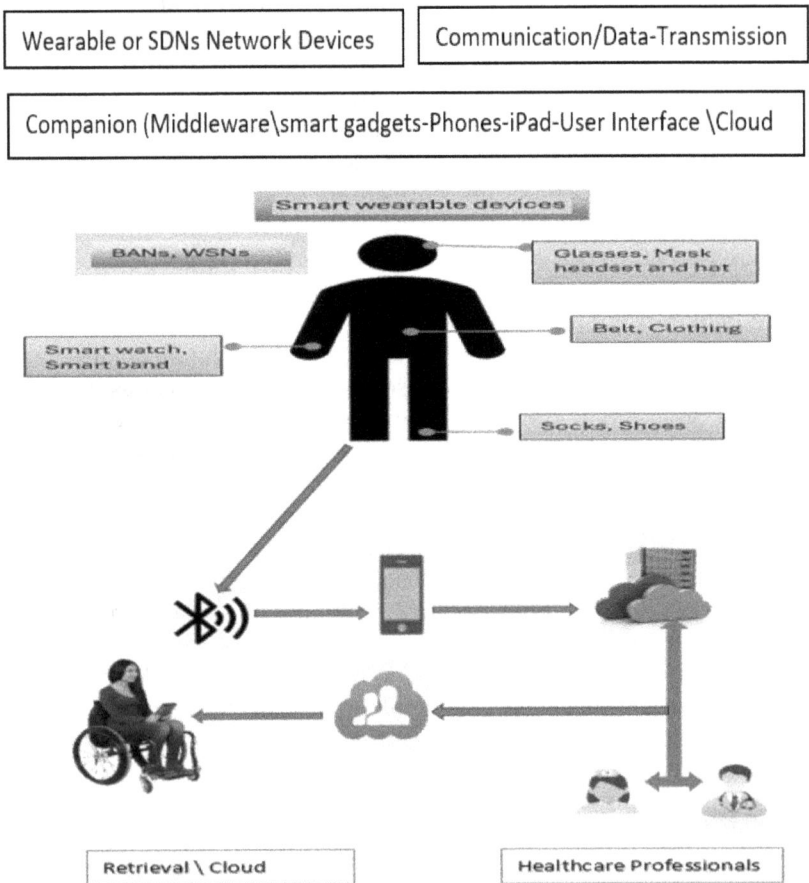

FIGURE 8.5
Smart wearable devices.

in the condition of the patient or individual with the implementation of machine learning methodologies and use of thresholding techniques in real-time and pre-management procedures for dementia care, system formulation or features can be figured on generic and customised basis of the patients or individuals. Moreover, combining smartwatch data with other wearable sensors (e.g., blood glucose monitors and fall detection devices) can provide a more comprehensive picture of a person's health. Algorithms can analyse health data to identify patterns and predict potential emergencies, enabling proactive interventions. Developing more sophisticated automation capabilities, such as automatic machine learning or semantic algorithm analysis, which can help future emergency services with imperative thresholds, general, generic, specific, or adaptive thresholds, and further contacting relevant healthcare providers based on specific health metrics. Furthermore, incorporating social features to allow users to connect with others in similar situations, share experiences, and provide support, which is also a social networking dimension among populations, with most of the social apps can be defined with increased awarding systems like achieving badges, accumulating stars, even competing with social teams and groups promoting more wearable sensor oriented social networking derivatives for goal achievements eventually culminating in health promotion and goal achievements for health and body welly or muscle wellness.

Extend frameworks on graphical user interface, IoT and oriented solutions, definitely require user-friendly interfaces, e.g., in the design of UI-UX special consideration has to be taken, from the beginning, how it can help and be friendly towards the older population, easily usable, scrolled or touch screen or added loud voice functions, as required or in any customisation process, a detailed study about user interfaces, given the rapid advancements in IoT and the growing demand for in-home monitoring as part of assisted-living strategies, there is a pressing need for scalable, interoperable applications that can connect new medical services to user interfaces [13], sensor devices, and healthcare resources. These applications must seamlessly function across existing communication infrastructure and existing technologies of provided network speeds for optimum results.

8.7 Use-Cases

8.7.1 Healthcare (e.g., Aged Care), Self-Health or External Scenarios

In healthcare, different settings are included to present an idea about how SDNs or IoT solutions can be applied efficiently for different living arrangements, like personalised care, external or self-healthcare settings, to achieve imperative requirements as monitoring devices [11].

8.7.2 Personalised Use-Case

With preference and thresholds, notifications, specific stakeholders, and regulations as advised if in healthcare settings or self-health or under the observation of a family member.

8.7.2.1 Home-Based Care – Internal Environments: Indoor Settings

This is a recent trend that originated within the housing and healthcare sector. Preference of patients has grown to practise self-health care or home-based care,[8] instead of adopting aged care homes or other smart rehabilitation facilities, especially elderly prefer home-based care. Some reasons can be attributed to high admittance costs and difficulty in adjusting to the environment. Moreover, a large number of non-elderly patients suffering from cardiovascular disorders, asthmatic conditions, and obesity problems prefer self-health care, rather than visiting clinical settings regularly, a similar situation applies to people living with dementia, especially younger groups or those below 60 years old and also people residing in rural communities for whom digital health might not be available or their attitudes of ignorance can form an illogical practice or culture, which has to be addressed by healthcare or social care workers. For this group of people, many technological solutions have been applied in the past in telehealth monitoring, e-healthcare solutions, and video consultation [14, 15], but none of these technologies can provide continuous monitoring and observation. Perhaps, round-the-clock observation of essential monitoring, specifically disparities or problem-solving, can be achieved through SDN solutions in real-time along with detailed interaction-related activities endured at a given time of the day or time with an everyday record of health-related data stored for future predictive diagnosis and directions. These devices can target specific features to implement thresholds, solutions, or ML algorithms for automated functioning in addition to other software or frameworks for real-time assistance in the form of continuous alarms or notifications to rectify dementia behaviour effectively and promote self-health management 24 hrs a day and respond on time during an emergency event. Other reasons, like associated costs of expensive monitoring systems, the service cost of doctors to attend patients when most required, can be well planned in time [11].

8.7.3 Universal Use Case

It can be applied to general patients or population, specifically in healthcare settings.

8.7.3.1 Healthcare and Aged-Care Centres

In aged-care centres, what purposes can these solutions implement, for example, they can meet patient needs very timely for staff, promoting healthcare responses, specifically for patients under observation or chronic dementia sufferers. As mentioned before, challenges related to health-care staff or shortage are high, due to the lack of trained personnel in the workforce, there are limited people to look after the populated aged-care facilities or limited staff take up night roles Therefore, dementia patients or elderly are at risk to be monitored or guided regularly, especially vul-nerable group of patients with dementia complications during nighttime. To meet such challenges or demands, SDN solutions form an integrated framework to implement real-time, sensor-based wearable dementia solu-tions that can observe different stages of dementia, eventually promot-ing regular patient monitoring mechanisms with defined features and ML algorithms for prediction with minimal involvement of staff and ubiqui-tous monitoring.

8.7.4 External Environments

External Environments: outdoor setting (expand with references)

Figure 8.6 presents data about people living with dementia in different living scenarios. Numerous people are living mostly in healthcare settings or scenarios; however, many people with disability live in self-care settings alone, and others live in shared accommodation. So, overall, two different use cases are essentially formulated for monitoring people suffering from dementia and other disabilities in SDN classification.

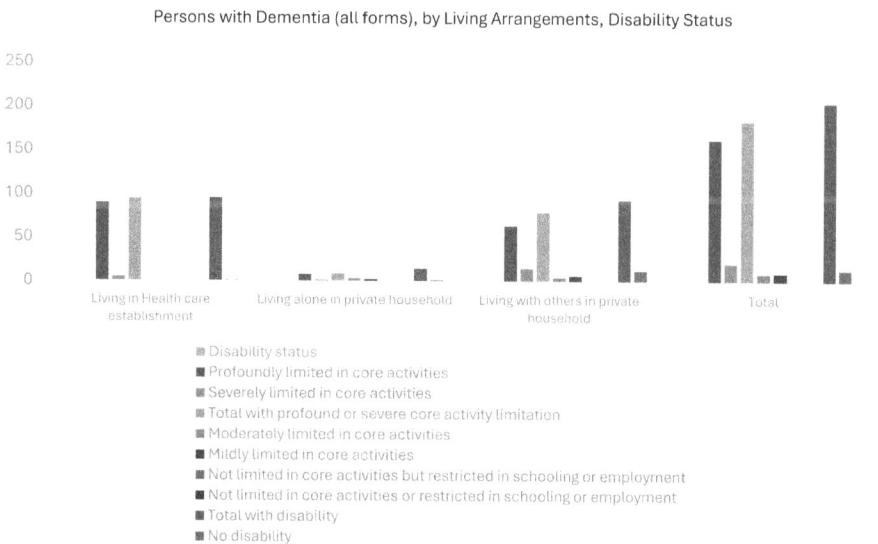

FIGURE 8.6
Persons with dementia by living arrangements and disability status.

8.8 Wearable Tracking

It is an important aspect or will present a considerable contribution, where machine learning or AI is taking the lead role in solving real-time solutions. However, constructive results are drawn based on data gathered, collected, generated, and analysed. To present a specific example, considering wearables, a large amount of data will be generated, which includes BMI, food logs, water intake or hydration, activity recognition, exercise goals, heart rate zones, etc. So, data collection, experimentation, and result analysis can lead the way to improve health and well-being among the wider community, raising red flags or monitoring activities or derailment of well-being among the wider population can be very beneficial and applicable on a broader scale. Also, to add, all the categories as mentioned earlier in semantic analysis can promote applicability towards real-time solutions and further effectiveness to benefit the general or specific population.

8.8.1 GPS Feature

Use, effectiveness, and applicability of this feature. Regulation, policy and common use among the population for location monitoring on smart devices, this feature is very imperative and be used on smartwatches, similarly can be integrated into smart systems or smart home environments and other SDN solutions with smart capabilities and which will help in tracing the patients or individuals in self-environments. During the onset of the episodes, which can be related to underlying reasons, leisure or hiking activities like camping, etc. and these activities are also much popular among older populations, nevertheless, even those suffer from dementia problems or similar underlying issues according to the different stages of the disease should be considered as a subject in these scenarios. Stages as defined medically or not, if not defined, it can be generalised by stating the reasons or it is effective in any underlying conditions, concerns, state of mind diseases, which are present in medical history or will progress in stages. Many individuals or patients go unreported, due to non-observation or denial of acceptance, privacy reasons, wearable tracking features, and personalised solutions can benefit these individuals. Some other underlying reasons can be stress, which can further instigate or abnormalise physiological parameters, there can be a **General and Specific Threshold** for every measurable or sensed feature, apart from worked or crafted algorithmic features like sleep, activities, etc.

8.8.2 GPS Tracking of the Dementia Patients

Use of this feature in external and internal environments can also detail the behaviour or GPS points of locations to study the onset or ongoing episode in more detail about the conditions or any external episode that triggers any data or information for the repetitive activities or location path. **Real-time Location Tracking:** GPS capabilities provide precise location data, enabling rapid dispatch of emergency services [16].

8.8.3 Emergency Response Handling or Emergency Response Procedures Existent with Integrated Systems – Early Detection of Emergencies

Abnormal physiological data can trigger alerts, potentially preventing adverse outcomes. **Enhanced Communication:** Direct contact with emergency services or other stakeholders to expedite assistance. **Remote Monitoring:** For patients in rehabilitation or under clinical supervision, it offers a layer of safety and security. **Pandemic Management (Dementia Patients Care):** It can aid in tracking and monitoring patient activity, supporting public health efforts, especially supporting dementia patients even during pandemics through IoT-driven smart solutions via sensor-based real-time data [17], regardless of other features or diseases that can impact the situation or can be threatening to humankind. During COVID, most elderly individuals, normal or patients, died in indoor settings. Like aged care homes, health monitoring smart homes, etc. So, to even cover this point during pandemics when dementia is in the top 10 causes of mortality according to U.N. Data, as specified earlier, these interventions are as important as to study, prevent, and produce solutions to counter pandemics, even there can be research or studies that can correlate any link of mortality between dementia and COVID.

8.8.4 Emergency Control Equipment

For patients or people with marginal, chronic, acute, and onset dementia. Numerous specific gadgets are prevalent in the care or market like emergency buttons or assistive technology gadgets [12]. These mechanisms have been serving people for a long time, though they help dispatch the alarm to the emergency carers stakeholders or law enforcement agencies. However, integrated features among more advanced or modern devices with multiple features and low cost make them viable and feasible for pre- or early management of emergency care, along with establishing predictive modelling from the data to study any patterns that are responsible for the onset or during the course or This is another recent trend originated within the healthcare sector. Preference of patients has grown to practise self-health care or home-based care,[9] instead of adopting aged care homes or other smart rehabilitation facilities, especially elderly prefer home-based care. Some reasons can be attributed to high admittance costs and difficulty in adjusting to the environment. Moreover, many non-elderly patients suffering from cardiovascular disorders, asthmatic conditions, and obesity problems prefer self-health care, rather than visiting clinical settings regularly, a similar situation applies to people living in rural communities. For this group of people, many technological solutions have been applied in the past in telehealth medicine, e-healthcare solutions, and video consultation [14, 15], but none of these technologies can provide continuous monitoring and observation. Perhaps, round-the-clock observation of vital sign monitoring specifically, IoT solutions action in real time [18], e.g., of the episode by collecting data through smart devices data collection and dispensing data batches to the cloud server or edge computing capabilities or other technological specifications to learn and implement solutions from historical data with real-time emergency management and precautionary obligation for the management of dementia among different age group people. Some of which require borderline treatments for early disease management.

8.8.5 Precise Tracking Systems-GPS [16]

SDNs can immensely contribute towards pre-management, which is onset of dementia, as discussed in the earlier sections. Secondly, during the ongoing episodes and at the time of aftereffects of dementia or Alzheimer's, like blushing, raised or decreased heart rate, or exhaustion, during different settings of livelihood or use cases. For example, if the person is in a self-health environment, rehabilitation or any other isolation setting (R) these precise smart gadgets like wearables, smartwatches and other smart devices can very well promote and dispense the GPS coordinates for the emergency services, for example, especially in the outdoor setting or external environment during rehabilitation or activities like walking, hiking, mountain climbing, etc. So, these context-aware devices can make it extremely convenient for people with underlying dementia causes. Moreover, as discussed earlier, these features can handle all three different use cases healthcare and aged-care centres, self-health, and external scenarios. We can discuss more on aged care scenarios, where activities to handle, train, and manage existing in an enclosed environment would be the hardest of all the scenarios to handle elderly with chronic dementia issues. Perhaps, integrated SDNs with enhanced features can help in their monitoring, observation, and timely medical attention at the right time with customised or personalised solutions or applications and preferred interfaces. Similarly, these smart networks like wearables, smartwatches, smart pendants even smart rings and other multiple featured smart customised the self or customised gadgets with specific features can certainly notify location coordinates, which was quite a sparse feature a decade ago, However, with the emergence of smart devices, it just became instantly prominent and part of every smart gadgets, which has helped on with increasing dementia problems by the use of general public and patients. Preciseness in GPS coordinates makes it the most preferred and effective approach to deal with any emergency.

Example of activity logs with GPS location live and very accurate GPS location protocol amid especially in the log's contributor time batch processing logs on data and accuracy portfolio presents context-aware location service. In the above GPS tracking through smartwatch here, we have used a Fitbit

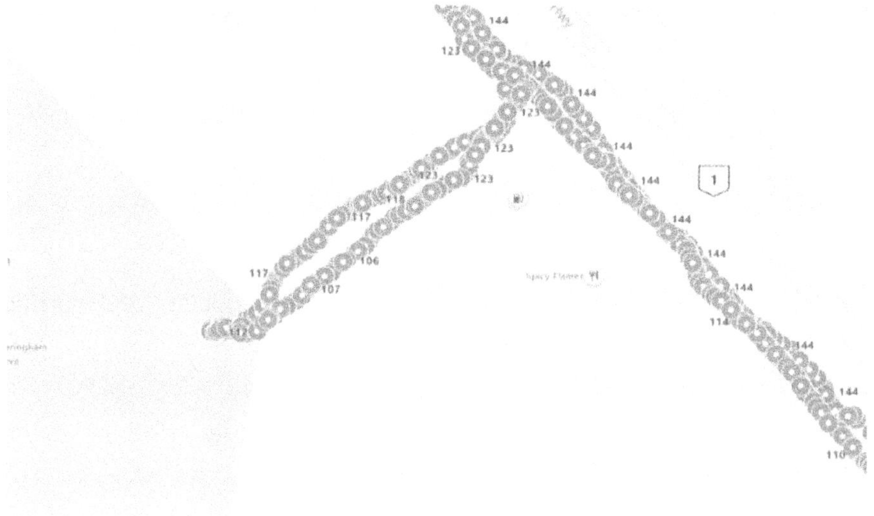

FIGURE 8.7
GPS coordinates.

smartwatch for activity or GPS location dashboard, as shown in Figure 8.7 both accuracy and exact points are provided with precise location services or can speak to the accuracy and every point if JGS A real-time activity tracking service is also available for tracking purposes, which can be implemented or installed on the design-side of health systems to monitor patient movements or activities. Also, GPS coordinates, for further assessment utilising **Location thresholds or network communication is very essential for sending** notifications, messaging or alarms, if required, because dementia patients living in self-health care can face challenges with proper or assistive equipment handy, However, if smart watches, wearable and other assistive technologies are not accompanying by any reason or due to dementias traits, it can be difficult, so wearable will help in severe or worse times, Some examples that can deliver this functionality in an application can be Splunk [19], etc.

8.9 Future Works: Cover All Three Points

8.9.1 Limitations

8.9.1.1 Considerations and Challenges

8.9.1.1.1 Battery Life

Ensuring sufficient battery life for extended periods, especially in emergencies, is crucial.

8.9.1.1.2 *Network Connectivity*

Reliable network coverage, especially in rural areas, is vital for effective communication.

8.9.1.1.3 *Cost*

The initial cost of the devices and ongoing subscription fees may be a barrier for some.

8.9.1.1.4 *User Acceptance*

Ensuring that users are comfortable with wearing the device and sharing their data is important in central use-case or self-health scenarios.

8.9.1.1.5 *False Alarms*

Minimising false alarms due to technical glitches or user errors is vital to prevent unnecessary disruptions.

8.9.2 Privacy Data Privacy

Protecting sensitive health and location data is essential to maintain trust.

8.9.3 Security

In the limitation section, include discussion and disadvantages. Include privacy and security reasons for robust solutions and designs.

8.10 Future Directions

How it can be effective, what outcomes or strategies should be used to enhance solution applicability or use-cases how will it benefit in integration with solutions with the home health system, if any in place or with aged care smart monitoring rooms, semantic analysis or historical data analysis with machine learning solutions along with area-based SDNs with improved coverage and response capabilities, in remote areas. Lastly, we also discuss the interoperability of healthcare systems for dementia networks along with emergency protocols to be followed in generalised care or aged care or other protective or carer homes, along with some self-health or other home-health environment scenarios. Solutions and look to fix limitations.

8.10.1 Potential Improvements and Future Directions

8.10.1.1 *Integration with Home Health Systems [8]*

Connecting the smartwatch to home health monitoring systems can provide a more comprehensive view of a patient's health.

8.10.1.1.1 Advanced Analytics

Using AI and machine learning to analyse data patterns can improve emergency prediction and response, so historical, semantic, and real-time data are very important.

8.10.1.1.2 Community-Based Networks

Leveraging community networks to enhance coverage and response capabilities in remote areas. It is important to utilise the in-depth or actual primary functionality of IoT systems or devices. Otherwise, lower speed and still use of the older generation network affect every feature of the system or solution, scalability problems, and robustness of the system.

8.10.1.1.3 Interoperability

Ensuring compatibility with various healthcare systems and emergency response protocols. This feature will eventually start to become very essential, as discussed earlier, this integration or merger will provide numerous advanced features.

8.11 Conclusion

IoT can help people with memory impairment to remember to do ADLs correctly and independently, reducing their dependence on others [20–22]. Studies have shown that using IoT technology can help people with memory impairment to perform activities such as daily walking independently and securely [20, 23, 24]. A study found a correlation of 0.597 between traditional memory tests (face-name test) and an IoT system, whereas the correlation between response time and face-name test was 0.341. This suggests that IoT systems can be used to measure memory abilities in people with Alzheimer's disease or dementia [24]. This chapter exhibits an approach for developing SDNs for designing wearable sensor oriented and technology solutions. These solutions are predictive and real-time to enhance context-aware and other location features. big data generated, by these networks can also be used for semantic, predictive health analytics and developing artificial intelligence applications that utilise machine learning methodologies, other factors for developing IoT solutions, their relationship and the role to serve diverse healthcare scenarios explained in section 6.2 like **Healthcare (e.g., aged care), Self-Health or External Scenarios, Personalised Use-case, Home-based care – Internal Environments: Indoor Settings** We also discuss generic or high-level IoT wearable framework including healthcare stakeholders to address dementia by reviewing some of their benefits and the underlying challenges concerning security and privacy issues regarding robust design and the development and implementation of health technology systems that serve distributed populations for cognitive enhancements.

Notes

1 https://www.dementia.org.au/about-dementia
2 https://www.prb.org/resources/fact-sheet-aging-in-the-united-states/
3 https://www.dementia.org.au/about-dementia/dementia-facts-and-figures
4 https://www.who.int/news-room/fact-sheets/detail/dementia
5 https://www.abs.gov.au/articles/dementia-australia
6 https://www.abs.gov.au/articles/dementia-australia
7 https://iris.who.int/bitstream/handle/10665/376869/9789240094703-eng.
  pdf?sequence=1
8 https://onthewards.org/4-emerging-healthcare-trends/
9 https://onthewards.org/4-emerging-healthcare-trends/

References

1. Carrera-Rivera, A., Larrinaga, F., and Lasa, G.: 'Context-awareness for the design of Smart-product service systems: Literature review', Computers in Industry, 2022, 142, p. 103730
2. Sepasgozar, S., Karimi, R., Farahzadi, L., Moezzi, F., Shirowzhan, S., Ebrahimzadeh, S.M., Hui, F., and Aye, L.: 'A systematic content review of artificial intelligence and the internet of things applications in smart home', Applied Sciences, 2020, 10, (9), p. 3074
3. Muñoz-Benítez, J., Molero-Castillo, G., and Benítez-Guerrero, E.: ' Data fusion as source for the generation of useful knowledge in context-aware systems', Journal of Intelligent & Fuzzy Systems, 2015, 34, pp. 1–12.
4. Millham, R.: 'Context-aware systems: A more appropriate response system to hurricanes and other natural disasters', Procedia Computer Science, 2014, 36, pp. 21–26
5. Geihs, K., Reichle, R., Wagner, M., and Khan, M.: 'Modeling of context-aware self-adaptive applications in ubiquitous and service-oriented environments', Lecture Notes in Computer Science 5525, pp. 146–163. https:doi.org/10.1007/978-3-642-02161-9_8
6. Hong, J.-y, Suh, E.-h, and Kim, S.-J.: 'Context-aware systems: A literature review and classification', Expert Systems with Applications, 2009, 36, (4), pp. 8509–8522
7. Daniels, K., and Bonnechère, B.: 'Harnessing digital health interventions to bridge the gap in prevention for older adults', Frontiers in Public Health, 2023, 11, p. 1281923
8. Philip, N.Y., Rodrigues, J.J., Wang, H., Fong, S.J., and Chen, J.: 'Internet of things for in-home health monitoring systems: Current advances, challenges and future directions', IEEE Journal on Selected Areas in Communications, 2021, 39, (2), pp. 300–310
9. Fröhlich, H., Bontridder, N., Petrovska-Delacréta, D., Glaab, E., Kluge, F., Yacoubi, M. E., ... and Klucken, J.: 'Leveraging the potential of digital technology

for better individualized treatment of Parkinson's disease', Frontiers in neurology, 2022, 13, p. 788427.

10. Gagnon, M.P., Ouellet, S., Attisso, E., Supper, W., Amil, S., Rhéaume, C., Paquette, J.S., Chabot, C., Laferrière, M.C., and Sasseville, M: 'Wearable devices for supporting chronic disease self-management: Scoping review', Interactive Journal of Medical Research, 2024,13, p. e55925. https://doi.org/10.2196/55925

11. Livingston, G., Huntley, J., Sommerlad, A., Ames, D., Ballard, C., Banerjee, S., Brayne, C., Burns, A., Cohen-Mansfield, J., Cooper, C., Costafreda, S.G., Dias, A., Fox, N., Gitlin, L.N., Howard, R., Kales, H.C., Kivimäki, M., Larson, E.B., Ogunniyi, A., Orgeta, V., Ritchie, K., Rockwood, K., Sampson, E.L., Samus, Q., Schneider, L.S., Selbæk, G., Teri, L., and Mukadam, N.: 'Dementia prevention, intervention, and care: 2020 report of the Lancet Commission', Lancet (London, England), 2020, 396, (10248), pp. 413–446

12. Sheikhtaheri, A., and Sabermahani, F.: 'Applications and outcomes of Internet of Things for patients with Alzheimer's disease/dementia: A scoping review', BioMed Research International, 2022, 2022, p. 6274185

13. Rodrigues, J.J.P.C., Wang, H., Fong, S.J., Philip, N.Y., and Chen, J.: 'Guest editorial: Internet of Things for in-home health monitoring', IEEE Journal on Selected Areas in Communications, 2021, 39, (2), pp. 295–299

14. Dang, S., Golden, A.G., Cheung, H.S., and Roos, B.A.: 'Chapter 128 – Telemedicine Applications in Geriatrics', in Fillit, H.M., Rockwood, K., and Woodhouse, K. (Eds.): 'Brocklehurst's Textbook of Geriatric Medicine and Gerontology (Seventh Edition)' (W.B. Saunders, 2010), pp. 1064–1069

15. Fensli, R., Gunnarson, E., and Gundersen, T.: 'A Wearable ECG-Recording System for Continuous Arrhythmia Monitoring in a Wireless Tele-Home-Care Situation', in Proceedings - IEEE Symposium on Computer-Based Medical Systems (2005), pp. 407–412.

16. Beauchamp, M., Kirkwood, R., Cooper, C., Brown, M., Newbold, K.B., Scott, D., and on behalf of the Mac, M.t.: 'Monitoring mobility in older adults using a Global Positioning System (GPS) smartwatch and accelerometer: A validation study', PLOS ONE, 2023, 18, (12), p. e0296159

17. Singh, G., Doss, R., and Adibi, S.: 'Wearable Tracking: An Effective Smartwatch Approach in Distributed Population Tracking During Pandemics': 'The Science behind the COVID Pandemic and Healthcare Technology Solutions' (Springer, 2022), pp. 235–250. https://doi.org/10.1007/978-3-031-10031-4_12

18. Akl, A., Snoek, J., and Mihailidis, A.: 'Unobtrusive detection of mild cognitive impairment in older adults through home monitoring', IEEE Journal of Biomedical and Health Informatics, 2015, 21, (2), pp. 339–348

19. Bruzzese, R.: 'An Analisys of Application Logs with Splunk: Developing an App for the Synthetic Analysis of Data and Security Incidents' (2019), pp. 1–20. https://doi.org/10.5121/csit.2019.91701

20. Pino, O., Bertoni, E., Diletto, P., Ferrari, L., Gaspari, M., and Pelosi, A.: 'Early detection of cognitive impairment in the general population through a digital tool targeting the prospective memory. A pilot study', Annals of Medicine, 2025, 57, (1), p. 2525389. https://doi.org/10.1080/07853890.2025.2525389

21. Alberdi, A., Weakley, A., Schmitter-Edgecombe, M., Cook, D.J., Aztiria, A., Basarab, A., and Barrenechea, M.: 'Smart home-based prediction of multidomain symptoms related to Alzheimer's disease', IEEE Journal of Biomedical and Health Informatics, 2018, 22, (6), pp. 1720–1731

22. Lazarou, I., Stavropoulos, T.G., Meditskos, G., Andreadis, S., Kompatsiaris, I.Y., and Tsolaki, M.: 'Long-term impact of intelligent monitoring technology on people with cognitive impairment: An observational study', Journal of Alzheimer's Disease, 2019, 70, (3), pp. 757–792

23. Nauha, L., Keränen, N.S., Kangas, M., Jämsä, T., and Reponen, J.: 'Assistive technologies at home for people with a memory disorder', Dementia, 2018, 17, (7), pp. 909–923

24. González-Landero, F., García-Magariño, I., Amariglio, R., and Lacuesta, R.: 'Smart cupboard for assessing memory in home environment', Sensors, 2019, 19, (11), p. 2552

9

Opportunities for Digital Health Solutions in Dementia Care: A Scoping Review

Ayesha Nilashini

9.1 Introduction

Chronic diseases, including diabetes, cardiovascular diseases, such as dementia, are among the leading causes of disability and death globally, presenting substantial challenges for healthcare systems. According to the World Health Organization (WHO), more than 55 million people currently live with dementia worldwide, with over 60% of these cases occurring in low- and middle-income countries. Each year, nearly 10 million new cases of dementia are reported, a number that is expected to grow significantly as populations age and lifestyle factors increase the prevalence of the disease. Dementia has become the seventh leading cause of death globally, contributing to a major public health burden. The impact of these chronic conditions extends beyond physical health, placing severe economic and psychological stress on individuals, families, caregivers, and society at large. On the other hand, in 2019, the global economic cost of dementia alone was estimated to reach US$1.3 trillion, with approximately half of this burden resulting from the informal care provided by family members and friends. On average, informal caregivers spend around five hours per day assisting and supervising those with dementia, further escalating the strain on healthcare systems and productivity losses.

In recent years, digital health solutions have emerged as capable tools to enhance chronic disease management. Leveraging advancements in technologies such as artificial intelligence (AI), 5th Generation (5G) connectivity, and wearable devices, these sophisticated and advanced solutions offer the potential to transform patient care by enabling early and accurate diagnosis (Loi et al., 2023), personalized treatment, and real-time monitoring (Duthie et al., 2024; Jones & Kerber, 2022). Digital health involves a broad range of applications, including AI-driven diagnostic tools, mobile health apps, and telemedicine platforms (Charchar et al., 2024; Gong et al., 2024; Matthews et al., 2020). The primary goal of these solutions is to enhance patient outcomes

DOI: 10.1201/9781003485681-9

and improve overall well-being, which has become increasingly critical in modern healthcare (Borna et al., 2024; Y. Zhang et al., 2024). Traditionally, diagnosis methods of dementia have involved a combination of clinical evaluations, cognitive assessments, and imaging techniques (Benjamin et al., 2021; Vodencarevic et al., 2022). Physicians begin by reviewing the patient's medical history and conducting physical and neurological exams to rule out other conditions (Zhang et al., 2024). However, these traditional methods are often identified as time-consuming and ineffective in diagnosing the disease at an early stage, often requiring observation over time to confirm a diagnosis, which highlights the need for more efficient, technology-driven solutions (Hophing et al., 2024).

Despite these potentials, the adoption of digital health solutions in chronic disease management faces several challenges. The key issues, such as digital literacy, data privacy, and the integration of new technologies into traditional healthcare systems, have slowed widespread implementation (Lim et al., 2022). Furthermore, socio-economic inequalities in technology access continue to create barriers, particularly for the populations in low- and middle-income countries (Stormacq et al., 2020). Addressing these challenges is critical to fully realizing the benefits of digital health innovations.

Grounded in the Diffusion of Innovation (DOI) theory (Rogers, 2003), this scoping review aims to explore the current application of digital health technologies in chronic disease management, with a particular focus on dementia considering published peer-reviewed studies. This study offers novel insights to understand the adoption of digital health solutions in dementia care. Unlike previous reviews, which often focus solely on the benefits of these technologies, this chapter takes a more comprehensive approach by evaluating both opportunities and barriers using a well-established theoretical framework. This perspective allows for a deeper understanding of how digital health solutions can be effectively integrated into real-world healthcare systems, particularly for dementia patients. By examining the opportunities, barriers, and enablers of these technologies, this review seeks to provide actionable insights for advancing the adoption of digital health solutions in healthcare. Specifically, this

This chapter attempts to address the following research questions:

- What are the key innovations in digital health that support the management of dementia?
- What are the primary barriers and enablers to adopting digital health solutions?
- How can emerging technologies such as AI and 5G enhance patient engagement and personalized care in the management of dementia?

Conducting this scoping review is timely and significant, as it offers a comprehensive examination of opportunities for how digital health solutions can address the growing challenges of chronic disease management. By identifying the current gaps and opportunities, this review provides a foundation for future research and development, ultimately contributing to more effective, patient-centered care for individuals living with chronic diseases.

9.2 Methodology

A scoping review of studies that examined digital health solutions, including AI-powered tools, 5G-enabled technologies, and wearable devices, for the management of chronic diseases, particularly dementia, was conducted using the databases MEDLINE, EMBASE, PubMed, SCOPUS, and Google Scholar. A search strategy was developed using keywords related to below core concepts and dividing the search into Digital Health, AI, Cognitive Training, and Telemedicine allows for a structured and comprehensive review of literature that targets both broad and specific aspects of digital health interventions (see Table 9.1).

- Digital health
- Dementia
- AI
- Cognitive training
- Telemedicine

TABLE 9.1

Keywords for Scoping Review

Concept	Keywords
Digital health	"Digital health" OR "mHealth" OR "eHealth" OR "mobile health" OR "telehealth" OR "telemedicine" OR "wearable devices" OR "remote monitoring" OR "digital solutions" OR "mobile applications" OR "health apps"
Dementia	"Dementia" OR "Alzheimer" OR "cognitive impairment" OR "memory loss" OR "cognitive decline" OR "intellectual impairment" OR "mental deficiency"
Artificial intelligence	"Artificial intelligence" OR "analytics"
Cognitive training	"Cognitive training" OR "cognitive apps" OR "memory training" OR "brain training" OR "cognitive function improvement"
Telemedicine	"Telemedicine" OR "telehealth" OR "remote consultation" OR "remote care" OR "virtual care" OR "video consultation") ("Telemedicine" OR "telehealth" OR "remote consultation" OR "remote care" OR "virtual care" OR "teleconsultation" OR "video consultation"

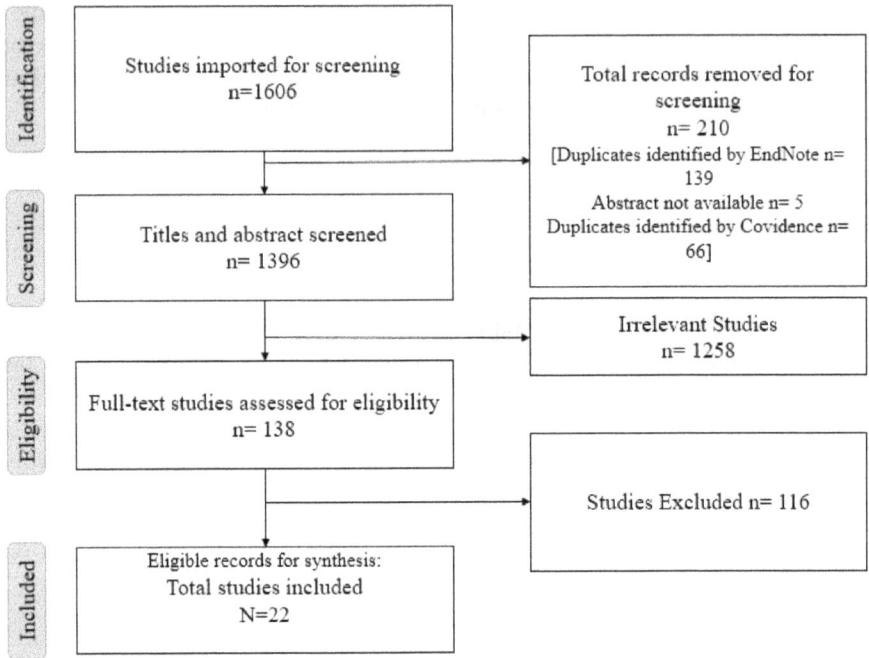

FIGURE 9.1
Scoping review flow diagram.

The search results were imported into EndNote to remove duplicates, after which the records were uploaded into Covidence software for screening. Each article's title and abstract were screened according to predefined inclusion and exclusion criteria (see Appendix A). Articles that passed the title and abstract screening underwent full-text review considering certain inclusion and exclusion criteria. Following this, data extraction from the included full-text articles was conducted using a data extraction form developed. Thematic analysis was employed to analyze the extracted data, focusing on the use of digital health innovations such as AI, telemedicine, and wearable devices, specifically in dementia care. The analysis also identified barriers and enablers to the adoption and implementation of these technologies. The scoping review was conducted in accordance with the Preferred Reporting Items for Systematic Reviews and Meta-Analyses (PRISMA) guidelines, as illustrated in Figure 9.1.

9.3 Analysis and Results

This section presents the key findings from the scoping review, focusing on digital health interventions that support the management of dementia, which serves as a case study for dementia management. The thematic analysis revealed key opportunities for digital health in dementia care, specifically in areas such as early diagnosis, patient engagement, caregiver support, and personalized care. Table 9.2 presents a summary of the characteristics of the included articles for this study.

Out of the 22 studies included in the review, 10 studies specifically focused on dementia as a disease. The included articles in this scoping review were published between 2020 and 2024. The trend indicates an increasing interest in the application of digital health and emerging technologies in dementia care over recent years. Approximately 55% of the articles were published in the last two years (2023–2024), reflecting a rising trend as research and technology in the field mature. The focus of these articles varied, with many exploring the use of AI, wearable devices, and telemedicine for dementia

TABLE 9.2

Overview of the Included Studies

Characteristics	Number of Studies (n = 22)
Year of Publication	
2020	5
2021	2
2022	3
2023	5
2024	7
Location	
High-income countries (HIC)	20
High-income countries/low-middle-income countries (HIC/ LMIC):	2
Dementia Focus	
Alzheimer's disease	4
Mixed dementia types	8
General dementia focus	10
Key Themes	
(1) Early Diagnosis and Monitoring Using AI	7
(2) Cognitive Training Apps for Dementia Management	5
(3) Caregiver Support via Telemedicine	6
(4) Barriers to Adoption of Digital Health in Dementia Care	9
Dementia Areas	
Diagnosis and Monitoring	13
Cognitive Training Applications	4
Caregiver Support and Telemedicine	7
Treatment and Intervention	4

care. Notably, most of the included studies were conducted in high-income countries, highlighting the gap in research contributions from low- and middle-income settings. The findings highlight an evolving emphasis on leveraging emerging technologies to improve dementia care and support.

9.3.1 Assessment of Digital Health Technologies in Dementia Care

Figure 9.2 presents an overview of the primary digital health technologies utilized in the included studies. Among the 22 studies, most focused on AI-powered diagnostic tools and cognitive support interventions for dementia care, reflecting a growing trend toward the adoption of digital technologies in healthcare. The studies were categorized into four major groups based on the technology type, early diagnosis and monitoring using AI, cognitive training applications, caregiver support via telemedicine, and barriers to adoption of digital health.

The technologies used in these studies are classified into three categories: AI-powered tools, cognitive training applications, and telemedicine.

AI-powered tools for diagnosis and monitoring were primarily used for early detection of dementia symptoms and included machine learning algorithms such as supervised and unsupervised learning. Supervised algorithms, such as decision trees and support vector machines, were commonly used for classification tasks to differentiate between various stages of dementia (Dumitrascu & Koronyo-Hamaoui, 2020; Jones et al., 2024). Principal Component Analysis (PCA), a commonly applied unsupervised learning algorithm, was used in some studies for reducing data dimensionality, which facilitated feature extraction from neuroimaging data (Carlson et al., 2022; Jones et al., 2024).

Cognitive training applications were implemented to enhance cognitive functioning and delay cognitive decline in patients diagnosed with dementia or those at risk of developing dementia. Apps and games aimed at cognitive enhancement, such as memory exercises, were frequently employed, and their effectiveness was assessed based on improvements in cognitive test scores (Azar et al., 2024; Harrell et al., 2023). These applications included AI-powered interventions specifically designed for memory and cognition, which showed benefits in enhancing cognitive performance among older adults (Kedar & Khazanchi, 2023). However, some studies highlighted barriers to wider adoption, such as usability challenges and the need for cultural adaptations (Azar et al., 2024).

Telemedicine, often integrated with wearable health monitoring devices (Artese et al., 2023), was a popular approach for providing support to dementia patients and their caregivers. Six studies focused on leveraging telehealth to maintain continuity of care, especially during the early to moderate stages of the disease (Jones et al., 2024; Puterman et al., 2021; Rosenlund et al., 2023). The use of wearable devices to collect real-time health data also supported telemedicine applications, improving caregiver involvement and

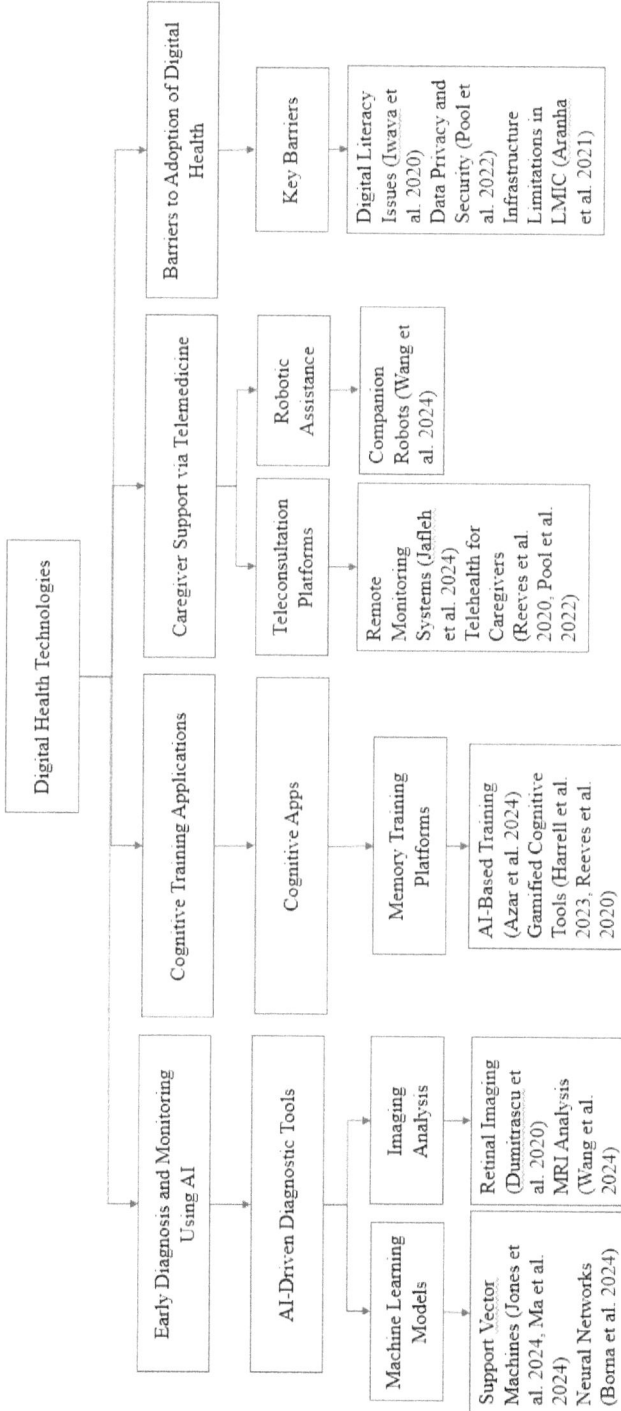

FIGURE 9.2
Overview of the primary digital health technologies used in the included studies.

reducing the burden of in-person visits (Chinese Society of Cardiology, 2024; Jafleh et al., 2024). These solutions were especially beneficial in facilitating patient management and providing resources for caregivers to better handle daily care demands (Borna et al., 2024).

Several challenges were frequently discussed across the studies, including digital literacy, data privacy concerns, and technology integration into existing healthcare systems. Digital literacy posed a significant barrier for older adults, limiting their ability to effectively use digital health tools (Grossman et al., 2020; Iwaya et al., 2020). Data privacy and security concerns were also highlighted as major challenges, particularly regarding how health data is managed and safeguarded (Pool et al., 2022). Studies emphasized the need for enhanced privacy frameworks and technology education programs to increase acceptance and usability among elderly patients, ensuring that technologies are accessible and user-friendly (Harrell et al., 2023; Yang et al., 2020) (see Table 9.3).

Figure 9.3 depicts the distribution of sample sizes across the studies. Most studies were conducted with fewer than 500 participants, which indicates a significant limitation regarding the generalizability of findings. Only two studies included more than 1000 participants, highlighting that sample size constraints remain a considerable barrier to validating the effectiveness of digital health interventions in dementia care.

The analysis of sample sizes in the reviewed studies shows considerable variability. Of the 22 studies, 2 had less than 50 participants, while 3 had between 50 and 100, and another 3 had between 101 and 500 participants. Only 1 study included 501–1000 participants, and 2 studies had more than 1000 participants. This variability indicates that while some research is scaling up, many studies remain limited, which impacts the generalizability of the findings. Future research should prioritize larger, well-defined sample sizes for more reliable conclusions.

9.3.2 Key Drivers for Adoption of Digital Health in Dementia Care

The successful adoption of digital health technologies in dementia care relies on several key drivers that influence their acceptance and use. These drivers are rooted in the benefits that digital health solutions provide to patients, caregivers, and healthcare systems. Table 9.4 outlines the key drivers for adopting digital health in dementia care, supported by recent literature.

9.4 Discussion

The novelty of this research lies in its combined use of emerging technologies like AI, 5G, and wearable devices, underpinned by the DOI Theory, to address specific barriers in dementia care. Unlike existing reviews, which focus on either the opportunities or the limitations of these technologies, this chapter

TABLE 9.3

Barriers to Digital Health Adoption

Barrier	Description	References	Cases from Data Extraction	Limitations
Low digital literacy	Low digital literacy among elderly users and caregivers hinders the effective use of digital health tools.	Rosenlund et al. (2023); Elaine C. Jones et al. (2024); Grossman et al. (2020); Harrell et al. (2023)	Rosenlund et al. and Elaine C. Jones et al. discussed the impact of low digital literacy on using telemedicine and mobile health apps, especially among elderly populations. Grossman et al. and Harrell et al. highlighted the need for extensive training, which is resource-intensive and often unfeasible.	Resource-intensive training requirements are often not feasible.
Privacy and data security concerns	Concerns over data privacy and security, particularly in AI and wearable devices, limit user adoption.	Iwaya et al. (2020); Puterman et al. (2021); Pool et al. (2022); Borna et al. (2024); Changsheng Ma et al. (2024)	Iwaya et al. and Pool et al. identified privacy as a major barrier to adoption, especially in wearable devices. Puterman et al. and Borna et al. emphasized users' concerns about personal data usage. Changsheng Ma et al. highlighted challenges in regulatory frameworks for managing patient data.	Lack of comprehensive data governance frameworks.
Connectivity and infrastructure limitations	Lack of high-speed internet and robust infrastructure limits the scalability and reach of digital health solutions.	Rosenlund et al. (2023); Elaine C. Jones et al. (2024)	Rosenlund et al. and Elaine C. Jones et al. pointed out that connectivity issues, especially in low-resource settings, hinder access to telemedicine and remote monitoring services. The lack of infrastructure for advanced technologies, such as real-time monitoring and cloud-based AI, is a significant barrier.	Limited scalability due to inadequate infrastructure.
Data accuracy and technical immaturity	Errors in data collection and the immaturity of AI diagnostic tools raise doubts about the reliability of digital health technologies.	Artese et al. (2023); Jafleh et al. (2024); Weixuan Wang et al. (2024); Dumitrascu & Koronyo-Hamaoui (2020)	Artese et al. and Jafleh et al. highlighted concerns regarding the accuracy of data generated by wearable devices. Weixuan Wang et al. and Dumitrascu & Koronyo-Hamaoui discussed the immaturity of AI diagnostic tools, particularly their reliability in clinical environments.	Data errors and concerns about AI reliability reduce trust among users and healthcare providers.

(Continued)

TABLE 9.3 (*Continued*)

Barriers to Digital Health Adoption

Barrier	Description	References	Cases from Data Extraction	Limitations
Cultural barriers	Lack of culturally adapted interventions limits the effectiveness of digital health solutions, particularly among diverse populations.	Azar et al. (2024)	Azar et al. emphasized that cultural factors, including varying expectations and norms, are significant barriers to the adoption of digital health technologies. Demographic factors such as age and socio-economic status further contribute to disparities in adoption.	Limited research on culturally adapted digital interventions.
User Engagement and Usability Challenges	Cognitive challenges, technical difficulties, and stigma hinder effective user engagement and usability of digital health solutions.	Hocking et al. (2022); Aranha et al. (2021); Grossman et al. (2020); Harrell et al. (2023)	Hocking et al. and Aranha et al. discussed usability challenges, including cognitive difficulties and lack of personalization. Grossman et al. and Harrell et al. noted that negative attitudes, forgetfulness, and technical challenges further reduce adherence to digital health solutions, especially among older adults and their caregivers.	Stigma and technical challenges reduce the adoption rates of digital health technologies.
Integration into Healthcare Workflows	Lack of standard protocols for integrating digital health tools with traditional healthcare systems impedes seamless adoption.	Kedar & Khazanchi (2023)	Bernardo et al. noted the absence of standard protocols for incorporating digital health tools into existing healthcare systems, making integration challenging. Kedar & Khazanchi highlighted the lack of training opportunities for healthcare professionals, further complicating effective integration.	Difficulty in integrating digital health tools into existing healthcare workflows.
Cost Barriers	High costs of wearable devices, AI-powered tools, and specialized training limit adoption, particularly in low-income settings.	Jafleh et al. (2024); Yang et al. (2020)	Jafleh et al. and Yang et al. highlighted the high costs of wearable devices and AI-powered applications as substantial barriers to adoption. This is particularly significant in low- and middle-income regions where financial resources are already limited.	High upfront and maintenance costs limit adoption in resource-constrained settings.
Lack of Comprehensive Evaluation	Absence of large-scale studies on the safety, efficacy, and long-term impact of digital health solutions reduces user trust and confidence.	Zhang et al. (2024); Yang et al. (2020); Carlson et al. (2022); Dumitrascu & Koronyo-Hamaoui (2020)	Zhang et al. and Yang et al. highlighted the lack of comprehensive evaluations of safety and long-term impact, affecting trust. Carlson et al. discussed issues like practice effects that limit the credibility of digital health assessment in trials. Dumitrascu & Koronyo-Hamaoui mentioned the variability in study designs that affects reliability.	Lack of established safety standards and evidence of long-term benefits.

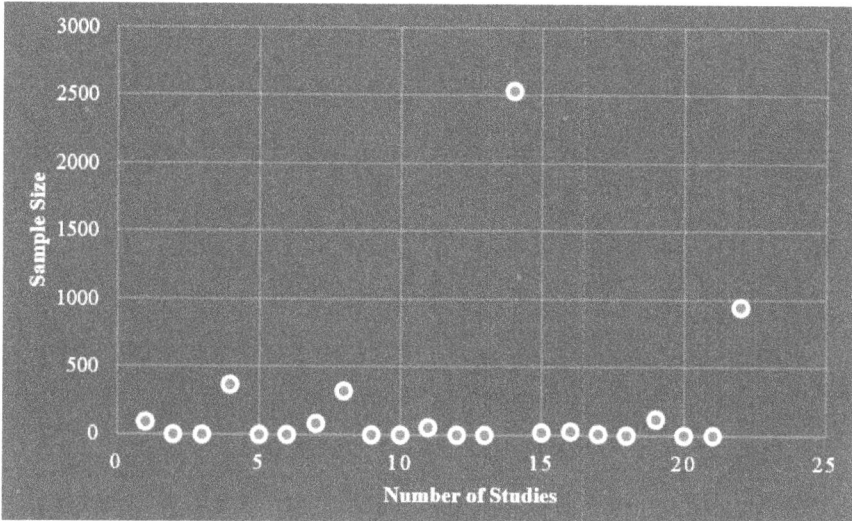

FIGURE 9.3
Distribution of the sample sizes.

integrates both perspectives, providing a holistic understanding of how to enhance dementia care. The focus on practical strategies for implementation adds a unique dimension not previously explored in existing literature.

The findings from this scoping review highlight the significant potential of digital health solutions to enhance dementia care. By exploring interventions such as cognitive training applications, AI-based monitoring tools, and telemedicine platforms, this review highlights how these technologies can contribute to improving patient outcomes, reducing caregiver burden, and facilitating early diagnosis. Despite these promising developments, several barriers must be addressed to ensure widespread adoption and effective implementation of these solutions in practice.

The findings from this review are particularly relevant in the post-COVID-19 era, where remote health monitoring and telemedicine have become essential components of care delivery. The pandemic has accelerated the adoption of digital health solutions, providing an opportunity to reimagine dementia care in a way that prioritizes accessibility, continuity, and patient-centered approaches. This context highlights the increasing importance of telehealth and wearable devices in managing chronic conditions like dementia.

9.4.1 Diffusion of Innovation Framework and Digital Health Solutions

In this study, the DOI theory provides a useful lens for understanding the adoption of digital health solutions, particularly in dementia care. DOI highlights five key factors: relative advantage, compatibility, complexity, trialability, and observability that influence how innovations diffuse within healthcare systems (see Table 9.5).

TABLE 9.4

Key Drivers for Adoption of Digital Health in Dementia Care

Enabler	Description	References	Cases from Data Extraction	Impact
Support for Self-Management and Access	Support for self-management and improved access to health services promote digital health adoption among patients and caregivers.	Rosenlund et al. (2023); Jafleh et al. (2024); Elaine C. Jones et al. (2024)	Rosenlund et al. highlighted improved accessibility through digital solutions, which enhances patient engagement and adherence. Jafleh et al. and Elaine C. Jones et al. discussed the convenience provided by remote access to health services through telemedicine, wearable devices, and mobile apps, reducing the need for frequent in-person visits.	Enhanced patient engagement and reduced healthcare burden.
Personalization of Digital Solutions	Personalized health recommendations and adaptable digital health solutions increase adherence and improve outcomes.	Puterman et al. (2021); Artese et al. (2024); Azar et al. (2024); Hocking et al. (2022)	Puterman et al. emphasized the significance of personalization in improving adherence. Artese et al. and Azar et al. discussed the importance of culturally adapted digital health solutions, while Hocking et al. highlighted customization features such as avatars to increase user engagement.	Increased adherence to health plans and improved health outcomes.
AI-Powered Tools for Diagnosis and Monitoring	AI tools that provide non-invasive imaging and monitoring enhance diagnostic accuracy and reduce clinician workload.	Dumitrascu & Koronyo-Hamaoui (2020); Borna et al. (2024)	Dumitrascu & Koronyo-Hamaoui discussed AI-based tools for non-invasive imaging, improving specificity and sensitivity in early diagnosis. Borna et al. highlighted AI tools' ability to support decision-making, reducing clinician burden.	Improved diagnostic accuracy and reduced clinician workload.
Improved Access, Cost Savings, and Flexibility	Remote monitoring systems provide real-time tracking of patient health, facilitating early interventions and promoting continuity of care.	Elaine C. Jones et al. (2024); Carlson et al. (2022); Zhang et al. (2024)	Elaine C. Jones et al. highlighted remote monitoring systems for early intervention. Carlson et al. discussed remote testing and digital phenotyping as convenient methods for cognitive health monitoring. Zhang et al. highlighted real-time health monitoring as a means to promote continuous care.	Facilitated early interventions and continuous monitoring of patient health.
Positive Perceptions and Support	Awareness of the benefits of digital health tools, healthcare provider encouragement, and social support foster positive attitudes toward technology adoption.	Kedar & Khazanchi (2023); Yang et al. (2020); Aranha et al. (2021)	Kedar & Khazanchi emphasized awareness and satisfaction with digital tools as a key enabler for adoption. Yang et al. discussed the positive perception of AI-powered tools, while Aranha et al. highlighted the importance of healthcare provider encouragement and social support in increasing technology adoption, especially among hesitant patients.	Improved user satisfaction and increased adoption rates.

Category	Description	References	Discussion	Outcome
Regulatory Frameworks	Data privacy and security regulations boost user confidence and promote ethical use of digital health technologies.	Pool et al. (2022); Changsheng Ma et al. (2024); Weixuan Wang et al. (2024)	Pool et al. highlighted the importance of privacy and informed consent practices. Changsheng Ma et al. and Weixuan Wang et al. emphasized the role of regulatory frameworks and industry standards in supporting secure healthcare ecosystems, thereby fostering greater adoption.	Enhanced user trust and confidence in digital health solutions.
Advances in Telemedicine and Wearables	Wearable devices and telemedicine enable real-time health monitoring, maintain continuity of care, and reduce caregiver burden.	Changsheng Ma et al. (2024); Puterman et al. (2021)	Changsheng Ma et al. highlighted wearable technologies for continuous health monitoring. Puterman et al. discussed the role of telemedicine in maintaining care continuity and reducing caregiver burden, allowing healthcare providers to make informed decisions based on real-time data.	Maintained continuity of care and reduced burden on caregivers.
Age-Specific Services	Age-specific digital health services improve usability for older adults and bridge the technology gap in dementia care.	Loi et al. (2023); Iwaya et al. (2020)	Loi et al. highlighted age-specific diagnostic tools that cater to older individuals, making digital health more user-friendly. Iwaya et al. emphasized context-sensitive services that ensure interventions are relevant within different healthcare settings.	Enhanced usability and improved health outcomes for older adults.
Adaptive Technologies	Adaptive technologies, such as reminder systems, enhance support for elderly users, helping to overcome cognitive challenges and forgetfulness.	Harrell et al. (2023); Zhang et al. (2024)	Harrell et al. highlighted adaptive reminder systems for elderly users. Zhang et al. discussed interactive communication features in remote monitoring systems that enhance user satisfaction and intervention efficacy.	Increased user satisfaction and effective health management support for elderly users.
Cultural Adaptations	Culturally adapted digital health solutions enhance inclusivity and improve intervention outcomes by addressing demographic diversity.	Azar et al. (2024)	Azar et al. discussed the importance of cultural adaptation for improving inclusivity and effectiveness of digital health interventions. Culturally informed interventions were found to be crucial for addressing barriers related to demographic diversity and ensuring all populations benefit from digital health innovations.	Increased inclusivity and improved health outcomes in diverse populations.

TABLE 9.5

Application of Diffusion of Innovation (DOI) Theory to Digital Health Solutions in Dementia Care

DOI Element	Description	Findings from the Review
Innovation	The degree to which a new technology is perceived as novel or advanced.	The innovations discussed included AI-powered diagnostic tools, cognitive training applications, and telemedicine. These were perceived as valuable for early diagnosis, personalized care, and enhanced caregiver support (Jones et al., 2024; Reeves et al., 2020). However, technology acceptance is hindered by privacy and digital literacy concerns (Dumitrascu & Koronyo-Hamaoui, 2020; Iwaya et al., 2020).
Compatibility	The extent to which an innovation aligns with the existing values, experiences, and needs of potential adopters.	Many studies highlighted compatibility with the needs of elderly patients and caregivers. Telemedicine and wearable devices fit well with current care practices but require adaptation to individual user capabilities, particularly for older adults with limited digital literacy (Harrell et al., 2023; Kedar & Khazanchi, 2023).
Complexity	The perceived difficulty of understanding and using the innovation.	The digital health solutions varied in complexity. Cognitive training apps were found to be relatively user-friendly, while AI-based monitoring tools required significant training for both healthcare providers and caregivers, indicating a higher perceived complexity (Azar et al., 2024; Pool et al., 2022).
Trialability	The opportunity to test the innovation before full adoption.	Few studies emphasized trialability. In several cases, digital health tools were piloted with small groups of users, allowing stakeholders to assess feasibility (Hocking et al., 2023; Yang et al., 2020). Limited trials were reported, especially for AI-driven tools, which might have reduced broader adoption willingness.
Observability	The extent to which the results of an innovation are visible to others.	Improvements in patient outcomes, such as enhanced cognitive function and better health monitoring, were documented in some studies, contributing to the observability of the benefits (Loi et al., 2023; Puterman et al., 2021). However, the lack of large-scale studies limited the broader visibility of successful outcomes (J. Zhang et al., 2024).
Relative advantage	The perceived benefits of the innovation compared to existing solutions.	AI tools and telemedicine demonstrated clear advantages over traditional diagnosis and caregiving methods. They provided timely, data-driven insights and remote care options, offering significant advantages in terms of accuracy and convenience over traditional care models (Jafleh et al., 2024; Rosenlund et al., 2023).

TABLE 9.5 *(Continued)*

Application of Diffusion of Innovation (DOI) Theory to Digital Health Solutions in Dementia Care

DOI Element	Description	Findings from the Review
Facilitators	Factors that promote adoption, such as training and support.	Facilitators for adoption included user training, caregiver involvement, and integration of clinician input during the design of technologies. Regulatory support and privacy frameworks were also noted as important enablers in increasing trust and facilitating the use of digital health tools (Kedar & Khazanchi, 2023).
Barriers	Challenges preventing adoption such as privacy and digital literacy concerns.	The key barriers included data privacy issues, limited digital literacy among older adults, and difficulties in integrating new technologies into existing healthcare systems. Such barriers were frequently highlighted, suggesting a need for educational initiatives and better regulatory standards to overcome these issues (Carlson et al., 2022; Reeves et al., 2020).

9.4.2 Ethical and Regulatory Considerations

The rapid integration of digital health solutions such as AI-powered diagnostic tools and wearable devices into dementia care raises important ethical and regulatory questions. As AI becomes more prevalent in healthcare, concerns about data privacy, algorithmic transparency, and patient autonomy must be addressed (Iwaya et al., 2020). Elderly dementia patients, who often have limited capacity to understand the complexities of digital health technologies, are particularly vulnerable. Ensuring informed consent and maintaining patient trust are critical. In addition, regulations such as the General Data Protection Regulation (GDPR) and the Health Insurance Portability and Accountability Act (HIPAA) govern the collection, storage, and sharing of sensitive health data, but further guidelines tailored specifically to AI applications are needed (Jafleh et al., 2024; Pool et al., 2022). To ensure the safe and ethical use of digital health technologies, developers must adhere to these regulations while incorporating robust security measures to protect patient data. Transparency in how AI algorithms make clinical decisions can help mitigate the "black box" problem and improve trust among both patients and healthcare providers. Moving forward, interdisciplinary collaboration between healthcare professionals, technologists, and policymakers will be essential to create an ethical framework that supports innovation without compromising patient rights.

The practical managerial implications of adopting digital health solutions in dementia care are significant. By enabling early diagnosis, continuous monitoring, and enhanced caregiver support, these technologies can alleviate the burden on healthcare professionals and optimize resource allocation.

Specifically, AI-powered diagnostic tools can streamline the initial screening process, allowing healthcare providers to focus on advanced care needs, while telemedicine platforms offer a means for maintaining continuity of care even in remote locations. Managers in healthcare settings can utilize these technologies to reduce operational costs, minimize hospital admissions, and improve overall patient satisfaction. Additionally, by understanding and addressing the barriers identified, such as data privacy and digital literacy, healthcare administrators can design targeted intervention programs to improve the accessibility and adoption of digital health technologies, particularly for elderly patients and caregivers.

9.4.3 Future Directions and Research Gaps

While the findings of this review focus on the potential of digital health solutions in dementia care, significant gaps remain for further exploration. One critical area for future research is the scalability of AI-powered diagnostic tools across diverse populations, particularly in low- and middle-income countries where access to advanced technologies may be limited. The potential of digital twins, which offer individualized simulations for patient care, is another promising avenue that should be explored more thoroughly in the context of dementia management. Additionally, research should focus on enhancing the accessibility of cognitive training apps for elderly patients, addressing digital literacy barriers through simplified interfaces and targeted education programs. Collaboration between healthcare providers and technologists will be essential to develop digital solutions that seamlessly integrate into existing clinical workflows. Lastly, as AI continues to evolve, there is a pressing need for longitudinal studies to evaluate the long-term effectiveness of these technologies in improving patient outcomes and reducing healthcare costs.

9.5 Conclusion

This scoping review explored the application of digital health solutions in dementia care, with a particular focus on cognitive training applications, AI-based monitoring tools, and telemedicine platforms. The review revealed that these digital health solutions hold significant potential to improve patient outcomes, alleviate caregiver burden, and promote early diagnosis in dementia care. However, the adoption of these innovations is still at an early stage, and barriers such as digital literacy, data privacy concerns, and resistance from healthcare professionals must be addressed.

The DOI framework provided valuable insights into the factors influencing the adoption of digital health solutions. It highlighted that while these innovations show clear relative advantages, their complexity and digital literacy requirements pose challenges to widespread adoption, particularly among elderly patients. Additionally, the review identified the potential for AI-powered tools to significantly enhance early diagnosis and continuous monitoring of dementia patients, but the implementation of these tools is limited by the small sample sizes and data availability in many studies.

Moreover, telemedicine platforms have proven to be highly beneficial in supporting caregivers, reducing their burden, and providing access to much-needed resources. This finding emphasizes the importance of expanding telemedicine solutions not only in dementia care but also in other chronic disease management settings, where caregivers play a crucial role in patient outcomes.

References

Artese, A., Rawat, R., & Sung, A. (2023). The use of commercial wrist-worn technology to track physiological outcomes in behavioral interventions. *Curr Opin Clin Nutr Metab Care, 26*(6), 534–540. https://doi.org/10.1097/MCO.0000000000000970

Azar, M., Stelmokas, J., Stringer, A., & Arias, F. (2024). Nonpharmacological treatment for older adults with mild cognitive impairment: Considerations for culturally informed clinical practice and research. *Neuropsychology, 38*(7), 609–621. https://doi.org/10.1037/neu0000965

Benjamin, E., Go, A., Desvigne-Nickens, P., Anderson, C., Casadei, B., Chen, L., Crijns, H., Freedman, B., Hills, M., Healey, J., Kamel, H., Kim, D.-Y., Link, M., Lopes, R., Lubitz, S., McManus, D., Noseworthy, P., Perez, M., Piccini, J., Schnabel, R., Singer, D., Tieleman, R., Turakhia, M., Van Gelder, I., Cooper, L., Al-Khatib, S. (2021). Research priorities in atrial fibrillation screening: A report from a national heart, lung, and blood institute virtual workshop. *Circulation, 143*(4), 372–388. https://doi.org/10.1161/CIRCULATIONAHA.120.047633

Bernardo, J., Apostolo, J., Loureiro, R., Santana, E., Yaylagul, N. K., Dantas, C., Ventura, F., Duque, F. M., Jøranson, N., & Zechner, M. (2022). eHealth platforms to promote autonomous life and active aging: A scoping review. *Int J Environ Res Public Health, 19*(23), 15940. https://mdpi-res.com/d_attachment/ijerph/ijerph-19-15940/article_deploy/ijerph-19-15940-v2.pdf?version=1669886062

Borna, S., Maniaci, M. J., Haider, C. R., Gomez-Cabello, C. A., Pressman, S. M., Haider, S. A., Demaerschalk, B. M., Cowart, J. B., & Forte, A. J. (2024). Artificial intelligence support for informal patient caregivers: A systematic review. *Bioengineering (Basel), 11*(5), 483. https://doi.org/10.3390/bioengineering11050483

Carlson, S., Kim, H., Devanand, D., & Goldberg, T. (2022). Novel approaches to measuring neurocognitive functions in Alzheimer's disease clinical trials. *Curr Opin Neurol, 35*(2), 240–248. https://doi.org/10.1097/WCO.0000000000001041

Charchar, F., Prestes, P., Mills, C., Ching, S., Neupane, D., Marques, F., Sharman, J., Vogt, L., Burrell, L., Korostovtseva, L., Zec, M., Patil, M., Schultz, M., Wallen, M., Renna, N., Islam, S., Hiremath, S., Gyeltshen, T., Chia, Y.-C.,

Gupta, A., Schutte, A., Klein, B., Borghi, C., Browning, C., Czesnikiewicz-Guzik, M., Lee, H.-Y., Itoh, H., Miura, K., Brunstrom, M., Campbell, N., Akinnibossun, O., Veerabhadrappa, P., Wainford, R., Kruger, R., Thomas, S., Komori, T., Ralapanawa, U., Cornelissen, V., Kapil, V., Li, Y., Zhang, Y., Jafar, T., Khan, N., Williams, B., Stergiou, G., & Tomaszewski, M. (2024). Lifestyle management of hypertension: International Society of Hypertension position chapter endorsed by the World Hypertension League and European Society of Hypertension. *J Hypertens*, 42(1), 23–49. https://doi.org/10.1097/HJH.0000000000003563

Chinese Society of Cardiology, C. (2024). Chinese Guidelines for the diagnosis and management of atrial fibrillation. *Cardiol Discov*, 4(2), 89–133. https://doi.org/10.1097/CD9.0000000000000123

Dumitrascu, O., & Koronyo-Hamaoui, M. (2020). Retinal vessel changes in cerebrovascular disease. *Curr Opin Neurol*, 33(1), 87–92. https://doi.org/10.1097/WCO.0000000000000779

Duthie, N., Ansari, K., Wang, M., & Ray, P. (2024). Design of a shared context-aware assistive robot for personalised aged-care services. *Digit. Med. 10*(1). https://doi.org/10.1097/DM-2023-00017

Gong, P., Chen, X., Zhou, T., Tian, Y., & Su, M. (2024). Digital twin prevalence in the medical caring fields: A bibliomatrics study and visualization analysis through CiteSpace. *Interdiscip Nurs Res*, 3(2), 126–134. https://doi.org/10.1097/NR9.0000000000000062

Grossman, J., Frumkin, M., Rodebaugh, T., & Lenze, E. (2020). mHealth assessment and intervention of depression and anxiety in older adults. *Harv Rev Psychiatry*, 28(3), 203–214. https://doi.org/10.1097/HRP.0000000000000255

Harrell, E., Roque, N., & Boot, W. (2023). Comparing the effectiveness of two theory-based strategies to promote cognitive training adherence. *J Exp Psychol Appl*, 29(4), 782–792. https://doi.org/10.1037/xap0000485

Hocking, J., Oster, C., Maeder, A., & Lange, B. (2023). Design, development, and use of conversational agents in rehabilitation for adults with brain-related neurological conditions: A scoping review. *JBI Evid Synth*, 21(2), 326–372. https://doi.org/10.11124/JBIES-22-00025

Hophing, L., Tse, T., Naimer, N., Masellis, M., Mirza, S., Izenberg, A., Khosravani, H., Kassardjian, C., & Mitchell, S. (2024). Virtual compared with in-person neurologic examination study. *Neurol Clin Pract*, 14(6), e200339. https://doi.org/10.1212/CPJ.0000000000200339

Iwaya, L. H., Ahmad, A., & Babar, M. A. (2020). Security and privacy for mHealth and uHealth systems: A systematic mapping study. *IEEE Access*, 8, 150081–150112.

Jafleh, E. A., Alnaqbi, F. A., Almaeeni, H. A., Faqeeh, S., Alzaabi, M. A., Al Zaman, K., Alnaqbi, F., Almaeeni, H., & Alzaabi, M. (2024). The role of wearable devices in chronic disease monitoring and patient care: A comprehensive review. *Cureus*, 16(9), e68921. https://doi.org/10.7759/cureus.68921.

Jones, D., & Kerber, K. (2022). Artificial intelligence and the practice of neurology in 2035: The neurology future forecasting series. *Neurology*, 98(6), 238–245. https://doi.org/10.1212/WNL.0000000000013200

Jones, E., F., Kummer, B., & Wilkinson, J. (2024). Teleneurology and artificial intelligence in clinical practice. *Continuum*, 30(3), 904–914. https://doi.org/10.1212/CON.0000000000001430

Kedar, S., & Khazanchi, D. (2023). Neurology education in the era of artificial intelligence. *Curr Opin Neurol, 36*(1), 51–58. https://doi.org/10.1097/WCO.0000000000001130

Lim, J., Hong, M., Lam, W., Zhang, Z., Teo, Z., Liu, Y., Ng, W., Foo, L., & Ting, D. (2022). Novel technical and privacy-preserving technology for artificial intelligence in ophthalmology. *Curr Opin Ophthalmol, 33*(3), 174–187. https://doi.org/10.1097/ICU.0000000000000846

Loi, S., Pijnenburg, Y., & Velakoulis, D. (2023). Recent research advances in young-onset dementia. *Curr Opin Psychiatry, 36*(2), 126–133. https://doi.org/10.1097/YCO.0000000000000843

Matthews, P., Block, V., & Leocani, L. (2020). E-health and multiple sclerosis. *Curr Opin Neurol, 33*(3), 271–276. https://doi.org/10.1097/WCO.0000000000000823

Pool, J., Akhlaghpour, S., Fatehi, F., & Gray, L. C. (2022). Data privacy concerns and use of telehealth in the aged care context: An integrative review and research agenda. *Int J Med Inform, 160*, 104707.

Puterman, E., Pauly, T., Ruissen, G., Nelson, B., & Faulkner, G. (2021). Move more, move better: A narrative review of wearable technologies and their application to precision health. *Health Psychol, 40*(11), 803–810. https://doi.org/10.1037/hea0001125

Reeves, S., Williams, V., Costela, F., Palumbo, R., Umoren, O., Christopher, M., Blacker, D., & Woods, R. (2020). Narrative video scene description task discriminates between levels of cognitive impairment in Alzheimer's disease. *Neuropsychology, 34*(4), 437–446. https://doi.org/10.1037/neu0000621

Rogers, E. M. (2003). *Diffusion of innovations* (5th ed.). Free Press.

Rosenlund, M., Kinnunen, U.-M., & Saranto, K. (2023). The use of digital health services among patients and citizens living at home: Scoping review. *J Med Internet Res, 25*, e44711.

Stormacq, C., Wosinski, J., Boillat, E., & Van den Broucke, S. (2020). Effects of health literacy interventions on health-related outcomes in socioeconomically disadvantaged adults living in the community: A systematic review. *JBI Evid Synth, 18*(7), 1389–1469. https://doi.org/10.11124/JBISRIR-D-18-00023

Vodencarevic, A., Weingartner, M., Caro, J., Ukalovic, D., Zimmermann-Rittereiser, M., Dipl-Ing, M. B. M., Schwab, S., Md, P., Kolominsky-Rabas, P., & Md, P. (2022). Prediction of recurrent ischemic stroke using registry data and machine learning methods: The Erlangen stroke registry. *Stroke, 53*(7), 2299–2306. https://doi.org/10.1161/STROKEAHA.121.036557

Yang, Y., Chen, H., Qazi, H. A., & Morita, P. P. (2020). Intervention and evaluation of mobile health (mHealth) technologies in chronic dialysis patient management: A scoping review. *JMIR Mhealth Uhealth, 8*, e15549.

Zhang, H., Jiao, L., Yang, S., Li, H., Jiang, X., Feng, J., Zou, S., Xu, Q., Gu, J., Wang, X., & Wei, B. (2024). Brain-computer interfaces: The innovative key to unlocking neurological conditions. *Int J Surg, 110*(9), 5745–5762. https://doi.org/10.1097/JS9.0000000000002022

Zhang, Y., Luo, L., & Wang, X. (2024). Aging with robots: A brief review on eldercare automation. *Interdiscip Nurs Res 3*(1), 49–56. https://doi.org/10.1097/NR9.0000000000000052

Zhang, J., Nie, X., Yang, X., Mei, Q., Xiang, X., & Cheng, L. (2024). A meta-analysis of effectiveness of mobile health interventions on health-related outcomes in patients with heart failure. *J Cardiovasc Med (Hagerstown), 25*(8), 587–600. https://doi.org/10.2459/JCM.0000000000001631

Appendix A

Criterion	Inclusion Criteria	Exclusion Criteria
Publication Type	Peer-reviewed journal articles, conference papers, or systematic/scoping reviews.	Grey literature (e.g., reports, theses, editorials, opinion pieces, or non-peer-reviewed sources).
Publication Date	Studies published between January 1, 2020, and October 7, 2025 (to capture recent advancements in digital health technologies).	Studies published before 2020.
Language	English.	Non-English articles.
Study Focus	Articles addressing digital health solutions (e.g., AI-powered tools, wearable devices, mobile health apps, telemedicine, or cognitive training platforms) applied to dementia care, management, or related chronic neurological conditions (e.g., Alzheimer's disease, mild cognitive impairment).	Studies not related to digital health or dementia (e.g., purely pharmacological interventions).
Population and Setting	Focus on adults (particularly older adults) with dementia or at risk of dementia, caregivers, or healthcare providers in home, clinical, or community settings.	Studies focused on pediatric populations
Geographic Scope	Studies from high-income (HIC) or low- and middle-income countries (LMIC), preferably highlighting global applicability.	–

10

Using Digital Tools to Detect Spatial Navigation Impairment in Early Alzheimer's Disease

Ming-Chyi Pai and Sheng-Hsiang Yang

10.1 The Need for a Screening Tool for Alzheimer's Disease

As the proportion of the elderly population continues to rise, the number and rate of individuals with dementia are also increasing. More than half of those with dementia suffer from Alzheimer's disease (AD). Recently, the advent of anti-amyloid monoclonal antibodies has launched a new era in AD treatment, leading to a raised demand for the early identification of cases with Alzheimer's biomarkers [1–3]. This demand is accelerating the clinical teams' shift from solely clinical judgments to biomarker-confirmed diagnoses. However, current biomarkers are still facing barriers related to cost (e.g., amyloid PET) or invasiveness (e.g., cerebrospinal fluid biomarkers). Blood-based biomarkers offer advantages such as ease of collection and relatively affordable costs, with their accuracy continually being validated [4–6]. Using blood-based biomarkers alone as a screening tool, however, still requires consideration of cost and capacity issues currently. Therefore, it is necessary to develop clinical screening tools for AD with high sensitivity and specificity, which can then be integrated with plasma biomarkers to create an appropriate diagnostic pipeline.

Although numerous neurocognitive tests are used as screening tools in the diagnostic process for AD, most lack the ability to distinguish individuals with AD from those without it at very early stages. As the demand for early diagnosis grows, the development of a reliable screening tool becomes increasingly essential.

10.2 Spatial Navigation: Distribution of Related Brain Areas and Their Association with Alzheimer's Disease

It is essential for animals to be aware of their current location and the distance relative to their target, continually check their heading direction, and update this information constantly. This knowledge is crucial for performing behaviors related to survival, such as forage, reproduction, social activity, and migration.

Humans are no exception. Despite significant advancements in technology and the availability of numerous assistive tools such as compasses, maps, and global positioning systems (GPS) that help maintain the correct path or navigate unfamiliar locations for travel or residence, we still primarily rely on our inherent spatial navigation abilities. These innate skills are essential for everyday tasks such as locating objects in a room, finding a car parked in a lot, discovering a nearby restaurant, or visiting friends and relatives in distant places.

Upon closer examination, individuals require sufficient attention and memory, and must continuously receive and process visual, auditory, olfactory, vestibular, proprioceptive, and other somatic sensations. They must then apply, store, and retrieve this information using numerous cognitive strategies to achieve successful navigation.

There are at least two perspectives or viewpoints in cognitive strategy during spatial navigation. One is egocentric, where one navigates from their own point of view, using their location as the reference point and performing numerous calculations for navigation. The frame of reference may shift over time due to continuous changes in relative position during movement, thus heavily relying on allothetic cues, including visual, auditory, and olfactory signals, as well as idiothetic cues, such as vestibular, proprioceptive, and other somatic sensations [7]. The ability to navigate using solely idiothetic cues is referred to as path integration ability. This concept was first postulated by Charles Darwin in his book, "Origin of Certain Instincts" [8]. Another strategy is allocentric navigation. Contrary to egocentric navigation, it employs a bird's eye view, using a relatively stable frame of reference and viewpoints that reference objects other than oneself, like a cognitive map. This approach utilizes the relative positions of multiple landmarks to anchor both the navigator's and the target's locations for navigation [7, 9]. Piaget and Inhelder proposed a theory suggesting that spatial navigation strategies are clearly divisible and hierarchical, with egocentric information being formed first and then translated into an allocentric cognitive map [10]. However, this model has been challenged by numerous theoretical and experimental studies. The most recent theory posits that egocentric pathways and allocentric topological knowledge coexist simultaneously and are interchangeable, adapting to meet the demands of varying situations [9, 11].

To date, the neurophysiological mechanisms and corresponding brain areas involved in spatial navigation remain subjects of ongoing research. In 1999, Aguirre and D'Esposito proposed a hypothesis that classifies spatial navigation abilities according to developmental and environmental-cognitive theories. They suggested that spatial navigation is facilitated by several sub-abilities, each provided by distinct brain regions, and proceeds through the cooperation of these areas. These brain areas and the abilities they provide include: [1] the posterior parietal cortex, involved in egocentric spatial orientation; [2] the retrosplenial cortex within the posterior cingulate gyrus, responsible for heading orientation; [3] the inferior temporal cortex, such as the lingual gyrus, specialized in the perception of landmarks; and [4] the medial temporal lobe, responsible for anterograde spatial orientation [12]. The hypothesis closely references the visual stream theory proposed by Ungerleider and Mishkin in 1982. According to this theory, the posterior parietal cortex and the retrosplenial cortex are components of the dorsal stream, responsible for processing spatial locations based on visual stimuli—often referred to as the "where" pathway. Meanwhile, the inferior temporal cortex is part of the ventral stream, which is responsible for identifying objects, thus addressing the "what" aspect of visual processing [9, 13].

Numerous brain lesion studies have demonstrated the functional roles of these areas. Subsequent research in animals, non-human primates, and humans has identified additional regions involved in spatial navigation, including the hippocampus, entorhinal cortex, and parahippocampal cortex. The precuneus within the parietal cortex, the frontal cortex, and subcortical structures such as the caudate nucleus and thalamus are also central to spatial navigation [14]. How do these brain areas operate? Contrary to the model proposed by Aguirre and D'Esposito, subsequent researches suggest that these areas do not function independently but require specific regions to serve as hubs, forming a network. This network enables the brain areas to operate simultaneously and coordinate actions to facilitate spatial navigation. This hypothesis has been substantiated by recent functional imaging studies [9, 11]. Several specialized neurons play crucial roles in the execution of spatial navigation. Place cells activate when individuals approach specific locations within a space [15, 16]. Grid cells partition an area into a grid-like lattice, increasing in activity as individuals approach the nodes of these lattices and decreasing as they move away. Adjacent grid cells correspond to adjacent lattice nodes and may activate when individuals approach nearby positions, thereby anchoring one's coordinate position [17]. Head direction cells increase in activity when the head is oriented toward specific directions [18]. Border cells activate when individuals approach the boundaries of an area [19, 20]. Speed cells are triggered according to the movement speed [21]. Conjunctive cells become active only under specific conditions and are believed to be linked to the conjunction of the cells mentioned above [9, 22].

When discussing the relationship between spatial navigation abilities and AD, it is necessary to refer to the Braak & Braak staging, which outlines the progression of Alzheimer's pathology in a temporal-spatial context. The tau pathology, closely associated with functional decline, aggregates in the entorhinal cortex at a very early stage, immediately following the transentorhinal cortex [23]. This suggests that the functional consequences of tau pathology in the entorhinal cortex may manifest at the earliest stages of AD. The entorhinal cortex is integral to spatial navigation; animal studies have shown that grid cells within this region play a crucial role in this process. This discovery led to May-Britt Moser and Edvard Moser being awarded the 2014 Nobel Prize in Physiology or Medicine [17]. Approximately 95% of neurons in the medial entorhinal cortex are related to spatial cognition. Similar neurons performing analogous functions have been identified in the entorhinal cortex of primates [24]. Additionally, grid cells with similar functions and arrangements have been found in the human posterior medial entorhinal cortex [25]. Recent studies also indicate that both the inhibition of grid cells and the aggregation of tau proteins can impair path integration abilities, which are essential for spatial navigation [26, 27]. Consequently, it is plausible to hypothesize that impairments in spatial navigation could be an early indicator of AD.

Spatial navigation is so widely and naturally utilized in daily life that impairments in this ability can lead to troublesome and even dangerous situations. These issues often emerge in the early stages of AD, corresponding to the initial involvement of related brain regions. Therefore, early detection of deficits in this domain is crucial for preventing incidents such as disorientation or getting lost. Furthermore, as our understanding of the underlying mechanisms improves, we can develop more precise tests to assess specific aspects of spatial navigation and their corresponding anatomical counterparts in the brain.

10.3 Methods for Detecting Impairments in Spatial Navigation

Spatial navigation or sense of location is elemental and essential in our daily life. However, as other cognitive functions, to get sufficient reliability and validity, it is necessary to use standardized scale, exam, or questionnaire for measuring this ability. Researchers have developed numerous exams for measuring the ability of spatial navigation in animals, with some of these being applied in human studies. Furthermore, as techniques keep evolving, various associated exams are available to meet this purpose. These exams can be classified into several groups by the interface used, which include functional assessments, pencil-paper tests, desktop virtual reality tests, immersive virtual reality tests, and real-world tests.

Pencil-and-paper tests and questionnaires offer the advantages of being easy to administer and requiring less time to complete. However, they also have inherent limitations due to their differences from real-world spatial navigation, including variations in settings, tasks, stimuli, and behavioral responses [28, 29].

In real-world tests, participants can access complete information necessary for spatial navigation, including vision, odor, proprioception, other somatic sensations, vestibular sensation, and auditory input without any loss. There are also confounding factors such as crowds, scenes, and sounds that change over time, however, which are not easily excluded. Additionally, environmental and weather conditions may present changes and dangers. Moreover, it is more challenging to manipulate associated variables [30–32]. Some tests restrict the experimental area to better control variables, such as within a specific campus or a laboratory setting. This approach may exclude some confounding factors and facilitate the control of experimental conditions. However, it limits the space available and precludes the performance of spatial navigation tests in larger areas. Moreover, replicating experiments in the same area under identical conditions may also be challenging [31–33]. Additionally, the mobility of participants may also pose a restrictive issue [30, 31].

Desktop spatial navigation tests can eliminate unnecessary interference and allow for the manipulation of experimental variables, thereby enhancing replicability. Additionally, the screen can be positioned within a magnetic resonance imaging (MRI) machine, facilitating simultaneous functional MRI studies [30]. The degree of concentration required for these tests, however, depends on the size of the screen and the environmental design. Moreover, there is a lack of vestibular sensation and proprioception, both of which are crucial for path integration [30, 32, 34–36]. Furthermore, for populations with limited exposure to Computers, Communications, and Consumer products, the unfamiliar interface may adversely affect the experimental results [36, 37].

Immersive virtual reality tests enhance participant focus within the virtual environment. Some methods involve occupying a larger visual angle, using large, curved, or room-sized screens to better engage participants in the conditions [36, 38]. As technologies continue to evolve, an increasing number of methods now employ head-mounted virtual reality goggles [31, 39–42]. To address the lack of vestibular and proprioceptive inputs, most methods utilize a defined space with fixed dimensions, employing sensors to track the location of participants. These coordinates are then translated into the virtual environment at a fixed ratio to enhance idiothetic sensory input. However, spatial limitations exist with these methods, leading some experiments to employ treadmills to simulate locomotion in real space [43, 44]. Cybersickness is more likely to occur when using head-mounted virtual reality goggles. Additionally, the difficulty in adaptation and the risk of falls associated with treadmill use should also be addressed, particularly in the elderly population [30].

Alongside tests that measure objective performance in spatial navigation, there are also assessments that evaluate subjective complaints of spatial

TABLE 10.1

Classification of Spatial Navigation Tests by Interface

Functional assessments	QuENA (Pai 2012) (46), Santa Barbara Sense of Direction Scale (SBSOD) (Hegarty 2002) (45), The Wayfinding Questionnaire (WQ) (van der Ham 2013) (68), Subjective Spatial Navigation Complaints Questionnaire (Hort, 2015) (47)
Traditional pencil-paper tests	Snellgrove Maze Test (SMT) (Snellgrove 2005) (69), Perspective Taking/Spatial Orientation Test (Hegarty & Waller 2004) (70), The Standardized Road-Map Test of Direction Sense (Money & Walker 1965) (71), Piagetian three-mountain task (Piaget 1956) (10), Mental rotation of two-dimensional shapes (Cooper 1975) (72), Mental Rotation of Three-Dimensional Objects (Shepard & Metzler 1971) (73), Table-top distance-estimation task (Klatzky & Pellegrino 1995) (74)
Desktop virtual reality assessments	Sea Hero Quest (SHQ) (Hyde 2016) (75), Virtual Y-maze strategy assessment (vYSA) (Roger 2012) (76), Virtual supermarket task (VST) (Tu 2015) (77), Virtual spatial navigation assessment (VSNA) (Ventura 2013) (78), Computerized spatial orientation test (Friedman & Hegarty 2019) (79), Spatial navigation task (Basso 2024) (80), Virtual reality town (Maguire & Burgess 1998) (81), Virtual Silcton (Weisberg 2014) (82), Concurrent spatial discrimination learning task (CSDLT) & 4-on-8 Virtual Maze (Dahmani & Bohbot 2020) (83), Minecraft Memory and Navigation task (Simon & Mednick 2022) (84), the Navigation Test Suite (Wiener et al 2019, Laczó et al 2021a) (85), Virtual 2-dimensional computer version of the Hidden Goal Task (HGT) or Blue Velvet Arena (Hort 2012) (86), CG Arena (Jacobs 2001) (87), The virtual environments navigation assessment (VIENNA) (Rekers 2023) (88), VR-Maze Test and VR-Road-Map Test (Morganti & Riva 2007) (89), Virtual Town (another) (Hartley 2003) (90), Dual-solution paradigm (DSP) (Marchette & Shelton 2011) (91), 2D virtual Morris water maze (Padilla & Cashdan 2016) (92), Virtual cities (Kraemer 2017) (93), Object-Location Memory Task (Stangl & Wolbers 2018) (94)
Real-world settings	Pai-Jan (PJ) device (Pai 2020) (95), Detour Navigation Test (DNT) (Puthusseryppady 2022) (96), Spatial orientation paradigms (Zwergal 2016) (97), The Hidden Goal Task (HGT) or Blue Velvet Arena (Hort 2007, Kalová & Bureš 2005) (98), Floor Maze Test (FMT) (Sanders 2008) (99), Bienwald forest and Sahara desert (Souman & Ernst 2009) (100), Triangle completion task (Loomis 1993) (101), ALZENTIA (another form of Hidden-Goal Tests, HGT) (Bažadona 2020) (102)
Immersive virtual reality settings	Pai-Jan Virtual Reality (PJVR) (Lai & Pai, 2024) (31), Immersive virtual reality triangle completion task (Howett 2019) (39), Loop closure task (Chrastil 2019) (103), Immersive Y-maze tasks (Bécu & Arleo 2023) (104), Virtual Ashmolean (Lazaridou & Psarra 2017) (105), Modified virtual version of the MWM-task (Iggena & Finke 2023) (40), Sunnybrook City (Zakzanis & Mraz 2009) (106), Seahaven (König 2021) (107), 7*7 pattern Minecraft (Thorp & Grassini 2024) (108), The virtual hedge maze (Warren & Ericson 2017) (109), Spatial Orientation in Immersive Virtual Environment Maze Test (SOIVET-Maze) (Silva & Pompeu, 2023) (110), VR-CogAssess (Ijaz & Calvo 2019) (111), Counter-strike map (Lim & Gilbert 2020) (112), Westgate Mall in Singapore (Li & Schinazi 2019) (113), No name virtual maze by Chance (Chance 1998) (42), Immersive VR in a physical laboratory (Ruddle & Lessels 2006) (114), Triangle completion task with treadmill (Harrotonian & Ekstrom 2020) (115), Virtual point-to-origin task (Barhorst-Cates & Creem-Regehr 2020) (41), Virtual triangle completion task in different situations (Kelly & Gilbert 2022) (116), The VENLab (Kearns & Tarr 2002) (117)
Others	Triangle Completion Tasks (TCTs, real-world setting plus desktop virtual reality) (Adamo 2012) (118), AudioMaze (Makoto Miyakoshi 2021 (50)

navigation impairments using questionnaires [45–47]. These questionnaires are designed to gauge individuals' subjective experiences of daily spatial navigation, with each questionnaire emphasizing different aspects of navigation. Some questionnaires are available in both self-reported and informant-reported versions. They are often brief and require less time to administer than objective tests, offering benefits in clinical applications. Although the accuracy of these questionnaires may be affected by imprecise subjective sensations, the informant-reported versions have been shown to effectively discriminate not only between cognitively normal and impaired individuals, but also between participants who are positive and negative for AD biomarkers [48]. Examples of methods for detecting impairments in spatial navigation are listed and classified in Table 10.1.

Depending on their distinct features, each spatial navigation test may excel in specific scenarios, such as distinguishing individuals with AD from others, or more accurately simulating daily activities to predict future incidents of getting lost. It is crucial to understand the specific aspect of spatial navigation that a test assesses in order to utilize these valuable tools effectively.

10.4 Variants of Immersive Virtual Reality Methods

The effective application of immersive virtual reality methods depends heavily on the equipment and settings used. Sensory inputs play a critical role in spatial navigation and can be selectively manipulated during assessments to better isolate specific aspects of navigational ability. For example, when using head-mounted virtual reality goggles, the type of sensory input can vary significantly between different methods of movement, such as using a joystick or controller while seated, walking around with a 1:1 distance ratio, or using an exercise or omnidirectional treadmill [36]. These variations are particularly noticeable in proprioception and movement inputs, such as speed. By obscuring inputs like landmarks or surface details, cues from landmarks and visual flow can be eliminated to test path integration abilities [39, 49]. Conversely, if the goal is to evaluate the phenomenal or physiological aspects of spatial navigation using allothetic cues, navigating with a joystick or controller in a seated position may be more appropriate. Additionally, some studies have eliminated visual inputs, using auditory cues for spatial navigation to mimic conditions encountered by visually impaired individuals and to analyze the corresponding neural networks involved. However, these studies employed distinct methods and techniques that may be categorized as "sparse augmented reality (AR)," which falls beyond the scope of this chapter [50–52].

The dimensions and scale of the virtual reality environment can influence the strategies that participants use during the navigation process. Spatial scale can be categorized into figural, vista, environmental, and geographical spaces [53]. Figural and geographical spaces are typically too small or too large, respectively, for practical experimentation [54]. Most spatial navigation studies are conducted in vista or environmental spaces, which differ not only in size but also in the visibility of landmarks or beacons [54]. Some studies have investigated the brain areas involved in navigating spaces of different scales and the specific abilities or strategies employed during such navigation [55–57]. This field of research is continually evolving.

Participants wearing head-mounted virtual reality goggles cannot be evaluated using functional brain MRI due to equipment incompatibility. However, several studies have utilized EEG during navigation in virtual environments to detect temporal functional changes in brain areas [58–61]. This approach may enhance our understanding of how the cortical network operates during spatial navigation. Like real-space tests, eye tracking can also be implemented during immersive virtual reality navigation to observe participants' visual behavior. This includes tracking what participants are looking at, how long they gaze at specific landmarks or beacons, and their level of concentration [62–64]. As technology continues to advance, the possibilities for such research are likely to expand and become less restricted in the future.

As technology continues to advance, there have been significant advances in spatial-computing techniques, as exemplified by devices like Apple Vision Pro, which enable seamless transitions between real space, augmented reality, virtual reality, and merged reality. Utilizing such technologies allows for more detailed manipulation and alleviation of certain restrictions during testing. Moreover, such techniques offer the potential not only to prevent individuals with spatial navigation impairments from getting lost or going missing but also to serve as tools for training spatial navigation abilities.

10.5 Using GPS Techniques to Detect Spatial Navigation Impairments

Several studies have utilized GPS techniques to track and record participants' daily activity trajectories for analysis, aiming to detect underlying spatial navigation impairments and indirectly differentiate AD cases from controls. Some of these studies have also incorporated machine learning methods to achieve this purpose [65–67].

In contrast to controlled laboratory settings, these techniques offer maximum ecological validity by testing spatial navigation in a more natural manner. Beyond differentiating AD cases from controls, these technologies may also have the potential to detect early changes in spatial navigation abilities.

This allows users or their families to take necessary precautions to prevent getting lost and, furthermore, to seek expert advice for possible underlying causes of spatial navigation impairments.

10.6 Conclusions

Given the early involvement of associated brain areas in AD, spatial navigation impairment has the potential to serve as a crucial behavioral marker for early detection of the disease. Numerous tests have been developed, and some have proven effective in distinguishing individuals with AD from those without. As technologies continue to advance, machine learning and artificial intelligence are poised to play significant roles in enhancing tools for detecting spatial navigation impairments, making the process more precise and efficient. With proper design, the application of these tools in both clinical and everyday life settings may prove to be promising in the future.

10.7 Discussion

Due to the early involvement of associated functional areas, spatial navigation may play a crucial role in the early detection of AD. Developing a suitable tool that can assess specific aspects of spatial navigation—particularly those corresponding to the early involvement of the posterior medial entorhinal cortex in AD—while minimizing unnecessary confounding factors is essential. For instance, avoiding the unintentional assessment of executive function, which may result from complex and non-intuitive methods, is critical for achieving accurate evaluations. Advancements in technology may contribute to this goal in two ways: by making assessment methods more controllable and intuitive through improved interfaces, or by enabling the extraction of meaningful information from ecologically valid yet complex data using machine learning and artificial intelligence. Moreover, given the interindividual differences in baseline spatial navigation ability, longitudinal follow-up assessments may help overcome the limitations of single-time-point testing. This approach can capture sequential changes at the earliest possible stage, facilitating timely intervention. As an essential ability in daily life, spatial navigation should be monitored closely, as impairments can lead to serious consequences, including disorientation, getting lost, and increased risks to personal safety. Such difficulties often result in lifestyle restrictions and subsequent social isolation. New technologies that support training, assist with navigation, and enable early detection of disorientation—when combined with other measures such as dementia-friendly environments—have the potential to enhance safety and improve the quality of life for older adults.

References

1. Rahman A, Hossen MA, Chowdhury MFI, Bari S, Tamanna N, Sultana SS, Haque SN, Al Masud A, Saif-Ur-Rahman KM. Aducanumab for the treatment of Alzheimer's disease: A systematic review. Psychogeriatr. 2023;23(3):512–22.
2. Sims JR, Zimmer JA, Evans CD, Lu M, Ardayfio P, Sparks J, Wessels AM, Shcherbinin S, Wang H, Monkul Nery ES, Collins EC, Solomon P, Salloway S, Apostolova LG, Hansson O, Ritchie C, Brooks DA, Mintun M, Skovronsky DM, Investigators T-A. Donanemab in early symptomatic Alzheimer disease: The TRAILBLAZER-ALZ 2 randomized clinical trial. JAMA. 2023;330(6):512–27.
3. Mahase E. Alzheimer's disease: Lecanemab gets full FDA approval and black box safety warning. BMJ. 2023;382:1580.
4. Mattsson-Carlgren N, Collij LE, Stomrud E, Pichet Binette A, Ossenkoppele R, Smith R, Karlsson L, Lantero-Rodriguez J, Snellman A, Strandberg O, Palmqvist S, Ashton NJ, Blennow K, Janelidze S, Hansson O. Plasma biomarker strategy for selecting patients with Alzheimer disease for antiamyloid immunotherapies. JAMA Neurol. 2024;81(1):69–78.
5. Rissman RA, Langford O, Raman R, Donohue MC, Abdel-Latif S, Meyer MR, Wente-Roth T, Kirmess KM, Ngolab J, Winston CN, Jimenez-Maggiora G, Rafii MS, Sachdev P, West T, Yarasheski KE, Braunstein JB, Irizarry M, Johnson KA, Aisen PS, Sperling RA, team AS. Plasma abeta42/abeta40 and phospho-tau217 concentration ratios increase the accuracy of amyloid PET classification in preclinical Alzheimer's disease. Alzheimers Dement. 2024;20(2):1214–24.
6. Jack Jr. CR, Andrews JS, Beach TG, Buracchio T, Dunn B, Graf A, Hansson O, Ho C, Jagust W, McDade E, Molinuevo JL, Okonkwo OC, Pani L, Rafii MS, Scheltens P, Siemers E, Snyder HM, Sperling R, Teunissen CE, Carrillo MC. Revised criteria for diagnosis and staging of Alzheimer's disease: Alzheimer's Association Workgroup. Alzheimers Dement. 2024;20(8):5143–69.
7. Klatzky RL. Allocentric and egocentric spatial representations: Definitions, distinctions, and interconnections. Spatial cognition. Lecture notes in computer science. 1404. Berlin, Heidelberg: Springer; 1998. p. 1–17.
8. Darwin C. Origin of certain instincts. Nature. 1873;7(179):417–18.
9. Ekstrom AD, Spiers HJ, Bohbot VD, Rosenbaum RS. Human spatial navigation. Human spatial navigation. Princeton, NJ: Princeton University Press; 2018. p. 45–101.
10. Piaget J, Inhelder B, Langdon FJ, Lunzer J. The child's conception of space/by Jean Piaget and Bärbel Inhelder; translated from the French by F.J. Langdon & J.L. Lunzer. New York; Routledge & Kegan Paul: London; printed in Great Britain; 1956. p. 1–490.

11. Ekstrom AD, Huffman DJ, Starrett M. Interacting networks of brain regions underlie human spatial navigation: A review and novel synthesis of the literature. J Neurophysiol. 2017;118(6):3328–44.
12. Aguirre GK, D'Esposito M. Topographical disorientation: A synthesis and taxonomy. Brain. 1999;122 (Pt 9):1613–28.
13. Mishkin M, Ungerleider LG, Macko KA. Object vision and spatial vision: Two cortical pathways. Trends Neurosci. 1983;6:414–17.
14. Coughlan G, Laczo J, Hort J, Minihane AM, Hornberger M. Spatial navigation deficits—overlooked cognitive marker for preclinical Alzheimer disease? Nat Rev Neurol. 2018;14(8):496–506.
15. O'Keefe J. Place units in the hippocampus of the freely moving rat. Exp Neurol. 1976;51(1):78–109.
16. Dudchenko PA, Wood ER. Place fields and the cognitive map. Hippocampus. 2015;25(6):709–12.
17. Hafting T, Fyhn M, Molden S, Moser MB, Moser EI. Microstructure of a spatial map in the entorhinal cortex. Nature. 2005;436(7052):801–6.
18. Taube JS, Muller RU, Ranck JB, Jr. Head-direction cells recorded from the postsubiculum in freely moving rats. I. Description and quantitative analysis. J Neurosci. 1990;10(2):420–35.
19. Barry C, Lever C, Hayman R, Hartley T, Burton S, O'Keefe J, Jeffery K, Burgess N. The boundary vector cell model of place cell firing and spatial memory. Rev Neurosci. 2006;17(1–2):71–97.
20. Lever C, Burton S, Jeewajee A, O'Keefe J, Burgess N. Boundary vector cells in the subiculum of the hippocampal formation. J Neurosci. 2009;29(31):9771–7.
21. Kropff E, Carmichael JE, Moser MB, Moser EI. Speed cells in the medial entorhinal cortex. Nature. 2015;523(7561):419–24.
22. Sargolini F, Fyhn M, Hafting T, McNaughton BL, Witter MP, Moser MB, Moser EI. Conjunctive representation of position, direction, and velocity in entorhinal cortex. Science. 2006;312(5774):758–62.
23. Braak H, Braak E. Neuropathological stageing of Alzheimer-related changes. Acta Neuropathol. 1991;82(4):239–59.
24. Killian NJ, Jutras MJ, Buffalo EA. A map of visual space in the primate entorhinal cortex. Nature. 2012;491(7426):761–4.
25. Jacobs J, Weidemann CT, Miller JF, Solway A, Burke JF, Wei XX, Suthana N, Sperling MR, Sharan AD, Fried I, Kahana MJ. Direct recordings of grid-like neuronal activity in human spatial navigation. Nat Neurosci. 2013;16(9):1188–90.
26. Gil M, Ancau M, Schlesiger MI, Neitz A, Allen K, De Marco RJ, Monyer H. Impaired path integration in mice with disrupted grid cell firing. Nat Neurosci. 2018;21(1):81–91.
27. Koike R, Soeda Y, Kasai A, Fujioka Y, Ishigaki S, Yamanaka A, Takaichi Y, Chambers JK, Uchida K, Watanabe H, Takashima A. Path integration deficits are associated with phosphorylated tau accumulation in the entorhinal cortex. Brain Commun. 2024;6(1):facd359.
28. Hegarty M, Montello DR, Richardson AE, Ishikawa T, Lovelace K. Spatial abilities at different scales: Individual differences in aptitude-test performance and spatial-layout learning. Intelligence. 2006;34(2):151–76.
29. Pinto JO, Dores AR, Peixoto B, Barbosa F. Ecological validity in neurocognitive assessment: Systematized review, content analysis, and proposal of an instrument. Appl Neuropsychol Adult. 2023;32(2):1–18.

30. Schoberl F, Zwergal A, Brandt T. Testing navigation in real space: Contributions to understanding the physiology and pathology of human navigation control. Front Neural Circuits. 2020;14:6.

31. Lai CH, Pai MC. The feasibility and practicality of auxiliary detection of spatial navigation impairment in patients with mild cognitive impairment due to Alzheimer's disease by using virtual reality. Heliyon. 2024;10(3):e24748.

32. Rizzo A, Schultheis M, Kerns K, Mateer C. Analysis of assets for virtual reality applications in neuropsychology. Neupsychol Rehabil. 2004;14(1):207–39.

33. Cogne M, Taillade M, N'Kaoua B, Tarruella A, Klinger E, Larrue F, Sauzeon H, Joseph PA, Sorita E. The contribution of virtual reality to the diagnosis of spatial navigation disorders and to the study of the role of navigational aids: A systematic literature review. Ann Phys Rehabil Med. 2017;60(3):164–76.

34. van der Ham IJ, Faber AM, Venselaar M, van Kreveld MJ, Loffler M. Ecological validity of virtual environments to assess human navigation ability. Front Psychol. 2015;6:637.

35. Taube JS, Valerio S, Yoder RM. Is navigation in virtual reality with fMRI really navigation? J Cogn Neurosci. 2013;25(7):1008–19.

36. Diersch N, Wolbers T. The potential of virtual reality for spatial navigation research across the adult lifespan. J Exp Biol. 2019;222(Pt Suppl 1):jeb187252. https://doi.org/10.1242/jeb.187252.

37. Hegarty M, He C, Boone AP, Yu S, Jacobs EG, Chrastil ER. Understanding differences in wayfinding strategies. Top Cogn Sci. 2023;15(1):102–19.

38. Tuena C, Serino S, Stramba-Badiale C, Pedroli E, Goulene KM, Stramba-Badiale M, Riva G. Usability of an embodied cave system for spatial navigation training in mild cognitive impairment. J Clin Med. 2023;12(5):1949.

39. Howett D, Castegnaro A, Krzywicka K, Hagman J, Marchment D, Henson R, Rio M, King JA, Burgess N, Chan D. Differentiation of mild cognitive impairment using an entorhinal cortex-based test of virtual reality navigation. Brain. 2019;142(6):1751–66.

40. Iggena D, Jeung S, Maier PM, Ploner CJ, Gramann K, Finke C. Multisensory input modulates memory-guided spatial navigation in humans. Commun Biol. 2023;6(1):1167.

41. Barhorst-Cates EM, Stefanucci JK, Creem-Regehr SH. A comparison of virtual locomotion methods in movement experts and non-experts: Testing the contributions of body-based and visual translation for spatial updating. Exp Brain Res. 2020;238(9):1911–23.

42. Chance SS, Gaunet F, Beall AC, Loomis JM. Locomotion mode affects the updating of objects encountered during travel: The contribution of vestibular and proprioceptive inputs to path integration. Presence: Teleoperators Virtual Environ. 1998;7(2):168–78.

43. Campos JL, Bülthoff HH. Multimodal integration during self-motion in virtual reality. In: Murray MM, Wallace MT, editors. The neural bases of multisensory processes. Boca Raton, FL: CRC Press/Taylor & Francis; 2012. p. 603–28.

44. Starrett MJ, McAvan AS, Huffman DJ, Stokes JD, Kyle CT, Smuda DN, Kolarik BS, Laczko J, Ekstrom AD. Landmarks: A solution for spatial navigation and memory experiments in virtual reality. Behav Res Methods. 2021;53(3):1046–59.

45. Hegarty M, Richardson AE, Montello DR, Lovelace KL, Subbiah I. Development of a self-report measure of environmental spatial ability. Intelligence. 2002;30(5): 425–47.

46. Pai MC, Lee CC, Yang YC, Lee YT, Chen KC, Lin SH, Jheng SS, Sun PW, Cheng PJ. Development of a questionnaire on everyday navigational ability to assess topographical disorientation in Alzheimer's disease. Am J Alzheimers Dis Other Demen. 2012;27(1):65–72.

47. Jan Laczó KS, Ivana Mokrisova MV, Ross Andel PT. Spatial navigation complaints are associated with anxiety regardless of the real performance in non-demented elderly. J Depress Anxiety. 2015;4(4):1000205.

48. Laczo M, Svatkova R, Lerch O, Martinkovic L, Zuntychova T, Nedelska Z, Horakova H, Vyhnalek M, Hort J, Laczo J. Spatial navigation questionnaires as a supportive diagnostic tool in early Alzheimer's disease. iScience. 2024;27(6):109832.

49. Castegnaro A, Ji Z, Rudzka K, Chan D, Burgess N. Overestimation in angular path integration precedes Alzheimer's dementia. Curr Biol. 2023;33(21):4650–61.e7.

50. Miyakoshi M, Gehrke L, Gramann K, Makeig S, Iversen J. The AudioMaze: An EEG and motion capture study of human spatial navigation in sparse augmented reality. Eur J Neurosci. 2021;54(12):8283–307.

51. Shikauchi Y, Miyakoshi M, Makeig S, Iversen JR. Bayesian models of human navigation behaviour in an augmented reality audiomaze. Eur J Neurosci. 2021;54(12):8308–17.

52. Gehrke L, Gramann K. Single-trial regression of spatial exploration behavior indicates posterior EEG alpha modulation to reflect egocentric coding. Eur J Neurosci. 2021;54(12):8318–35.

53. Montello DR. Scale and multiple psychologies of space. In: Frank, UA, Campari, Irene, editors. Spatial Information Theory: A Theoretical Basis for GIS; Sep. 19–22, 1993; Berlin, Heidelberg: Springer Berlin Heidelberg; 1993. p. 312–21.

54. Wolbers T, Wiener JM. Challenges for identifying the neural mechanisms that support spatial navigation: The impact of spatial scale. Front Hum Neurosci. 2014;8:571.

55. Peer M, Ron Y, Monsa R, Arzy S. Processing of different spatial scales in the human brain. ELife. 2019;8:e47492.

56. Anastasiou C, Baumann O, Yamamoto N. Does path integration contribute to human navigation in large-scale space? Psychon Bull Rev. 2023;30(3):822–42.

57. Huffman DJ, Ekstrom AD. An important step toward understanding the role of body-based cues on human spatial memory for large-scale environments. J Cogn Neurosci. 2021;33(2):167–79.

58. Chrastil ER, Rice C, Goncalves M, Moore KN, Wynn SC, Stern CE, Nyhus E. Theta oscillations support active exploration in human spatial navigation. Neuroimage. 2022;262:119581.

59. Do TN, Lin CT, Gramann K. Human brain dynamics in active spatial navigation. Sci Rep. 2021;11(1):13036.

60. Gramann K, Hohlefeld FU, Gehrke L, Klug M. Human cortical dynamics during full-body heading changes. Sci Rep. 2021;11(1):18186.

61. Wunderlich A, Gramann K. Eye movement-related brain potentials during assisted navigation in real-world environments. Eur J Neurosci. 2021;54(12): 8336–54.

62. Batsis JA, Boateng GG, Seo LM, Petersen CL, Fortuna KL, Wechsler EV, Peterson RJ, Cook SB, Pidgeon D, Dokko RS, Halter RJ, Kotz DF. Development and usability assessment of a connected resistance exercise band application for strength-monitoring. World Acad Sci Eng Technol. 2019;13(5):340–48.

63. Davis R. The feasibility of using virtual reality and eye tracking in research with older adults with and without Alzheimer's disease. Front Aging Neurosci. 2021;13:607219.

64. Walter JL, Schmidt V, König SU, König P. Navigating virtual worlds: Examining spatial navigation using a graph theoretical analysis of eye tracking data recorded in virtual reality. 2023 Symposium on Eye Tracking Research and Applications. p. 1–2. https://doi.org/10.1145/3588015.3590124

65. Bayat S, Babulal GM, Schindler SE, Fagan AM, Morris JC, Mihailidis A, Roe CM. GPS driving: A digital biomarker for preclinical Alzheimer disease. Alzheimers Res Ther. 2021;13(1):115.

66. Ghosh A, Puthusseryppady V, Chan D, Mascolo C, Hornberger M. Machine learning detects altered spatial navigation features in outdoor behaviour of Alzheimer's disease patients. Sci Rep. 2022;12(1):3160.

67. Puthusseryppady V, Morrissey S, Aung MH, Coughlan G, Patel M, Hornberger M. Using GPS tracking to investigate outdoor navigation patterns in patients with Alzheimer disease: Cross-sectional study. JMIR Aging. 2022;5(2):e28222.

68. Ham I, Kant N, Postma A, Visser-Meily J. Is navigation ability a problem in mild stroke patients? Insights from self-reported navigation measures. J Rehabil Med. 2013;45(5):429–33.

69. Snellgrove CA. Cognitive screening for the safe driving competence of older people with mild cognitive impairment or early dementia. In: Bureau ATS, editor. Canberra: Australian Transport Safety Bureau; 2005. p. 1–33.

70. Hegarty M. A dissociation between mental rotation and perspective-taking spatial abilities. Intelligence. 2004;32(2):175–91.

71. Money JW, Duane A, Walker HT. A standardized road-map test of direction sense. Baltimore, MD: Johns Hopkins Press; 1965. p. 1–32.

72. Cooper LA. Mental rotation of random two-dimensional shapes. Cogn Psychol. 1975;7(1):20–43.

73. Shepard RN, Metzler J. Mental rotation of three-dimensional objects. Science. 1971;171(3972):701–03.

74. Klatzky RL, Golledge RG, Loomis JM, Cicinelli JG, Pellegrino JW. Performance of blind and sighted persons on spatial tasks. Journal Visual Impair Blin. 1995;89:70–82.

75. Spiers H, Coutrot A, Hornberger M. Explaining world-wide variation in navigation ability from millions of people: Citizen Science Project Sea Hero Quest. Topics Cogn Sci. 2021;15. https://doi.org/10.1111/tops.12590.

76. Rodgers MK, Sindone JA, Moffat SD. Effects of age on navigation strategy. Neurobiol Aging. 2012;33(1):202.e15–22.

77. Tu S, Wong S, Hodges JR, Irish M, Piguet O, Hornberger M. Lost in spatial trans-lation—a novel tool to objectively assess spatial disorientation in Alzheimer's disease and frontotemporal dementia. Cortex. 2015;67:83–94.

78. Ventura M, Shute V, Wright T, Zhao W. An investigation of the validity of the virtual spatial navigation assessment. Front Psychol. 2013;4:852.

79. Friedman A, Kohler B, Gunalp P, Boone AP, Hegarty M. A computerized spatial orientation test. Behav Res Methods. 2019;52(2):799–812.

80. Smith AJ, Tasnim N, Psaras Z, Gyamfi D, Makani K, Suzuki WA, Basso JC. Assessing human spatial navigation in a virtual space and its sensitivity to exercise. J Vis Exp. 2024(203):e65332.

81. Maguire EA, Burgess N, Donnett JG, Frackowiak RSJ, Frith CD, O'Keefe J. Knowing where and getting there: A human navigation network. Science. 1998;280(5365):921–4.

82. Weisberg SM, Schinazi VR, Newcombe NS, Shipley TF, Epstein RA. Variations in cognitive maps: Understanding individual differences in navigation. J Exp Psychol Learn Mem Cogn. 2014;40(3):669–82.

83. Dahmani L, Bohbot VD. Habitual use of GPS negatively impacts spatial memory during self-guided navigation. Sci Rep. 2020;10(1):6310.

84. Simon KC, Clemenson GD, Zhang J, Sattari N, Shuster AE, Clayton B, Alzueta E, Dulai T, de Zambotti M, Stark C, Baker FC, Mednick SC. Sleep facilitates spatial memory but not navigation using the Minecraft Memory and Navigation Task. Proc Natl Acad Sci U S A. 2022;119(43):e2202394119.

85. Wiener JM, Carroll D, Moeller S, Bibi I, Ivanova D, Allen P, Wolbers T. A novel virtual-reality-based route-learning test suite: Assessing the effects of cognitive aging on navigation. Behav Res Methods. 2019;52(2):630–40.

86. Nedelska Z, Andel R, Laczó J, Vlcek K, Horinek D, Lisy J, Sheardova K, Bureš J, Hort J. Spatial navigation impairment is proportional to right hippocampal volume. Proc Natl Acad Sci U S A. 2012;109(7):2590–94.

87. Thomas KGF, Hsu M, Laurance HE, Nadel L, Jacobs WJ. Place learning in virtual space iii: Investigation of spatial navigation training procedures and their application to fMRI and clinical neuropsychology. Behav Res Meth Ins C. 2001;33(1): 21–37.

88. Rekers S, Finke C. Translating spatial navigation evaluation from experimental to clinical settings: The virtual environments navigation assessment (Vienna). Behav Res Methods. 2023;56(3):2033–48.

89. Morganti F, Gaggioli A, Strambi L, Rusconi ML, Riva G. A virtual reality extended neuropsychological assessment for topographical disorientation: A feasibility study. J Neuroeng Rehabil. 2007;4(1):26.

90. Hartley T, Maguire EA, Spiers HJ, Burgess N. The well-worn route and the path less traveled distinct neural bases of route following and wayfinding in humans. Neuron. 2003;37(5):877–88.

91. Marchette SA, Bakker A, Shelton AL. Cognitive mappers to creatures of habit: Differential engagement of place and response learning mechanisms predicts human navigational behavior. J Neurosci. 2011;31(43):15264–68.

92. Padilla LM, Creem-Regehr SH, Stefanucci JK, Cashdan EA. Sex differences in virtual navigation influenced by scale and navigation experience. Psychon Bull Rev. 2016;24(2):582–90.

93. Kraemer DJM, Schinazi VR, Cawkwell PB, Tekriwal A, Epstein RA, Thompson-Schill SL. Verbalizing, visualizing, and navigating: The effect of strategies on encoding a large-scale virtual environment. J Exp Psychol Learn Mem Cogn. 2017;43(4):611–21.

94. Stangl M, Achtzehn J, Huber K, Dietrich C, Tempelmann C, Wolbers T. Compromised grid-cell-like representations in old age as a key mechanism to explain age-related navigational deficits. Curr Biol. 2018;28(7):1108–15.e6.

95. Pai M-C, Jan S-S. Have I been here? Sense of location in people with Alzheimer's disease. Front Aging Neurosci. 2020;12:582525.

96. Puthusseryppady V, Morrissey S, Spiers H, Patel M, Hornberger M. Predicting real world spatial disorientation in Alzheimer's disease patients using virtual reality navigation tests. Sci Rep. 2022;12(1):13397.

97. Zwergal A, Schöberl F, Xiong G, Pradhan C, Covic A, Werner P, Trapp C, Bartenstein P, la Fougère C, Jahn K, Dieterich M, Brandt T. Anisotropy of human horizontal and vertical navigation in real space: Behavioral and PET correlates. Cereb Cortex. 2016;26(11):4392–404.

98. Kalová E, Vlček K, Jarolímová E, Bureš J. Allothetic orientation and sequential ordering of places is impaired in early stages of Alzheimer's disease: Corresponding results in real space tests and computer tests. Behav Brain Res. 2005;159(2):175–86.

99. Sanders AE, Holtzer R, Lipton RB, Hall C, Verghese J. Egocentric and exocentric navigation skills in older adults. J Gerontol A Biol Sci Med Sci. 2008; 63(12):1356–63.

100. Souman JL, Frissen I, Sreenivasa MN, Ernst MO. Walking straight into circles. Curr Biol. 2009;19(18):1538–42.

101. Loomis JM, Klatzky RL, Golledge RG, Cicinelli JG, Pellegrino JW, Fry PA. Nonvisual navigation by blind and sighted: Assessment of path integration ability. J Exp Psychol Gen. 1993;122(1):73–91.

102. Bažadona D, Fabek I, Babić Leko M, Bobić Rasonja M, Kalinić D, Bilić E, Raguž JD, Mimica N, Borovečki F, Hof PR, Šimić G. A non-invasive hidden-goal test for spatial orientation deficit detection in subjects with suspected mild cognitive impairment. J Neurosci Methods. 2020;332:108547.

103. Chrastil ER, Nicora GL, Huang A. Vision and proprioception make equal contributions to path integration in a novel homing task. Cognition. 2019; 192:103998.

104. Bécu M, Sheynikhovich D, Ramanoël S, Tatur G, Ozier-Lafontaine A, Authié CN, Sahel J-A, Arleo A. Landmark-based spatial navigation across the human lifespan. ELife. 2023;12:e81318.

105. Lazaridou A, Psarra S. Spatial navigation in real and virtual multi-level museums. 11th Space Syntax Symposium; Lisbon, Portugal 2017. p. 14.1–14.18.

106. Zakzanis KK, Quintin G, Graham SJ, Mraz R. Age and dementia related differences in spatial navigation within an immersive virtual environment. Med Sci Monit. 2009;15(4):CR140–50.

107. König SU, Keshava A, Clay V, Rittershofer K, Kuske N, König P. Embodied spatial knowledge acquisition in immersive virtual reality: Comparison to map exploration. Front Virtual Real. 2021;2:625548.

108. Thorp SO, Rimol LM, Lervik S, Evensmoen HR, Grassini S. Comparative analysis of spatial ability in immersive and non-immersive virtual reality: The role of sense of presence, simulation sickness and cognitive load. Front Virtual Real. 2024;5:1343872.

109. Warren WH, Rothman DB, Schnapp BH, Ericson JD. Wormholes in virtual space: From cognitive maps to cognitive graphs. Cognition. 2017;166:152–63.

110. Silva JMd, Santos MDd, Costa RQMd, Moretto EG, Viveiro LAPd, Lopes RdD, Brucki SMD, Pompeu JE. Applicability of an immersive virtual reality system to assess egocentric orientation of older adults. Arq Neuropsiquiatr. 2023;81(1):019–26.

111. Ijaz K, Ahmadpour N, Naismith SL, Calvo RA. An immersive virtual reality platform for assessing spatial navigation memory in predementia screening: Feasibility and usability study. JMIR Ment Health. 2019;6(9):e13887.

112. Lim AF, Kelly JW, Sepich NC, Cherep LA, Freed GC, Gilbert SB. Rotational self-motion cues improve spatial learning when teleporting in virtual environments. 2020 Symposium on Spatial User Interaction; Virtual Event, Canada. p. 1–7. https://www.youtube.com/watch?v=u5jP9k6FA_4

113. Li H, Thrash T, Hölscher C, Schinazi VR. The effect of crowdedness on human wayfinding and locomotion in a multi-level virtual shopping mall. J Environ Psychol. 2019;65:101320.

114. Ruddle RA, Lessels S. For efficient navigational search, humans require full physical movement, but not a rich visual scene. Psychol Sci. 2006;17(6):460–5.

115. Battaglia FP, Harootonian SK, Wilson RC, Hejtmánek L, Ziskin EM, Ekstrom AD. Path integration in large-scale space and with novel geometries: Comparing vector addition and encoding-error models. PLoS Comput Biol. 2020; 16(5):e1007489.

116. Kelly JW, Doty TA, Cherep LA, Gilbert SB. Boundaries reduce disorientation in virtual reality. Front Virtual Real. 2022;3:882526.

117. Kearns MJ, Warren WH, Duchon AP, Tarr MJ. Path integration from optic flow and body senses in a homing task. Perception. 2002;31:349–74.

118. Adamo DE, Briceño EM, Sindone JA, Alexander NB, Moffat SD. Age differences in virtual environment and real world path integration. Front Aging Neurosci. 2012;4:26.

11

Digital Solutions to Empower Multicultural Families Impacted by Dementia

Josefine Antoniades and Joyce Siette

11.1 Introduction

As of 2024, the average internet user worldwide spends 6 hours and 36 minutes online each day. In the United States, that number climbs to over 7 hours—almost a full workday dedicated to screens [1]. Globally, people spend an average of 2.3 hours daily on social media alone. But these numbers tell only part of the story, especially when considering ethnically diverse communities and diasporas.

In India, one of the world's largest mobile markets, there are now over 1 billion smartphone users, with individuals spending an average of 7 hours daily online and 2.6 hours on social media platforms like WhatsApp, YouTube, and Facebook [1]. Similarly, migrant communities globally are increasingly reliant on smartphones, with over 80% using mobile devices as their primary tool for accessing information, healthcare services, and maintaining cultural ties in their host countries [2,3].

For many, these digital tools are more than just a way to stay connected—they are essential lifelines for navigating healthcare systems, accessing critical health information, and staying engaged with their cultural heritage. As digital technologies continue to transform how healthcare is delivered, particularly for marginalized and ethnically diverse populations, understanding these patterns of multimedia use is key to ensuring equitable access and culturally sensitive care [4].

Digital technologies have become embedded at all layers of society and have been transformative in the way we communicate, businesses operate, services are provided, how medicine is practiced and healthcare is delivered, not to mention the impact on education, the sciences, and arts [5,6].

In the realm of healthcare, these technologies have enabled rapid advancements, offering tools that improve diagnostic precision, treatment delivery, and patient engagement. However, alongside these benefits, the accelerated uptake of digital health technologies has also amplified existing inequities,

DOI: 10.1201/9781003485681-11

particularly among already disadvantaged groups. Factors such as ethnicity, geographic location, educational attainment, digital literacy, and financial disadvantage continue to influence who benefits from these technological innovations [7].

In the context of dementia, digital technologies are also enthusiastically employed to innovate across the spectrum of needs related to dementia from prodromal identification and precision diagnosis to different uses for care, support as well as education and health promotion [8–10].

Digital biomarkers, for instance, offer promising avenues for early detection of cognitive decline, while telehealth platforms and mobile health applications facilitate access to different types of educational programs, care, and support. These innovations are ideal as they can potentially offer low-cost solutions, and high-impact programs to, e.g., raise awareness about dementia, address stigmatizing attitudes, and educate carers with the ability to have a broad reach, depending on the program, may be upscaled, and can be tailored to cultural contexts to empower families and communities enabling them to take proactive measures for dementia prevention and care [11]. The rise of mobile technology and social media platforms, such as WhatsApp, has enabled the rapid dissemination of health information, allowing diverse communities to engage with content that is culturally relevant and easily accessible.

Digital technologies can have a key role in bridging gaps in dementia knowledge and support to ethnically diverse communities in migrant-receiving communities, and in low- and middle-income countries (LMICs). In the LMIC context, access to formal care is often scarce, and digital resources may provide an accessible, low-cost solution to offer some level of support to improve care for the person living with dementia and reduce carer burden [12].

Despite these advancements, a significant gap persists in ensuring these technologies are inclusive and representative of ethnically diverse populations [13].

In this chapter, we delve into digital innovations in healthcare, using dementia care as a key example to explore the application and potential of these technologies in ethnically diverse communities. While digital tools such as cognitive assessment apps, remote monitoring devices, and telehealth platforms are increasingly integrated into dementia care, their potential to improve early detection, diagnosis, and ongoing support is clear [14]. However, the needs and culturally specific contexts of ethnically diverse communities are often overlooked in the development of digital innovations among most other research [13].

Ethnically diverse populations remain underrepresented in dementia research, limiting the generalizability and effectiveness of digital tools for these groups [15]. This lack of representation contributes to disparities in diagnosis and access to care, particularly for non-English-speaking individuals who may experience unique challenges, such as reverting to their primary language during dementia progression [15]. We further highlight how digital media can be leveraged to bridge these gaps, explore how to culturally tailor digital resources for diverse family carers, and provide some examples of how inclusive design can enhance the accessibility and relevance of dementia care tools [1]. By focusing on co-design, multilingual support, and community engagement, digital innovations can be transformed into effective resources for all communities.

11.2 Defining Diversity

The use of varied terms such as "ethnically diverse," "Culturally and Linguistically Diverse (CALD)," and "Black, Asian, and Minority Ethnic (BAME)" highlights the complexities involved in categorizing diverse populations globally. The absence of an international consensus on terminology arises from the different historical, social, and political contexts in which these terms are employed. Each term carries its own connotations and is shaped by the specific needs of a particular region or country, aiming to address unique demographic realities.

For example, "CALD" is a term commonly used in Australia to encompass cultural and linguistic diversity beyond racial classifications, focusing on communities that may require specific support due to language or cultural differences [16]. In contrast, "BAME" is mainly used in the UK to describe racial minority groups and to emphasize intersections of race and ethnicity. The relevance and acceptance of these terms vary across contexts; what may be seen as inclusive terminology in one country may not carry the same meaning in another.

Furthermore, the fluid nature of identity and cultural understanding means that fixed terminology may not adequately represent the lived experiences of those it aims to describe. This has resulted in a constantly evolving landscape of terms attempting to capture complex identities and communities without achieving a universal standard. Additionally, these terms are frequently contested within their respective contexts [17], as communities advocate for language that accurately reflects their experiences and challenges without reinforcing stereotypes or causing erasure.

In this chapter, "ethnically diverse" refers to individuals whose cultural and linguistic backgrounds differ from those of predominantly English-speaking countries, such as the UK, USA, Australia, New Zealand, and Canada. This includes people from countries where English is spoken but accompanied by unique cultural and linguistic distinctions. For instance, a person from Nigeria living in Australia would be considered part of an ethnically diverse group.

11.3 Inclusion of Ethnically Diverse Communities in Research

The World Health Organization (WHO) underscores the critical need for culturally sensitive and inclusive dementia resources globally, especially in LMICs where over two-thirds of people with dementia reside [18]. This call is supported by multiple studies highlighting barriers and challenges faced by diverse communities in accessing dementia care.

Mukadam's work illuminates these disparities, revealing that genetic risk scores (GRS) for predicting dementia risk are predominantly based on data from individuals of European ancestry, with minimal testing in other groups. This underrepresentation limits the applicability of these tools to diverse populations [19] and many digital health tools lack meaningful and authentic stakeholder engagement from ethnically diverse communities, reducing their relevance and accessibility [20]. Moreover, research highlights that stigma relating to dementia, especially in multicultural societies, stymies early diagnosis and help-seeking behaviors [21,22].

Globally, there is a pressing need for better data collection practices to accurately reflect population diversity in dementia research [13,23]. Without accounting for racial, ethnic, and cultural diversity in epidemiological assumptions, population-based data may fail to accurately reflect the true health landscape [23]. This lack of specificity can lead to misleading conclusions about the burden of diseases like dementia or diagnostic rates within certain ethnic communities. As a result, such data may not serve as a reliable foundation for guiding public policy, potentially perpetuating health disparities and overlooking the unique needs of underrepresented groups. Ensuring that epidemiological models incorporate cultural and demographic variability is essential for developing equitable and effective public health strategies [13,23].

11.4 Digital Innovation in the Context of Dementia

The proliferation of digital technologies has revolutionized how clinical and care services are delivered, health promotion campaigns delivered, and indeed how entire healthcare systems are organized to leverage new innovations to improve efficiency and health outcomes (e.g., with respect to chronic disease management and cost-effectiveness [24–26], as well as self-management and monitoring [27] or to reduce health inequities [28], mobile solutions, apps, and telemedicine, to mention but just a few possibilities, can play a big role).

11.5 Digital Biomarkers

Digital biomarkers defined as physiological and behavioral data collected via digital devices, are emerging as tools to be used in early detection and management of cognitive impairments and dementia. In a world with an ageing population and a general rise in dementia and mild cognitive impairment (MCI), continues to rise, the search for precise, sensitive, accessible, and scalable diagnostic tools is ongoing [29] Digital cognitive biomarkers from e.g. computerized tests, wearables, and mobile applications may have superior diagnostic precision relative to paper-and-pencil neuropsychological tests, while valuable, often lack the sensitivity to detect subtle cognitive changes in preclinical stages, they further offer continuous monitoring, and the potential for remote assessments [14].

Significant advances are being made in this field and a myriad of digital biomarkers are being explored [30,31] ranging from physiological markers to neuropsychological assessments. For example, one study found that digital data from wayfinding exercises could predict the development of dementia in individuals with subjective cognitive decline [30], highlighting the potential of spatial navigation tasks as early markers of cognitive impairment. Similarly, eye movement analysis has been proposed as a non-invasive, sensitive tool for the early detection of Alzheimer's disease, offering insights into attentional and memory-related deficits that may precede clinical symptoms [32,33].

Furthermore, digital cognitive assessments have demonstrated superior predictive power compared to traditional biomarkers, such as amyloid-beta and tau PET scans, in identifying individuals at risk for mild cognitive impairment and future cognitive decline. In particular, deficits in mnemonic discrimination—a person's ability to distinguish between similar but distinct memories—have been identified as critical indicators, underscoring the value of digital tools in detecting subtle cognitive changes that may signal early-stage Alzheimer's disease [34].

While it is outside the scope of this chapter to review the extensive literature, it suffices to say that digital avenues for prodromal detection and dementia diagnosis are rapidly evolving, with significant advancements in digital biomarkers, mobile applications, and machine learning tools, however, there is a way to go these digital advances become part of the everyday toolkit in clinical practice [35]. The use of such technologies for early detection of dementia has a cadre of challenges that will need to be progressed, such as standardization, validation, and the representativeness of the technologies, as diverse populations are frequently underrepresented in development, data sets, and trials [36,37].

Indeed, as highlighted by Ford et al. [37] a significant challenge in adopting digital tools, such as artificial intelligence (AI) and biomarkers, lies in the limitations of existing datasets. These datasets often lack diversity, leading to biases that compromise their applicability to real-world clinical populations.

The authors highlight the critical need for inclusive datasets that account for the cultural, social, and economic factors influencing clinical care. Integrating these variables ensures AI models are better suited to reflect the realities of diverse communities, fostering equitable and effective applications in dementia diagnosis and management. Similarly, Brijnath et al. [13] stress the underrepresentation of ethnic minorities in dementia research and advocate for consistent recruitment strategies and data collection practices that reflect the needs of multicultural communities. Achieving this inclusivity, however, requires substantial funding commitments and a strong understanding of the importance of reducing biases in research paradigms.

Further, concerns have been raised about potential discrimination arising from the early detection of dementia risk markers [37]. As Brijnath et al. (2022) point out, culturally informed approaches in dementia research can mitigate such risks by ensuring that diagnostic tools and interventions are developed with sensitivity to diverse populations' unique needs and preferences.

Continued research and collaboration with stakeholders are essential to harness the full potential of these digital innovations in dementia care. By prioritizing cultural diversity and inclusivity, researchers can design solutions that benefit all populations, advancing equity and the ethical imperative of reducing health disparities.

11.6 Digital Programs-Co-Designed to Engage and Be Culturally Relevant

Digital technologies offer great opportunities to engage via different types of media to deliver interventions and programs related to all aspects of dementia directly to consumers, e.g., help improve dementia awareness. Via digital media, especially smartphones, community members and families can access bitesize information about dementia in a non-threatening, palatable format, that can be accessed immediately or downloaded for offline use.

Working with diverse communities, researchers, and public health professionals employ digital technologies and co-design methods to create culturally relevant and engaging health information. A systematic review has highlighted that culturally adapted psychological interventions are more effective than non-adapted ones [38], and integrating culturally relevant images, narratives, and entertainment-education formats is critical for effective health education programs [7]. Indeed, digital programs may help address the challenges that people from ethnically diverse backgrounds face including stigma, language, accessibility issues, delayed diagnosis, poor access and uptake of treatment and services, and lack of culturally relevant support [23,39–41], to mention a few, by making dementia-related information more relatable and accessible [21]. By further applying techniques such as visual storytelling that has the potential to deeply engage ethnically diverse communities by reflecting on THEIR lived experiences, traditions, and identities.

Indeed, storytelling is part of human development throughout our history, and provides the means to share histories and implicit customs, and cultural norms, and strengthen community bonds [42–44]. Storytelling has been leveraged with great success in different health settings for use in health promotion [45]. As described by Fiddian-Green and colleagues [46] storytelling is a powerful tool for global public health practice, and it can incorporate, e.g., films, photovoice, comics, and participatory theater.

To effectively connect with multicultural audiences, digital programs leveraging storytelling can be co-designed in collaboration with the end-users and empower ethnically diverse communities by repositioning them as co-producers of knowledge, fostering engagement and collaboration in the storytelling process [47].

The *Moving Pictures* project exemplifies this approach by using short films co-produced with carers from ethnically diverse communities in Australia [48]. Based on lived experience video interviews with carers of persons living with dementia conducted in nine community languages, the short films focus on dementia detection, timely diagnosis, navigating aged care systems, and promoting self-care. The short films were co-produced and tailored to resonate with the target communities by allowing the voices of participants to convey the key messages. Similarly, the *ADAPT* project leveraged digital animations to raise awareness and encourage dementia prevention in ethnically diverse communities. Animations and storylines were co-created with community members to make sure that the final resource was culturally appropriate, while also engaging [18]. In the United States, leveraging telenovelas—a staple of Latino culture—has shown significant promise in promoting dementia awareness. Telenovelas integrate educational content into emotionally engaging narratives, enhancing knowledge and behavioral intentions among Latino communities. One such notable example is Webnovela Mirela, an online Spanish-language telenovela designed to help Hispanic dementia caregivers cope with stress and develop effective caregiving strategies [49].

By integrating digital technologies and culturally resonant media formats, such as short digital videos based on lived experience voices, telenovelas, and animated films, these programs address the specific needs of ethnically diverse communities in ways that are engaging, culturally relevant, and importantly, reach the target audiences.

11.7 Conclusion

The pervasive use of digital technologies worldwide presents both opportunities and challenges in the realm of healthcare, including in the context of dementia. Digital information has become part and parcel of health information in most countries in the West across the globe both in Western countries, but increasingly so in LMIC regions as well.

Digital innovations in dementia care, such as digital biomarkers, telehealth platforms, and mobile health applications, offer promising avenues for early detection, education, and ongoing support. These technologies can be tailored to cultural contexts, raising awareness, addressing stigma, and empowering carers and families to take proactive measures in dementia prevention and care.

However, the accelerated adoption of digital health technologies has also amplified existing inequities. Factors like ethnicity, geographic location, digital literacy, and financial disadvantage continue to influence who benefits from these innovations. Ethnically diverse populations remain underrepresented in dementia research, limiting the generalizability and effectiveness of digital tools. To bridge these gaps, it is crucial to focus on inclusive design, multilingual support, and community engagement, ensuring that digital innovations in dementia care are accessible, culturally sensitive, and effective for all communities. By integrating culturally sensitive digital interventions, healthcare systems can better serve ethnically diverse populations, ultimately contributing to more equitable and effective dementia care globally.

References

1. Statistica. Time spent online worldwide 2024. *Statista* https://www.statista.com/statistics/1380282/daily-time-spent-online-global/.
2. Pew Research Center. Social Media and News Fact Sheet. *Pew Research Center* https://www.pewresearch.org/journalism/fact-sheet/social-media-and-news-fact-sheet/ (2024).
3. Hong, Y. A., Juon, H.-S. & Chou, W.-Y. S. Social Media Apps Used by Immigrants in the United States: Challenges and Opportunities for Public Health Research and Practice. *mHealth* 7, 52 (2021).
4. United Nations Development Programme. *Access to Empowerment: Digital Inclusion in a Dynamic World.* (2024).
5. Stoumpos, A. I., Kitsios, F. & Talias, M. A. Digital Transformation in Healthcare: Technology Acceptance and Its Applications. *Int. J. Environ. Res. Public. Health* 20, 3407 (2023).
6. Madina, M., Dinara, Z. & Sholpan, J. Digital Society and Social Conflicts: A Science Map of the Field. In *Modeling and Simulation of Social-Behavioral Phenomena in Creative Societies* (eds. Agarwal, N., Sakalauskas, L. & Tukeyev, U.) 46–57 (Springer Nature Switzerland, Cham, 2024). doi:10.1007/978-3-031-72260-8_4.
7. Yao, R. *et al.* Inequities in Health Care Services Caused by the Adoption of Digital Health Technologies: Scoping Review. *J. Med. Internet Res.* 24, e34144 (2022).

8. Lott, S. A. *et al.* Digital Health Technologies for Alzheimer's Disease and Related Dementias: Initial Results from a Landscape Analysis and Community Collaborative Effort. *J. Prev. Alzheimers Dis.* **11**, 1480–1489 (2024).

9. Muirhead, K. *et al.* Establishing the Effectiveness of Technology-Enabled Dementia Education for Health and Social Care Practitioners: A Systematic Review. *Syst. Rev.* **10**(1), 252 (2021).

10. Goodall, G., Taraldsen, K. & Serrano, J. A. The Use of Technology in Creating Individualized, Meaningful Activities for People Living with Dementia: A Systematic Review. *Dement. Lond. Engl.* **20**, 1442–1469 (2020).

11. Talbot, C. V. & Briggs, P. The Use of Digital Technologies by People with Mild-to-Moderate Dementia during the COVID-19 Pandemic: A Positive Technology Perspective. *Dementia* **21**, 1363–1380 (2022).

12. Brijnath, B. *et al.* Using Digital Media to Improve Dementia Care in India: Protocol for a Randomized Controlled Trial. *JMIR Res. Protoc.* **11**, e38456 (2022).

13. Brijnath, B., Croy, S., Sabates, J., Thodis, A., Ellis, S., de Crespigny, F., Moxey, A., Day, R., Dobson, A., Elliott, C., Etherington, C., Geronimo, M. A., Hlis, D., Lampit, A., Low, L. F., Straiton, N. & Temple, J. Including Ethnic Minorities in Dementia Research: Recommendations from a Scoping Review. *Alzheimers Dement. (N Y).* **8**(1), e12222 (2022)

14. Piau, A., Wild, K., Mattek, N. & Kaye, J. Current State of Digital Biomarker Technologies for Real-Life, Home-Based Monitoring of Cognitive Function for Mild Cognitive Impairment to Mild Alzheimer Disease and Implications for Clinical Care: Systematic Review. *J. Med. Internet Res.* **21**, e12785 (2019).

15. Low, L., Barcenilla-Wong, A. L. & Brijnath, B. Including Ethnic and Cultural Diversity in Dementia Research. *Med. J. Aust.* **211**, 345 (2019).

16. Pham, T. T. L. *et al.* Definitions of Culturally and Linguistically Diverse (CALD): A Literature Review of Epidemiological Research in Australia. *Int. J. Environ. Res. Public. Health* **18**, 737 (2021).

17. Gill, S. *"We Are No Longer Using the Term BAME"*: A Qualitative Analysis Exploring How Activists Position and Mobilize Naming of Minority Ethnic Groups in Britain. *Commun. Cult. Crit.* **17**, 9–16 (2024).

18. World Health Organization. *Global Status Report on the Public Health Response to Dementia* (World Health Organization, Geneva, 2021).

19. Mukadam, N., Giannakopoulou, O., Bass, N., Kuchenbaecker, K. & McQuillin, A. Genetic Risk Scores and Dementia Risk across Different Ethnic Groups in UK Biobank. *PLoS One* **17**, e0277378 (2022).

20. Cassidy, J. *et al.* Engaging a Diverse Patient and Care Partner Council to Refine Dementia Care Digital Health Tools. *Innov. Aging* **6**, 777–777 (2025) Jungo, K. T., Choudhry, N. K., Marcantonio, E. R., Bhatkhande, G., Crum, K. L., Haff, N., Hanken, K. E. & Lauffenburger, J. C. Feasibility and Acceptability of Engaging Care Partners of Persons Living With Dementia With Electronic Outreach for Deprescribing. *Gerontologist.* **65**(4), gnaf028 (2025). https://doi.org/10.1093/geront/gnaf028

21. Mukadam, N., Cooper, C. & Livingston, G. Improving Access to Dementia Services for People from Minority Ethnic Groups. *Curr. Opin. Psychiatry* **26**, 409–414 (2013).

22. Mukadam, N., Waugh, A., Cooper, C. & Livingston, G. What Would Encourage Help-Seeking For Memory Problems among UK-Based South Asians? A Qualitative Study. *BMJ Open* **5**, e007990 (2015).

23. Hazan, J., Liu, K. Y., Isaacs, J. D. & Mukadam, N. Dementia Diagnosis Rates and the Impact of Ethnicity, Rurality and Deprivation. *Aging Ment. Health* **29**, 138–144 (2025).

24. Dale, L. P. *et al.* Text Message and Internet Support for Coronary Heart Disease Self-Management: Results from the Text4Heart Randomized Controlled Trial. *J. Med. Internet Res.* **17**, e4944 (2015).

25. Eze, N. D., Mateus, C. & Hashiguchi, T. C. O. Telemedicine in the OECD: An Umbrella Review of Clinical and Cost-Effectiveness, Patient Experience and Implementation. *PLoS One* **15**, e0237585 (2020).

26. Leo, D. G. *et al.* Interactive Remote Patient Monitoring Devices for Managing Chronic Health Conditions: Systematic Review and Meta-Analysis. *J. Med. Internet Res.* **24**, e35508 (2022).

27. Creber, A. *et al.* Use of Telemonitoring in Patient Self-Management of Chronic Disease: A Qualitative Meta-Synthesis. *BMC Cardiovasc. Disord.* **23**, 469 (2023).

28. Salisbury, C., Quigley, A., Hex, N. & Aznar, C. Private Video Consultation Services and the Future of Primary Care. *J. Med. Internet Res.* **22**, e19415 (2020).

29. Ding, Z., Lee, T. & Chan, A. S. Digital Cognitive Biomarker for Mild Cognitive Impairments and Dementia: A Systematic Review. *J. Clin. Med.* **11**, 4191 (2022).

30. Marquardt, J. *et al.* Identifying Older Adults at Risk for Dementia Based on Smartphone Data Obtained during a Wayfinding Task in the Real World. *PLOS Digit. Health* **3**, e0000613 (2024).

31. Wang, Y. *et al.* A New Smart 2-Min Mobile Alerting Method for Mild Cognitive Impairment Due to Alzheimer's Disease in the Community. *Brain Sci.* **13**, 244 (2023).

32. Almario, G. & Piñero, D. P. Impact of Alzheimer's Disease in Ocular Motility and Visual Perception: A Narrative Review. *Semin. Ophthalmol.* **37**, 436–446 (2022).

33. Wang, X. *et al.* Machine Learning Based on Optical Coherence Tomography Images as a Diagnostic Tool for Alzheimer's Disease. *CNS Neurosci. Ther.* **28**, 2206–2217 (2022).

34. Vanderlip, C. R., Stark, C. E. L., & Alzheimer's Disease Neuroimaging Initiative. Digital Cognitive Assessments as Low-Burden Markers for Predicting Future Cognitive Decline and Tau Accumulation across the Alzheimer's Spectrum. *BioRxiv Prepr. Serv. Biol.* 2024.05.23.595638 (2024) doi:10.1101/2024.05.23.595638.

35. Guideline Adaptation Committee. *Clinical Practice Guidelines and Principles of Care for People with Dementia* (2016) doi:ISBN Online: 978-0-9945415-0-5.

36. Birkenbihl, C., Salimi, Y., Fröhlich, H., for the Japanese Alzheimer's Disease Neuroimaging Initiative, & the Alzheimer's Disease Neuroimaging Initiative. Unraveling the Heterogeneity in Alzheimer's Disease Progression across Multiple Cohorts and the Implications For Data-Driven Disease Modeling. *Alzheimers Dement.* **18**, 251–261 (2022).

37. Ford, E., Milne, R. & Curlewis, K. Ethical Issues When Using Digital Biomarkers and Artificial Intelligence for the Early Detection of Dementia. *WIREs Data Min. Knowl. Discov.* **13**, e1492 (2023).

38. Chowdhary, N. *et al.* The Methods and Outcomes of Cultural Adaptations of Psychological Treatments for Depressive Disorders: A Systematic Review. *Psychol. Med.* **44**, 1131–1146 (2014).

39. Kenning, C., Daker-White, G., Blakemore, A., Panagioti, M. & Waheed, W. Barriers and Facilitators in Accessing Dementia Care by Ethnic Minority Groups: A Meta-Synthesis of Qualitative Studies. *BMC Psychiatry* **17**, 316 (2017).

40. Shatnawi, E., Steiner-Lim, G. Z. & Karamacoska, D. Cultural Inclusivity and Diversity in Dementia Friendly Communities: An Integrative Review. *Dement. Lond. Engl.* **22**, 2024–2046 (2023).

41. Sagbakken, M., Spilker, R. S. & Ingebretsen, R. Dementia and Migration: Family Care Patterns Merging with Public Care Services. *Qual. Health Res.* **28**, 16–29 (2018).

42. Briant, K. J., Halter, A., Marchello, N., Escareño, M. & Thompson, B. The Power of Digital Storytelling as a Culturally Relevant Health Promotion Tool. *Health Promot. Pract.* **17**, 793–801 (2016).

43. Rieger, K. L. *et al.* Elevating the Uses of Storytelling Methods within Indigenous Health Research: A Critical, Participatory Scoping Review. *Int. J. Qual. Methods* **22**, 16094069231174764 (2023).

44. Gallo, C. Storytelling to Inspire, Educate, and Engage. *Am. J. Health Promot.* **33**, 469–472 (2019).

45. Lohr, A. M. *et al.* The Use of Digital Stories as a Health Promotion Intervention: A Scoping Review. *BMC Public Health* **22**, 1180 (2022).

46. Fiddian-Green, A., Gubrium, A. & Hill, A. Digital Storytelling: Public Health Storytelling as a Method and Tool for Empathy, Equity, and Social Change. In *Handbook of Social Sciences and Global Public Health* (ed. Liamputtong, P.) 877–898 (Springer International Publishing, Cham, 2023). doi:10.1007/978-3-031-25110-8_61.

47. Elers, P., Elers, S., Dutta, M. J. & Torres, R. Applying the Culture-Centered Approach to Visual Storytelling Methods. *Rev. Commun.* **21**, 33–43 (2021).

48. Brijnath, B. *et al.* Moving Pictures: Raising Awareness of Dementia in Cald Communities through Multimedia. *Innov. Aging* **3**, S452–S452 (2019).

49. Kajiyama, B., Fernandez, G., Carter, E. A., Humber, M. B. & Thompson, L. W. Helping Hispanic Dementia Caregivers Cope with Stress Using Technology-Based Resources. *Clin. Gerontol.* **41**, 209–216 (2018).

12

Digital Solutions in Dementia Treatment, Care, and Support

Upasana Baruah and Zara Page

12.1 Introduction

Dementia, a progressive neurological disorder affecting millions world-wide, presents substantial challenges in public health. It is estimated that the number of people with dementia would increase from 57.4 million cases globally in 2019 to 152.8 million cases in 2050 (Nichols et al., 2022). As populations around the world continue to age, the incidence of dementia is increasing, necessitating innovative strategies for effective management and care (Arvanitakis, Shah, & Bennett, 2019). This rise in dementia prevalence, combined with global shortages of healthcare workers, geographical con-straints, and mobility challenges, underscores the urgent need for scalable and accessible diagnostic and care solutions (Alzheimer's Association, 2024). In response, digital technologies have emerged as crucial tools in addressing these pressing issues. The COVID-19 pandemic further highlighted the trans-formative potential of digital solutions, as widespread lockdowns and social distancing measures required a shift to online and remote service delivery (Cuffaro et al., 2020; Sacco, Lléonart, Simon, Noublanche, & Annweiler, 2020). This period effectively served as a natural experiment, demonstrating the feasibility and advantages of digital engagement even among individuals with cognitive impairments.

Consequently, there is a growing recognition of the necessity for a "digi-tal revolution" in dementia care, wherein digital diagnostic tools, telecare, and assistive technologies assume a pivotal role (Mok et al., 2020). These technological innovations not only facilitate greater access to care and pro-mote autonomy and independent living among older adults, but they also enhance communication and coordination among patients, carers, and healthcare providers. The adoption of digital solutions to support the diag-nosis and monitoring of cognitive changes is gaining popularity across both research and clinical settings, exemplified by digital cognitive assessments and the emergence of new digital biomarkers (Öhman, Hassenstab, Berron,

Schöll, & Papp, 2021). Additionally, a variety of care technologies, such as socially assistive robots and eHealth applications, have been developed to address the unique challenges posed by an aging population (Leonardsen et al., 2023).

This chapter will delve into the integration of digital solutions in the treatment, care, and support of individuals with dementia, emphasizing their potential to be woven into everyday healthcare practices. By doing so, these technologies hold promise for significantly improving the quality of life (QOL) for those living with dementia and their carers.

12.2 Digital Solutions in Dementia Treatment and Care

Digital solutions in dementia care encompass a diverse array of technologies, including digital cognitive assessments, telemedicine, wearable devices, mobile applications, and artificial intelligence (AI). Each of these technologies plays a unique and vital role in addressing the multifaceted challenges associated with dementia care. Digital cognitive testing facilitates early detection and diagnosis by providing efficient, accurate, and accessible tools to assess cognitive function, while telemedicine offers a platform for remote consultations, enabling continuous monitoring and management of the condition, regardless of geographical barriers (Staffaroni, Tsoy, Taylor, Boxer, & Possin, 2020). Wearable devices, such as smartwatches and health trackers, provide real-time data on patients' physical and physiological states, assisting in monitoring daily activities, detecting falls, tracking heart rate, and alerting carers or healthcare providers to potential emergencies (Masoumian Hosseini, Masoumian Hosseini, Qayumi, Hosseinzadeh, & Sajadi Tabar, 2023). Mobile applications are designed to support both patients and carers by offering reminders for medication, scheduling, and managing daily routines, thereby promoting independence and enhancing QOL (Wang, Newman, Martin, & Lapum, 2022; Zgonec, 2021). AI algorithms contribute to personalized treatment plans by analyzing vast amounts of data to identify patterns and predict disease progression, as well as to provide tailored interventions that cater to the specific needs of each individual with dementia (Angelucci, Ai, Piendel, Cerman, & Hort, 2024). Moreover, AI-powered tools, including social assistive robots, offer companionship and engage patients in therapeutic activities, thereby addressing social and emotional needs (Padhan, Mohapatra, Ramasamy, & Agrawal, 2023). Together, these digital solutions represent a comprehensive approach to dementia care, covering the entire spectrum from early diagnosis and ongoing monitoring to personalized treatment and support for both patients and their carers.

12.3 Early Diagnosis and Monitoring

Early diagnosis of dementia and mild cognitive impairment (MCI) is crucial for effective management. Early or timely diagnosis supports the well-being of both people living with dementia and their families by facilitating access to care and treatment services (Livingston et al., 2024). Digital tools are a growing component of diagnostic and monitoring approaches and provide an opportunity for more equitable and widespread access to these services. Key digital solutions related to diagnosis of MCI and dementia include digital cognitive tests and digital biomarkers.

12.3.1 Digital Cognitive Tests

Digital cognitive tests are an emerging alternative to traditional pencil-and-paper tests for the diagnosis and monitoring of cognitive decline. Generally, digital cognitive tests are brief tasks that assess a range of cognitive domains. The format and administration of digital cognitive tests vary widely. Tests may be supervised (requiring trained staff) or unsupervised (self-administered) in a range of settings, including in clinic or at home, and may be administered on a range of devices (e.g., computer, tablet, or smartphone) (Staffaroni, Tsoy, Taylor, Boxer, & Possin, 2020). Many digital tests also include automatic scoring, which may reduce the time burden for clinicians. The digital format of tests more readily allows for the generation and administration of alternate test items, which is especially important for long-term and repeated assessment. When considered in combination with the shorter administration time and cost-effectiveness, digital cognitive tests are advantageous to assess more individuals efficiently in the case of large-scale trials or studies and clinically to improve access to diagnostic services, especially for those in remote areas, when delivered appropriately. The utility of remote assessment via digital technologies is further underscored by the COVID-19 pandemic, where traditional in-clinic pencil-and-paper assessment was severely limited. Evidence supports comparable diagnostic performance of digital cognitive tests to traditional pencil-and-paper tests for detection of MCI and dementia (Chan, Yau, Kwok, & Tsoi, 2021; Ding, Lee, & Chan, 2022). Digital cognitive tests are not restricted to computerized equivalents of traditional paper versions of tests. A novel approach to digital testing is computerized cognitive games, which purport to assess multiple domains via tasks in either 2D or 3D scenarios (Bottiroli et al., 2021; Valladares-Rodriguez et al., 2017). Virtual reality (VR) is another emerging digital technology to assess cognition in more naturalistic settings, such as simulating daily activities (Eraslan Boz et al., 2020; Rapp et al., 2018). These novel applications of technology present an interesting direction for future test approaches; however, considerable work on the development and validation of these formats is necessary before such technologies are widely used (Cubillos & Rienzo, 2023). Computerized testing also allows for the parallel collection of a range of digital biomarkers.

12.3.2 Digital Biomarkers

Digital biomarkers are objective behavioral and/or physiological data that may be actively or passively collected by wearable devices or sensors that indicate normal or pathogenic biological processes and capture therapeutic or intervention response (Piau, Wild, Mattek, & Kaye, 2019). These technologies allow for a more ecologically valid and continuous assessment over a longer term, compared to more traditional assessments conducted at discrete time points (Piau, Wild, Mattek, & Kaye, 2019). They are a lower-cost and scalable approach for the early detection of cognitive changes and monitoring of cognition when compared to traditional cognitive tests and biological biomarkers. Commonly reported digital biomarkers include activities of daily living (ADLs), gait/movement, and speech. Speech-based digital biomarkers are a compelling example of novel digital solutions to address early diagnosis as objective data can be remotely captured in naturalistic settings via unobtrusive tasks or methods (Robin et al., 2020). Speech-based digital biomarkers are also an example of how digital cognitive testing practices may be extended to optimize the technology and delivery mode by collecting additional data points alongside the test itself, i.e., natural language processing analyses could be conducted using AI from a recording of a story-recall task.

Passively collected digital biomarkers require no additional time or demand on clinicians, patients, or their carers, which is critical for the widespread implementation and large-scale adoption of such technologies. Passive digital biomarkers that analyze already collected data in electronic health records (EHRs) present a promising digital solution that integrates technology into existing and everyday healthcare processes to monitor people with dementia and evaluate their care plans. Whilst there is preliminary evidence to support the performance of such algorithms in the detection and monitoring of Alzheimer's disease and related dementias (ADRD) (Ford, Milne, & Curlewis, 2023), caution is warranted in selecting the most appropriate digital biomarkers based on factors such as the quality of the source data and its structure (i.e., structured vs unstructured EHR data) and the similarity of the cohorts in which the algorithms were developed and validated (Taylor, Barboi, & Boustani, 2023). This approach of analyzing EHR data in clinical settings may also be applied to research contexts, such as in large cohort studies to further develop and validate such digital biomarkers. Further, wearable devices and sensors play a significant role in monitoring cognitive and physical health. These devices track vital signs, movement patterns, and sleep quality, providing continuous data that can indicate changes in the individual's condition (Kourtis, Regele, Wright, & Jones, 2019). Remote monitoring through these devices allows healthcare providers to intervene promptly, when necessary, potentially delaying the progression of dementia. In-home sensors are another proposed digital solution to assess and monitor functional performance of individuals in real-life settings, and have shown some promise in discriminating between healthy controls and individuals with MCI (Akl, Taati, & Mihailidis, 2015). Similar to in-home sensors, in-car sensors allow for an individual's driving performance and behaviors to be passively captured and monitored, for the purposes of detecting early-stage dementia (Bayat et al., 2021) or to inform whether it is suitable for the person with dementia to continue driving independently.

Digital tools such as AI algorithms and machine learning models that analyze medical data can also be applied to biological and imaging biomarkers, including brain scans and genetic information, to identify early signs of dementia. For example, AI-powered imaging techniques can detect subtle changes in brain structure, facilitating earlier and more accurate diagnoses. Machine learning, specifically deep learning approaches, is widely reported in the literature with some evidence for highly accurate discrimination between healthy controls and patients with MCI and dementia (Ahmed et al., 2019; Pellegrini et al., 2018). Nevertheless, these approaches are only available to patients who are seen in specialist settings and have access to imaging (Ford, Milne, & Curlewis, 2023), limiting wide scale adoption of such an approach in lower resource settings.

However, many of these digital solutions and technologies are in their infancy and require further development and validation with more diverse populations in various settings and evaluation of cost-effectiveness and economic viability as large-scale solutions. Further work is essential to ensure the usability and acceptability for people living with dementia for successful implementation to be achieved.

12.4 Personalized Treatment in Dementia

Digital technologies enable the creation of individualized treatment plans that cater to the unique needs of each person with dementia. Mobile applications and online platforms provide cognitive training exercises aimed at improving memory, attention, and problem-solving skills. These exercises are designed to adapt to the user's performance, offering a customized experience that optimizes cognitive outcomes. VR and augmented reality (AR) technologies offer immersive experiences that enhance cognitive functioning. For example, VR simulations can recreate familiar environments, aiding individuals in recalling memories and navigating daily tasks more effectively. AR applications, on the other hand, can overlay digital information onto the real world, assisting with activities such as medication management and navigation.

A wide range of digital tools has been investigated to create meaningful and individualized activities for people living with dementia, addressing key challenges such as memory support, behavior management, engagement, and communication (Goodall, Taraldsen, & Serrano, 2020). These technologies can be grouped into four main categories aligned with the needs of individuals with dementia: reminiscence therapy and memory support, behavior management, engagement and activity facilitation, and communication and language support.

12.4.1 Reminiscence Therapy and Memory Stimulation

Digital tools such as multimedia applications and digital life storybooks have been developed to support reminiscence and memory recall for individuals with dementia (Critten & Kucirkova, 2019; Laird et al., 2018; Ryan et al., 2020). These tools often use personal photographs, videos, and audio recordings familiar to the individual, providing both a comforting and cognitively stimulating experience. For instance, digital life storybooks allow users to revisit significant life events, which can enhance memory recall and provide emotional comfort. Lancioni et al. (2016) examined two technology-aided interventions designed to enhance verbal reminiscence and physical activity in individuals with moderate Alzheimer's disease. The first intervention employed videos and photographs to stimulate verbal engagement, while the second used personalized songs and images to encourage arm-raising activities. The findings indicated significant improvements in both verbal and physical activity, highlighting the potential of technology-aided reminiscence in dementia care (Lancioni et al., 2016).

12.4.2 Behavior Management

Technologies like social robots and personalized multimedia devices have been used to manage behaviors associated with dementia, such as agitation and anxiety (Leng et al., 2019; Lu et al., 2021; Park et al., 2020). These tools offer customized interventions that can help calm individuals during periods of distress. For example, social robots can engage with users in a soothing manner, providing companionship and alleviating feelings of loneliness. Pet robots, like Person Al Robot, which is an animated robotic baby seal that uses sensors and authentic seal sounds to engage with people, have been shown to improve mood and reduce agitation in people with dementia (Jones et al., 2018; Moyle et al., 2017).

12.4.3 Engagement and Activity Facilitation

Encouraging engagement in meaningful activities is essential for the well-being of people with dementia. Digital solutions, including VR and interactive applications, have been developed to stimulate cognitive and sensory engagement (Tortora et al., 2024; Zhu et al., 2022). These technologies offer immersive experiences that can capture the attention of individuals with dementia, promoting active participation and mental stimulation. For example, VR applications can simulate familiar environments, enabling individuals to explore places they once knew, which helps maintain cognitive functions.

12.4.4 Communication and Language Support

Digital tools also play a crucial role in facilitating communication between individuals with dementia and their carers. Devices such as speech-generating tools and communication apps can help bridge the gap caused by cognitive decline, allowing individuals to express their needs and emotions more effectively (Ambegaonkar, Ritchie, & de la Fuente Garcia, 2021). These tools can be tailored to the user's specific communication abilities, providing accessible means for interaction. However, evidence indicates that communication applications require substantial improvement, as key features like text-to-speech, two-way communication, and personalized content are often missing, limiting their effectiveness for target users (Wilson, Cochrane, Mihailidis, & Small, 2020).

Most studies examining these technologies have taken place in the homes of community-dwelling individuals, with family members frequently acting as facilitators. The involvement of another person, such as a family member, professional carer, or therapist, has often been essential for the successful use of these technologies. Even in cases where individuals with dementia are encouraged to use the devices independently, carer support is typically available. Training on how to use these digital tools is provided to both individuals with dementia and their carers, though the extent and depth of training can vary across studies. For instance, in research involving the InspireD app, both dementia patients and their family members received training from an IT assistant, which included reminiscence training (Boyd, Bond, Ryan, Goode, & Mulvenna, 2021). In other cases, such as with the personalized multimedia touchscreen devices, participants received individualized training sessions based on spaced retrieval learning principles to help them effectively use the technology (Davison et al., 2016). However, some participants encountered difficulties due to cognitive or sensory impairments, highlighting the importance of personalized support and thoughtful design considerations.

Facilitation of these technologies has varied, from professional carers having complete control to joint use by individuals with dementia and their family members, and in some cases, more independent use by the individuals themselves. For example, lifelogging technologies like the SenseCam and smartphone lanyards were worn by people with dementia throughout the day but still required support from another person to manage the data (Karlsson, Zingmark, Axelsson, & Sävenstedt, 2017; Silva et al., 2017). This collaborative approach not only assists the person with dementia but also enhances the overall caregiving experience by fostering a cooperative care environment.

12.5 Support for People Living with Dementia and Their Carers

Caring for individuals with dementia presents significant physical, emotional, and psychological challenges. Digital assistive technologies (DATs) have emerged as valuable tools to ease the burden of caregiving and enhance the well-being of both carers and people living with dementia. These technologies provide crucial support by facilitating the management of daily routines, promoting autonomy and dignity, and improving the overall QOL for people living with dementia (Chen, Ding, & Wang, 2023).

DATs encompass a broad range of technologies designed to support education, rehabilitation, and participation in everyday activities, while also enhancing cognitive, sensory, and motor functions. They empower individuals with functional limitations to engage more fully in daily activities, educational opportunities, work, and leisure pursuits (Margot-Cattin et al., 2024; Schneider, Nißen, Kowatsch, & Vinay, 2024). Recent advancements have led to the development of devices and applications that leverage sensory data specifically tailored for people living with dementia. Examples include smartphones and wearable devices that monitor physical activity and provide in-home care support, as well as location tracking systems to manage wandering behavior (Chen, Ding, & Wang, 2023; Ehn, Richardson, Landerdahl Stridsberg, Redekop, & Wamala-Andersson, 2021).

Moreover, the integration of AI has enabled the creation of social assistive robots, such as the robotic seal PARO, designed to offer companionship and engage users in therapeutic activities (Kelly et al., 2021). These technologies extend beyond basic assistance by fostering social interaction, supporting memory, facilitating engagement in leisure activities, and enhancing overall health monitoring (Koo & Vizer, 2019; Lee, Chung, Kim, & Nam, 2022).

Ensuring a high quality of life for people living with dementia is essential and involves physical, mental, social, and emotional dimensions, such as emotional well-being, social inclusion, and self-esteem (Appel et al., 2021). Research indicates that DATs can positively impact these aspects by promoting autonomy, enhancing engagement and social interaction, supporting health monitoring, and facilitating ADLs. They also help manage behavioral and psychological symptoms of dementia (BPSD) and ensure safety (Schneider, Nißen, Kowatsch, & Vinay, 2024). DATs have the potential to enable people living with dementia to age in place, live independently, and preserve their dignity by maintaining or regaining their ability to engage in daily activities and social interactions, thereby improving cognitive function, general well-being, and safety.

However, some studies have identified potential negative effects of DATs on the QOL of people living with dementia, including increased anxiety, concerns over negative outcomes, aggression toward the technology, and, in some cases, an exacerbation of BPSD (Flynn et al., 2022; Koh, Ang, & Casey, 2021; Ong, Tang, & Tam, 2021; Yu, Sommerlad, Sakure, & Livingston, 2022).

12.6 Well-Being and Engagement

Digital interventions play a crucial role in enhancing the well-being and engagement of people with dementia and their carers, offering innovative solutions that address the unique challenges posed by cognitive decline and caregiving demands and could be categorized into robot-based, experience-based, and reminiscence interventions (Bradley, Shanker, Murphy, Fenge, & Heward, 2023).

12.6.1 Robot-Based Interventions

include assistive, pet, and social robots. Assistive robots or homecare robots could offer both practical and therapeutic benefits, such as functional support (help with daily tasks), monitoring physical and psychological well-being, and providing therapeutic interventions (Begum, Huq, Wang, & Mihailidis, 2015; Darragh et al., 2017). Begum, Huq, Wang, and Mihailidis (2015) observed a teleoperated robot assisting a person with dementia in completing a tea-making task. The robot prompted the person and asked questions, later guiding them back to their carer. This pilot study highlighted both benefits and challenges, suggesting the need for larger studies to understand the needs of people with dementia and to develop an intelligent robot control interface capable of effective collaboration. Social robots like Sophie and Jack, two baby-faced robots, delivered diversion therapy services, including face recognition, emotion recognition, and entertainment activities like singing and dancing, and were found to enhance social engagement and QOL (Chu, Khosla, Khaksar, & Nguyen, 2017). Another robot named Eva, which incorporated conversational strategies to enable interactions without human intervention, led to more sustained conversations with people with dementia, underscoring the importance of integrating such strategies in future robot designs (Cruz-Sandoval & Favela, 2019). Similarly, Feng, Barakova, Yu, Hu, and Rauterberg (2020) showed that using a robotic sheep to facilitate interactions with a simulated farm environment reduced apathy and promoted purposeful engagement, further underscoring the value of social robots in dementia care.

12.6.2 Experience-Based Interventions

Experience-based interventions focus on providing recreational, sensory, and social networking opportunities through digital technologies. Studies explored the use of digital technology to enhance recreational leisure activities for individuals with cognitive impairment and suggest that VR and touchscreen interfaces can provide immersive and engaging activities (D'Cunha et al., 2021; Lazar, Demiris, & Thompson, 2016). D'Cunha et al. (2021) investigated a group VR cycling experience in aged care facilities, where residents engaged in physical activity by cycling along pre-recorded videos of local paths. The experience was found to be immersive and challenging, promoting environmental stimulation and reminiscence about past cycling experiences. This suggests that virtual cycling could serve as an engaging alternative to traditional activities, potentially increasing physical activity levels in aged care settings. Lazar, Demiris, and Thompson (2016) examined a touchscreen-based system designed to support the physical and mental well-being of older adults with memory impairments. The system facilitated social interaction, entertainment, motor engagement, and cognitive training. While the system was reported to enhance enjoyment, social connections, and mental stimulation, challenges such as technical and ethical concerns were also noted. Sensory interventions, such as the SENSE-GARDEN, a multi-sensory experience designed to promote narrative identity and relationships through individualized and meaningful activities, help preserve narrative identity and foster relationships (Goodall, André, Taraldsen, & Serrano, 2021). People living with dementia, supported by care workers and family, could interact with sensory stimuli, including familiar scents, scenic imagery, and personalized videos. SENSE-GARDEN could stimulate emotional experiences and foster interpersonal relationships, highlighting the importance of a holistic approach in dementia care. Social networking through platforms like Friendsource, a closed Facebook support group for carers of people with Alzheimer's disease has also been found to reduce carer stress and enhance support networks (Wilkerson, Brady, Yi, & Bateman, 2018).

12.6.3 Reminiscence Interventions

Reminiscence interventions utilize technology to support memory and improve relationships between people with dementia and their carers and increase engagement and physical activity. An example is the InspireD app, which has been used to facilitate technology-supported reminiscence in the homes of people with dementia. The 12-week program, which included 5 training sessions, resulted in statistically significant improvements in mutuality, relationship quality, and subjective well-being for participants with dementia (Laird et al., 2018).

12.7 Education and Training

Digital solutions have become increasingly vital in dementia education and training, particularly for informal carers who play a crucial role in care provision. Education that focuses on dementia knowledge, care strategies, self-care, and burnout prevention has been shown to improve care management and social support-seeking behavior among carers (Jensen, Agbata, Canavan, & McCarthy, 2015). Importantly, digital education offers the advantage of remote, asynchronous learning, which is particularly beneficial for carers in rural areas with limited access to services. Systematic reviews and meta-analyses have demonstrated that digitally delivered dementia education can positively impact carer depression, distress, burden, and overall caregiving experience (Frias et al., 2020; Scerbe et al., 2023).

Various technology-based interventions, including websites, mobile apps, VR, and telephone-based learning, have been developed to deliver dementia education. Online platforms offer a wealth of educational resources and training programs that equip carers with the knowledge and skills necessary to provide effective care (Klimova, Valis, Kuca, & Masopust, 2019). These resources cover a wide array of topics, including dementia progression, communication strategies, and behavior management techniques, the WHO iSupport program is an example (Pot et al., 2019). Interactive modules and video tutorials enhance learning by allowing carers to engage with content at their own pace, which facilitates the practical application of newly acquired skills in real-world settings. Additionally, these digital resources can be customized to address specific challenges faced by carers, making them more relevant and practical for diverse caregiving scenarios.

Despite the advantages of digital education, its adoption remains limited, and disparities in access to quality education persist. Carers express mixed opinions about dementia technologies, with concerns about technical skills, privacy, and over-reliance on technology (Brookman et al., 2023; Wang, Newman, Martin, & Lapum, 2022). Addressing these challenges requires strengthening carers' digital competencies and ensuring equitable access to educational resources.

The integration of technology into dementia education aligns with global initiatives, such as the WHO's Global Action Plan and national dementia strategies, which emphasize the need to equip carers with the knowledge and skills to utilize digital tools effectively. However, current training programs for lay carers are underdeveloped, with significant variability in quality and content. To maximize the benefits of dementia technologies, it is essential to address gaps in carer education, promote transparency, and ensure the ethical deployment of technology that aligns with carers' values and needs (Martin, Tam, & Robillard, 2024).

12.8 Communication and Coordination

Effective communication and coordination among carers, healthcare providers, and other stakeholders are crucial for high-quality dementia care. Mobile apps and online platforms facilitate this by enabling the sharing of health data, care plans, and daily updates (Wang, Newman, Martin, & Lapum, 2022). Telemedicine has become an indispensable tool, allowing carers to consult with healthcare professionals remotely, which is especially beneficial in rural or underserved areas (Angelopoulou et al., 2022). Social media and online support groups provide carers with a sense of community, offering spaces to share experiences, seek advice, and find emotional support (Wilkerson, Brady, Yi, & Bateman, 2018). These virtual communities can reduce feelings of isolation and provide emotional relief, crucial given the demanding nature of caregiving.

A wide range of technological devices, including tablet computers and social robots, are employed to enhance social interactions for people living with dementia. Tablet-based interventions, often centered around reminiscence activities, have been shown to support communication between people living with dementia and their carers, whether in nursing facilities or home-based environments (Laird et al., 2018). Social robots, such as PARO, have been effective in facilitating communication by providing a focal point for interaction and reducing the pressure on conversation partners (Moyle et al., 2017). Computer systems, though more complex, offer tailored interventions for people living with dementia, supporting social interactions through cognitive stimulation and reminiscence (Davison et al., 2016; Lazar, Demiris, & Thompson, 2016). Other innovative technologies, such as 3D-printed objects for autobiographical reminiscence, are emerging as tools to enhance communication and connectedness.

These technologies not only foster better understanding between carers and people living with dementia but also alleviate the conversational burden on carers, making interactions more meaningful and less stressful. However, the design and implementation of these digital solutions must involve people living with dementia, their families, and care professionals to ensure they are adaptive, personalized, and effective in supporting well-being.

12.9 Ethical and Practical Considerations

While digital solutions offer numerous benefits in dementia care, their implementation must navigate several ethical and practical challenges. The paramount concern is privacy and data security, especially given the sensitive nature of medical information. These technologies capture immense amounts of personal data, necessitating robust measures to protect against breaches and unauthorized access (Perakslis & Ginsburg, 2021). Digital biomarkers represent a promising future direction for the detection and monitoring of ADRD. They are scalable and utilize technologies that are often already integrated into everyday life. However, the early detection of dementia, particularly in pre-symptomatic stages, raises significant ethical concerns. The ease of access to digital solutions allows individuals in the community to engage with these technologies independently of clinicians, often without clinical guidance, adding a new layer to the ethical debate (Ford, Milne, & Curlewis, 2023). While there is no consensus on how to best address these challenges, the following principles have been proposed to guide the use and regulation of these evolving technologies (Ford, Milne, & Curlewis, 2023). Ethical early detection of dementia using digital tools should align with screening criteria and focus on accurately predicting progression from MCI to dementia. Implementation at the population level is only justified if there is an effective early treatment, reliable predictive accuracy, minimally invasive and cost-effective detection methods, and adequate healthcare support. Additionally, early detection should be voluntary, confidential, and assessed for potential psychosocial harm while ensuring equitable access to avoid exacerbating health inequalities (Ford, Milne, & Curlewis, 2023).

The widespread availability of digital devices highlights the ease of access and cost-effectiveness of digital solutions, particularly for rural and remote communities with limited access to traditional face-to-face specialist services. However, it is crucial to consider the inequities faced by communities outside the global north when accessing digital solutions for dementia treatment, care, and support. The economic evidence on the cost-effectiveness of mobile health (mHealth) interventions for older adults with chronic conditions in homecare settings is inconsistent (Iribarren, Cato, Falzon, & Stone, 2017). While some interventions have not proven cost-effective, others have shown favorable outcomes. Yet, comprehensive evidence of cost-effectiveness for mHealth use among older adults, particularly those with MCI or dementia, remains limited (Ghani et al., 2022). Differences in intervention characteristics—such as the learning curve for healthcare professionals and patients, the level of professional engagement, and participant adherence—further complicate the generalization of cost-effectiveness findings across the mHealth field.

Accessibility and usability are critical factors in the successful adoption of digital tools. Digital accessibility should not be viewed merely as a technical issue; instead, it is an ongoing, dynamic process influenced by technological cycles, which are shaped by trade-offs with social, economic, and technical consequences (Botelho, 2021). These trade-offs are reflected in laws such as patents, copyrights, and consumer protections, which are influenced by societal values. Understanding the processes, structures, and values that impact accessibility is crucial for developing effective and sustainable initiatives to enhance this fundamental human right. User-friendly interfaces, clear instructions, accommodation of individuals with varying levels of digital literacy, and ongoing technical support are essential to ensure widespread use and effectiveness of digital technologies (Anawade, Sharma, & Gahane, 2024; Fitzpatrick, 2023).

12.10 Future Directions

Looking ahead, the integration of digital solutions in dementia care is expected to become even more sophisticated. Future advancements may include AI-driven predictive models that not only diagnose but also forecast the progression of dementia, enabling more personalized and proactive care (Arafah et al., 2023). The development of smart environments, powered by the Internet of Things (IoT), could further enhance the safety and independence of individuals with dementia, creating living spaces that adapt to their needs in real time (Dorri, Zabolinezhad, & Sattari, 2023; Sheikhtaheri & Sabermahani, 2022). There is a pressing need for continued dialogue among individuals with dementia, carers, and professionals in the development and adaptation of digital technologies to meet specific needs (Bradley, Shanker, Murphy, Fenge, & Heward, 2023). Future research should focus on refining these approaches to create inclusive technologies that are accessible to diverse populations, including those with varying levels of cognitive impairment (Darragh et al., 2017; Lazar, Demiris, & Thompson, 2016; Wang, Newman, Martin, & Lapum, 2022). Collaboration between technologists, healthcare professionals, and end-users will be key to developing tools that are both effective and practical in real-world settings. Further research should explore how multiple DAT devices can work together or be combined to better support individuals with dementia and their carers, rather than focusing solely on the capabilities of individual devices. Co-designing DAT solutions with those who have lived experience of the challenges of dementia, including carers, is essential (Brookman et al., 2023; Wang, Marradi, Albayrak, & van der Cammen, 2019). The ability of a carer to problem-solve should also be considered when prescribing and using DAT. Technology should match the needs of the person requiring its use, rather than forcing the person to adapt to the available technology.

12.11 Conclusion

Digital solutions are transforming dementia treatment, care, and support, offering innovative ways to enhance the lives of individuals with dementia and their carers. These technologies, ranging from early diagnosis and personalized treatment to carer education and support, provide valuable tools for managing the complexities of dementia. As we advance further into the digital age, the integration of these solutions will play an increasingly vital role in addressing the global challenge of dementia. They hold significant potential to improve accessibility, enhance the precision of diagnoses and interventions, and ultimately promote the well-being of those affected by the condition.

Advances in IoT technologies allow for continuous monitoring of vital health indicators, such as heart rate, respiratory rate, physical activity, and mood, with data transmitted in real-time to multidisciplinary healthcare teams for more responsive care (Dorri, Zabolinezhad, & Sattari, 2023; Sheikhtaheri & Sabermahani, 2022). Wearable devices within IoT systems support aging in place by enabling individuals to maintain independence while receiving appropriate care. Machine learning and data analytics further enhance IoT capabilities by facilitating early dementia detection, monitoring disease progression, and supporting advanced care planning. Utilizing existing healthcare records, these technologies help develop and monitor dementia risk scores, aiding clinical decision-making (Dorri, Zabolinezhad, & Sattari, 2023; Sheikhtaheri & Sabermahani, 2022). Data and text mining also offer new methods for identifying individuals at risk of dementia (Sucharitha, Chakraborty, Srinivasa Rao, & Reddy, 2021). Tools like dashboard systems improve healthcare productivity, care quality, and visualization of disease progression (Esquer Rochin, Gutierrez-Garcia, Rosales, & Rodriguez, 2021). However, their effective use requires flexible adaptation to the needs of both healthcare professionals and patients.

Equally important is the role of digital solutions in supporting carers, who are often the backbone of dementia care. Online platforms, mobile apps, and telehealth services provide carers with essential resources, including education, emotional support, and tools for managing daily caregiving tasks. These technologies not only alleviate the burden on carers but also empower them with the knowledge and confidence to provide better care (Scerbe et al., 2023). By connecting carers with healthcare professionals and peer support networks, digital solutions foster a collaborative care environment that benefits both carers and those they care for.

The successful design, development, deployment, and adoption of digital solutions for dementia care depend on overcoming key barriers while leveraging facilitating factors. Major challenges include limited digital literacy among older adults and carers, concerns over data privacy and security, high implementation costs, and the complexities of integrating new technologies into existing healthcare systems. Additionally, disparities in access to technology, particularly in low-resource settings, and the lack of standardized regulatory frameworks hinder equitable adoption. Ethical considerations, such as ensuring informed consent and minimizing potential psychosocial harms, must also be carefully addressed.

Conversely, several facilitators enhance the feasibility and effectiveness of digital solutions. Advances in AI, wearable technologies, and remote monitoring have expanded opportunities for innovative care models. Increased policy support, stakeholder engagement in co-design processes, and integration of digital tools into mainstream healthcare further promote their adoption. Ensuring user-friendly interfaces, robust technical support, and clear ethical guidelines will be crucial in mitigating barriers and fostering success-ful implementation.

While digital interventions such as virtual care and mobile technologies hold promise for improving QOL and reducing caregiving burdens, cur-rent evidence on their effectiveness and cost-effectiveness remains lim-ited (Ghani et al., 2022; Iribarren, Cato, Falzon, & Stone, 2017). A hybrid approach that integrates digital and traditional care methods could achieve more equitable and accessible dementia care. Engaging with various stakeholders—including healthcare professionals, patients, carers, and technology users—is crucial for the development of effective and meaning-ful digital solutions (Brookman et al., 2023; Wang, Marradi, Albayrak, & van der Cammen, 2019). Participatory design methods, involving stakeholders in the creation and implementation process, ensure that technologies are user-centered and address real-world challenges. Early involvement of stakeholders can also help overcome adoption barriers related to accep-tance, cost, ethics, and usability, while promoting educational practices that support the seamless integration of these technologies into primary care. Addressing these challenges while capitalizing on existing opportunities will be essential for realizing the full potential of digital innovations in dementia care.

In conclusion, the future of dementia care lies in the thoughtful integra-tion of digital solutions that are responsive to the needs of all stakeholders. By leveraging the power of IoT, machine learning, and data analytics, and prioritizing stakeholder engagement in the design process, we can create a more effective, compassionate, and personalized approach to dementia care. This will ensure that both individuals with dementia and their carers are supported every step of the way.

References

Ahmed, M. R., Zhang, Y., Feng, Z., Lo, B., Inan, O. T., & Liao, H. (2019). Neuroimaging and machine learning for dementia diagnosis: Recent advancements and future prospects. *IEEE Rev Biomed Eng, 12*, 19–33. doi:10.1109/rbme.2018.2886237

Akl, A., Taati, B., & Mihailidis, A. (2015). Autonomous unobtrusive detection of mild cognitive impairment in older adults. *IEEE Trans Biomed Eng, 62*(5), 1383–1394. doi:10.1109/TBME.2015.2389149

Alzheimer's Association. (2024). Alzheimer's disease facts and figures. *Alzheimers Dement, 20*(5), 3708–3821.

Ambegaonkar, A., Ritchie, C., & de la Fuente Garcia, S. (2021). The use of Mobile applications as communication aids for people with dementia: Opportunities and limitations. *J Alzheimers Dis Rep, 5*(1), 681–692. doi:10.3233/adr-200259

Anawade, P. A., Sharma, D., & Gahane, S. (2024). A comprehensive review on explor-ing the impact of telemedicine on healthcare accessibility. *Cureus, 16*(3), e55996. doi:10.7759/cureus.55996

Angelopoulou, E., Papachristou, N., Bougea, A., Stanitsa, E., Kontaxopoulou, D., Fragkiadaki, S., & ... Papageorgiou, S. (2022). How telemedicine can improve the quality of care for patients with Alzheimer's disease and related dementias? A narrative review. *Medicina (Kaunas), 58*(12). doi:10.3390/medicina58121705

Angelucci, F., Ai, A. R., Piendel, L., Cerman, J., & Hort, J. (2024). Integrating AI in fighting advancing Alzheimer: Diagnosis, prevention, treatment, monitoring, mechanisms, and clinical trials. *Curr Opin Struct Biol, 87*, 102857. https://doi.org/10.1016/j.sbi.2024.102857

Appel, L., Ali, S., Narag, T., Mozeson, K., Pasat, Z., Orchanian-Cheff, A., & Campos, J. L. (2021). Virtual reality to promote wellbeing in persons with dementia: A scoping review. *J Rehabil Assist Technol Eng, 8*, 20556683211053952. doi:10.1177/20556683211053952

Arafah, A., Khatoon, S., Rasool, I., Khan, A., Rather, M. A., Abujabal, K. A., & ... Rehman, M. U. (2023). The future of precision medicine in the cure of Alzheimer's disease. *Biomedicines, 11*(2). doi:10.3390/biomedicines11020335

Arvanitakis, Z., Shah, R. C., & Bennett, D. A. (2019). Diagnosis and management of dementia: Review. *Jama, 322*(16), 1589–1599. doi:10.1001/jama.2019.4782

Bayat, S., Babulal, G. M., Schindler, S. E., Fagan, A. M., Morris, J. C., Mihailidis, A., & Roe, C. M. (2021). GPS driving: A digital biomarker for preclinical Alzheimer disease. *Alzheimers Res Ther, 13*(1), 115. doi:10.1186/s13195-021-00852-1

Begum, M., Huq, R., Wang, R., & Mihailidis, A. (2015). Collaboration of an assistive robot and older adults with dementia. *Gerontechnology, 13*(4), 405–419.

Botelho, F. H. F. (2021). Accessibility to digital technology: Virtual barriers, real opportunities. *Assist Technol, 33*(sup1), 27–34. doi:10.1080/10400435.2021.1945705

Bottiroli, S., Bernini, S., Cavallini, E., Sinforiani, E., Zucchella, C., Pazzi, S., & ... Tassorelli, C. (2021). The smart aging platform for assessing early phases of cognitive impairment in patients with neurodegenerative diseases. *Front Psychol, 12*, 635410. doi:10.3389/fpsyg.2021.635410

Boyd, K., Bond, R., Ryan, A., Goode, D., & Mulvenna, M. (2021). Digital reminiscence app co-created by people living with dementia and carers: Usability and eye gaze analysis. *Health Expect, 24*(4), 1207–1219. doi:10.1111/hex.13251

Bradley, L., Shanker, S., Murphy, J., Fenge, L. A., & Heward, M. (2023). Effectiveness of digital technologies to engage and support the wellbeing of people with dementia and family carers at home and in care homes: A scoping review. *Dementia (London), 22*(6), 1292–1313. doi:10.1177/14713012231178445

Brookman, R., Parker, S., Hoon, L., Ono, A., Fukayama, A., Matsukawa, H., & Harris, C. B. (2023). Technology for dementia care: What would good technology look like and do, from carers' perspectives? *BMC Geriatrics, 23*(1), 867. doi:10.1186/s12877-023-04530-9

Chan, J. Y. C., Yau, S. T. Y., Kwok, T. C. Y., & Tsoi, K. K. F. (2021). Diagnostic performance of digital cognitive tests for the identification of MCI and dementia: A systematic review. *Ageing Res Rev, 72*, 101506. https://doi.org/10.1016/j.arr.2021.101506

Chen, C., Ding, S., & Wang, J. (2023). Digital health for aging populations. *Nat Med, 29*(7), 1623–1630. doi:10.1038/s41591-023-02391-8

Chu, M. T., Khosla, R., Khaksar, S. M., & Nguyen, K. (2017). Service innovation through social robot engagement to improve dementia care quality. *Assist Technol, 29*(1), 8–18. doi:10.1080/10400435.2016.1171807

Critten, V., & Kucirkova, N. (2019). "It brings it all back, all those good times; It makes me go close to tears". Creating digital personalised stories with people who have dementia. *Dementia (London)*, *18*(3), 864–881. doi:10.1177/1471301217691162

Cruz-Sandoval, D., & Favela, J. (2019). Incorporating conversational strategies in a social robot to interact with people with dementia. *Dement Geriatr Cogn Disord*, *47*(3), 140–148. doi:10.1159/000497801

Cubillos, C., & Rienzo, A. (2023). Digital cognitive assessment tests for older adults: Systematic literature review. *JMIR Ment Health*, *10*, e47487. doi:10.2196/47487

Cuffaro, L., Di Lorenzo, F., Bonavita, S., Tedeschi, G., Leocani, L., & Lavorgna, L. (2020). Dementia care and COVID-19 pandemic: A necessary digital revolution. *Neurol Sci*, *41*(8), 1977–1979. doi:10.1007/s10072-020-04512-4

D'Cunha, N. M., Isbel, S. T., Frost, J., Fearon, A., McKune, A. J., Naumovski, N., & Kellett, J. (2021). Effects of a virtual group cycling experience on people living with dementia: A mixed method pilot study. *Dementia (London)*, *20*(5), 1518–1535. doi:10.1177/1471301220951328

Darragh, M., Ahn, H. S., MacDonald, B., Liang, A., Peri, K., Kerse, N., & Broadbent, E. (2017). Homecare robots to improve health and well-being in mild cognitive impairment and early stage dementia: Results from a scoping study. *J Am Med Dir Assoc*, *18*(12), 1099.e1091–1099.e1094. doi:10.1016/j.jamda.2017.08.019

Davison, T. E., Nayer, K., Coxon, S., de Bono, A., Eppingstall, B., Jeon, Y. H., … & O'Connor, D. W. (2016). A personalized multimedia device to treat agitated behavior and improve mood in people with dementia: A pilot study. *Geriatr Nurs*, *37*(1), 25–29. doi:10.1016/j.gerinurse.2015.08.013

Ding, Z., Lee, T.-l, & Chan, A. S. (2022). Digital cognitive biomarker for mild cognitive impairments and dementia: A systematic review. *J Clin Med*, *11*(14). Retrieved from doi:10.3390/jcm11144191

Dorri, S., Zabolinezhad, H., & Sattari, M. (2023). The application of Internet of Things for the elderly health safety: A systematic review. *Adv Biomed Res*, *12*, 109. doi:10.4103/abr.abr_197_22

Ehn, M., Richardson, M. X., Landerdahl Stridsberg, S., Redekop, K., & Wamala-Andersson, S. (2021). Mobile safety alarms based on GPS technology in the care of older adults: Systematic review of evidence based on a general evidence framework for digital health technologies. *J Med Internet Res*, *23*(10), e27267. doi:10.2196/27267

Eraslan Boz, H., Limoncu, H., Zygouris, S., Tsolaki, M., Giakoumis, D., Votis, K., & … Yener, G. G. (2020). A new tool to assess amnestic mild cognitive impairment in Turkish older adults: Virtual supermarket (VSM). *Aging Neuropsychol Cogn*, *27*(5), 639–653. doi:10.1080/13825585.2019.1663146

Esquer Rochin, M. A., Gutierrez-Garcia, J. O., Rosales, J. H., & Rodriguez, L. F. (2021). Design and evaluation of a dashboard to support the comprehension of the progression of patients with dementia in day centers. *Int J Med Inform*, *156*, 104617. doi:10.1016/j.ijmedinf.2021.104617

Feng, Y., Barakova, E. I., Yu, S., Hu, J., & Rauterberg, G. W. M. (2020). Effects of the level of interactivity of a social robot and the response of the augmented reality display in contextual interactions of people with dementia. *Sensors (Basel)*, *20*(13). doi:10.3390/s20133771

Fitzpatrick, P. J. (2023). Improving health literacy using the power of digital communications to achieve better health outcomes for patients and practitioners. *Front Digit Health*, *5*, 1264780. doi:10.3389/fdgth.2023.1264780

Flynn, A., Healy, D., Barry, M., Brennan, A., Redfern, S., Houghton, C., & Casey, D. (2022). Key stakeholders' experiences and perceptions of virtual reality for older adults living with dementia: Systematic review and thematic synthesis. *JMIR Serious Games, 10*(4), e37228. doi:10.2196/37228

Ford, E., Milne, R., & Curlewis, K. (2023). Ethical issues when using digital biomarkers and artificial intelligence for the early detection of dementia. *Wiley Interdiscip Rev Data , 13*(3), e1492. doi:10.1002/widm.1492

Frias, C. E., Garcia-Pascual, M., Montoro, M., Ribas, N., Risco, E., & Zabalegui, A. (2020). Effectiveness of a psychoeducational intervention for caregivers of people with dementia with regard to burden, anxiety and depression: A systematic review. *J Adv Nurs, 76*(3), 787–802. doi:10.1111/jan.14286

Ghani, Z., Saha, S., Jarl, J., Andersson, M., Berglund, J. S., & Anderberg, P. (2022). Short term economic evaluation of the digital platform "Support Monitoring and Reminder Technology for Mild Dementia" (SMART4MD) for people with mild cognitive impairment and their informal caregivers. *J Alzheimers Dis, 86*(4), 1629–1641. doi:10.3233/jad-215013

Goodall, G., André, L., Taraldsen, K., & Serrano, J. A. (2021). Supporting identity and relationships amongst people with dementia through the use of technology: A qualitative interview study. *Int J Qual Stud Health Well-Being, 16*(1), 1920349. doi:10.1080/17482631.2021.1920349

Goodall, G., Taraldsen, K., & Serrano, J. A. (2020). The use of technology in creating individualized, meaningful activities for people living with dementia: A systematic review. *Dementia, 20*(4), 1442–1469. doi:10.1177/1471301220928168

Iribarren, S. J., Cato, K., Falzon, L., & Stone, P. W. (2017). What is the economic evidence for mHealth? A systematic review of economic evaluations of mHealth solutions. *PLoS One, 12*(2), e0170581. doi:10.1371/journal.pone.0170581

Jensen, M., Agbata, I. N., Canavan, M., & McCarthy, G. (2015). Effectiveness of educational interventions for informal caregivers of individuals with dementia residing in the community: Systematic review and meta-analysis of randomised controlled trials. *Int J Geriatr Psychiatry, 30*(2), 130–143. doi:10.1002/gps.4208

Jones, C., Moyle, W., Murfield, J., Draper, B., Shum, D., Beattie, E., & Thalib, L. (2018). Does cognitive impairment and agitation in dementia influence intervention effectiveness? Findings from a cluster-randomized-controlled trial with the therapeutic robot, PARO. *J Am Med Dir Assoc, 19*(7), 623–626. doi:10.1016/j.jamda.2018.02.014

Karlsson, E., Zingmark, K., Axelsson, K., & Sävenstedt, S. (2017). Aspects of self and identity in narrations about recent events: Communication with individuals with Alzheimer's disease enabled by a digital photograph diary. *J Gerontol Nurs, 43*(6), 25–31. doi:10.3928/00989134-20170126-02

Kelly, P. A., Cox, L. A., Petersen, S. F., Gilder, R. E., Blann, A., Autrey, A. E., & MacDonell, K. (2021). The effect of PARO robotic seals for hospitalized patients with dementia: A feasibility study. *Geriatr Nurs, 42*(1), 37–45. doi:10.1016/j.gerinurse.2020.11.003

Klimova, B., Valis, M., Kuca, K., & Masopust, J. (2019). E-learning as valuable caregivers' support for people with dementia—a systematic review. *BMC Health Serv Res, 19*(1), 781. doi:10.1186/s12913-019-4641-9

Koh, W. Q., Ang, F. X. H., & Casey, D. (2021). Impacts of low-cost robotic pets for older adults and people with dementia: Scoping review. *JMIR Rehabil Assist Technol, 8*(1), e25340. doi:10.2196/25340

Koo, B. M., & Vizer, L. M. (2019). Examining Mobile technologies to support older adults with dementia through the Lens of personhood and human needs: Scoping review. *JMIR Mhealth Uhealth, 7*(11), e15122. doi:10.2196/15122

Kourtis, L. C., Regele, O. B., Wright, J. M., & Jones, G. B. (2019). Digital biomarkers for Alzheimer's disease: The mobile/wearable devices opportunity. *npj Digit Med, 2*(1), 9. doi:10.1038/s41746-019-0084-2

Laird, E. A., Ryan, A., McCauley, C., Bond, R. B., Mulvenna, M. D., Curran, K. J., & ... Gibson, A. (2018). Using mobile technology to provide personalized reminiscence for people living with dementia and their carers: Appraisal of outcomes from a quasi-experimental study. *JMIR Ment Health, 5*(3), e57. doi:10.2196/mental.9684

Lancioni, G. E., Singh, N. N., O'Reilly, M. F., Sigafoos, J., D'Amico, F., Renna, C., & Pinto, K. (2016). Technology-aided programs to support positive verbal and physical engagement in persons with moderate or severe Alzheimer's disease. *Front Aging Neurosci, 8*, 87. doi:10.3389/fnagi.2016.00087

Lazar, A., Demiris, G., & Thompson, H. J. (2016). Evaluation of a multifunctional technology system in a memory care unit: Opportunities for innovation in dementia care. *Inform Health Soc Care, 41*(4), 373–386. doi:10.3109/17538157.2015.1064428

Lee, H., Chung, M. A., Kim, H., & Nam, E. W. (2022). The effect of cognitive function health care using artificial intelligence robots for older adults: Systematic review and meta-analysis. *JMIR Aging, 5*(2), e38896. doi:10.2196/38896

Leng, M., Liu, P., Zhang, P., Hu, M., Zhou, H., Li, G., & ... Chen, L. (2019). Pet robot intervention for people with dementia: A systematic review and meta-analysis of randomized controlled trials. *Psychiatry Res, 271*, 516–525. doi:10.1016/j.psychres.2018.12.032

Leonardsen, A. L., Hardeland, C., Helgesen, A. K., Bååth, C., Del Busso, L., & Grøndahl, V. A. (2023). The use of robotic technology in the healthcare of people above the age of 65—a systematic review. *Healthcare (Basel), 11*(6). doi:10.3390/healthcare11060904

Livingston, G., Huntley, J., Liu, K. Y., Costafreda, S. G., Selbæk, G., Alladi, S., ... & Mukadam, N. (2024). Dementia prevention, intervention, and care: 2024 report of the Lancet Standing Commission. *The Lancet, 404*(10452), 572–628. doi:10.1016/S0140-6736(24)01296-0

Lu, L. C., Lan, S. H., Hsieh, Y. P., Lin, L. Y., Lan, S. J., & Chen, J. C. (2021). Effectiveness of companion robot care for dementia: A systematic review and meta-analysis. *Innov Aging, 5*(2), igab013. doi:10.1093/geroni/igab013

Margot-Cattin, I., Deblock-Bellamy, A., Wassmer, J., Ledgerd, R., von Zweck, C., & World Federation of Occupational Therapists, W. (2024). Worldwide survey on Digital Assistive Technology (DAT) provision. *Occup Ther Int, 2024*, 9536020. doi:10.1155/2024/9536020

Martin, S. E., Tam, M. T., & Robillard, J. M. (2024). Technology in dementia education: An ethical imperative in a digitized world. *J Alzheimers Dis, 97*(3), 1105–1109. doi:10.3233/jad-230612

Masoumian Hosseini, M., Masoumian Hosseini, S. T., Qayumi, K., Hosseinzadeh, S., & Sajadi Tabar, S. S. (2023). Smartwatches in healthcare medicine: Assistance and monitoring; a scoping review. *BMC Med Inform Decis Mak, 23*(1), 248. doi:10.1186/s12911-023-02350-w

Mok, V. C. T., Pendlebury, S., Wong, A., Alladi, S., Au, L., Bath, P. M., & Scheltens, P. (2020). Tackling challenges in care of Alzheimer's disease and other dementias amid the COVID-19 pandemic, now and in the future. *Alzheimers Dement*, *16*(11), 1571–1581. doi:10.1002/alz.12143

Moyle, W., Jones, C. J., Murfield, J. E., Thalib, L., Beattie, E. R. A., Shum, D. K. H., … & Draper, B. M. (2017). Use of a robotic seal as a therapeutic tool to improve dementia symptoms: A cluster-randomized controlled trial. *J Am Med Dir Assoc*, *18*(9), 766–773. doi:10.1016/j.jamda.2017.03.018

Nichols, E., Steinmetz, J. D., Vollset, S. E., Fukutaki, K., Chalek, J., Abd-Allah, F., … & Vos, T. (2022). Estimation of the global prevalence of dementia in 2019 and forecasted prevalence in 2050: An analysis for the Global Burden of Disease Study 2019. *The Lancet Public Health*, *7*(2), e105–e125. doi:10.1016/S2468-2667(21)00249-8

Öhman, F., Hassenstab, J., Berron, D., Schöll, M., & Papp, K. V. (2021). Current advances in digital cognitive assessment for preclinical Alzheimer's disease. *Alzheimers Dement (Amst)*, *13*(1), e12217. doi:10.1002/dad2.12217

Ong, Y. C., Tang, A., & Tam, W. (2021). Effectiveness of robot therapy in the management of behavioural and psychological symptoms for individuals with dementia: A systematic review and meta-analysis. *J Psychiatr Res*, *140*, 381–394. doi:10.1016/j.jpsychires.2021.05.077

Padhan, S., Mohapatra, A., Ramasamy, S. K., & Agrawal, S. (2023). Artificial Intelligence (AI) and robotics in elderly healthcare: Enabling independence and quality of life. *Cureus*, *15*(8), e42905. doi:10.7759/cureus.42905

Park, S., Bak, A., Kim, S., Nam, Y., Kim, H. S., Yoo, D. H., & Moon, M. (2020). Animal-assisted and pet-robot interventions for ameliorating behavioral and psychological symptoms of dementia: A systematic review and meta-analysis. *Biomedicines*, *8*(6). doi:10.3390/biomedicines8060150

Pellegrini, E., Ballerini, L., Hernandez, M., Chappell, F. M., González-Castro, V., Anblagan, D., … & Wardlaw, J. M. (2018). Machine learning of neuroimaging for assisted diagnosis of cognitive impairment and dementia: A systematic review. *Alzheimers Dement (Amst)*, *10*, 519–535. doi:10.1016/j.dadm.2018.07.004

Perakslis, E., & Ginsburg, G. S. (2021). Digital health-the need to assess benefits, risks, and value. *Jama*, *325*(2), 127–128. doi:10.1001/jama.2020.22919

Piau, A., Wild, K., Mattek, N., & Kaye, J. (2019). Current state of digital biomarker technologies for real-life, home-based monitoring of cognitive function for mild cognitive impairment to mild Alzheimer disease and implications for clinical care: Systematic review. *J Med Internet Res*, *21*(8), e12785. doi:10.2196/12785

Pot, A. M., Gallagher-Thompson, D., Xiao, L. D., Willemse, B. M., Rosier, I., Mehta, K. M., … & Dua, T. (2019). iSupport: A WHO global online intervention for informal caregivers of people with dementia. *World Psychiatry*, *18*(3), 365–366. doi:10.1002/wps.20684

Rapp, S. R., Barnard, R. T., Sink, K. M., Chamberlain, D. G., Wilson, V., Lu, L., & Ip, E. H. (2018). Computer simulations for assessing cognitively intensive instrumental activities of daily living in older adults. *Alzheimer's Dement Diagn Assess Dis Monit*, *10*(1), 237–244. https://doi.org/10.1016/j.dadm.2018.01.008

Robin, J., Harrison, J. E., Kaufman, L. D., Rudzicz, F., Simpson, W., & Yancheva, M. (2020). Evaluation of speech-based digital biomarkers: Review and recommendations. *Digital Biomarkers*, *4*(3), 99–108. doi:10.1159/000510820

Ryan, A. A., McCauley, C. O., Laird, E. A., Gibson, A., Mulvenna, M. D., Bond, R., ... & Ferry, F. (2020). There is still so much inside': The impact of personalised reminiscence, facilitated by a tablet device, on people living with mild to moderate dementia and their family carers. *Dementia (London)*, 19(4), 1131–1150. doi:10.1177/1471301218795242

Sacco, G., Lléonart, S., Simon, R., Noublanche, F., & Annweiler, C. (2020). Communication technology preferences of hospitalized and institutionalized frail older adults during COVID-19 confinement: Cross-sectional survey study. *JMIR Mhealth Uhealth*, 8(9), e21845. doi:10.2196/21845

Scerbe, A., O'Connell, M. E., Astell, A., Morgan, D., Kosteniuk, J., Panyavin, I., ... & Webster, C. (2023). Digital tools for delivery of dementia education for caregivers of persons with dementia: A systematic review and meta-analysis of impact on caregiver distress and depressive symptoms. *PLoS One*, 18(5), e0283600. doi:10.1371/journal.pone.0283600

Schneider, C., Nißen, M., Kowatsch, T., & Vinay, R. (2024). Impact of digital assistive technologies on the quality of life for people with dementia: A scoping review. *BMJ Open*, 14(2), e080545. doi:10.1136/bmjopen-2023-080545

Sheikhtaheri, A., & Sabermahani, F. (2022). Applications and outcomes of Internet of Things for patients with Alzheimer's disease/dementia: A scoping review. *Biomed Res Int*, 2022, 6274185. doi:10.1155/2022/6274185

Silva, A. R., Pinho, M. S., Macedo, L., Moulin, C., Caldeira, S., & Firmino, H. (2017). It is not only memory: Effects of sensecam on improving well-being in patients with mild Alzheimer disease. *Int Psychogeriatr*, 29(5), 741–754. doi:10.1017/s104161021600243x

Staffaroni, A. M., Tsoy, E., Taylor, J., Boxer, A. L., & Possin, K. L. (2020). Digital cognitive assessments for dementia: Digital assessments may enhance the efficiency of evaluations in neurology and other clinics. *Pract Neurol (Fort Wash Pa)*, 2020, 24–45.

Sucharitha, M., Chakraborty, C., Srinivasa Rao, S., & Reddy, V. S. K. (2021). Early Detection of Dementia Disease Using Data Mining Techniques. In C. Chakraborty, A. Banerjee, M. H. Kolekar, L. Garg, & B. Chakraborty (Eds.), *Internet of Things for Healthcare Technologies* (pp. 177–194). Singapore: Springer Singapore.

Taylor, B., Barboi, C., & Boustani, M. (2023). Passive digital markers for Alzheimer's disease and other related dementias: A systematic evidence review. *J Am Geriatr Soc*, 71(9), 2966–2974. https://doi.org/10.1111/jgs.18426

Tortora, C., Di Crosta, A., La Malva, P., Prete, G., Ceccato, I., Mammarella, N., ... & Palumbo, R. (2024). Virtual reality and cognitive rehabilitation for older adults with mild cognitive impairment: A systematic review. *Ageing Res Rev, 93*, 102146. https://doi.org/10.1016/j.arr.2023.102146

Valladares-Rodriguez, S., Perez-Rodriguez, R., Facal, D., Fernandez-Iglesias, M. J., Anido-Rifon, L., & Mouriño-Garcia, M. (2017). Design process and preliminary psychometric study of a video game to detect cognitive impairment in senior adults. *PeerJ, 5*, e3508. doi:10.7717/peerj.3508

Wang, G., Marradi, C., Albayrak, A., & van der Cammen, T. J. M. (2019). Co-designing with people with dementia: A scoping review of involving people with dementia in design research. *Maturitas, 127*, 55–63. https://doi.org/10.1016/j.maturitas.2019.06.003

Wang, A. H., Newman, K., Martin, L. S., & Lapum, J. (2022). Beyond instrumental support: Mobile application use by family caregivers of persons living with dementia. *Dementia (London)*, 21(5), 1488–1510. doi:10.1177/14713012211073440

Wilkerson, D. A., Brady, E., Yi, E.-H., & Bateman, D. R. (2018). Friendsourcing peer support for Alzheimer's caregivers using Facebook social media. *J Technol Hum Serv*, *36*(2–3), 105–124.

Wilson, R., Cochrane, D., Mihailidis, A., & Small, J. (2020). Mobile Apps to support caregiver-resident communication in long-term care: Systematic search and content analysis. *JMIR Aging*, *3*(1), e17136. doi:10.2196/17136

Yu, C., Sommerlad, A., Sakure, L., & Livingston, G. (2022). Socially assistive robots for people with dementia: Systematic review and meta-analysis of feasibility, acceptability and the effect on cognition, neuropsychiatric symptoms and quality of life. *Ageing Res Rev*, *78*, 101633. doi:10.1016/j.arr.2022.101633

Zgonec, S. (2021). Mobile Apps supporting people with dementia and their carers: Literature review and research agenda. *IFAC-PapersOnLine*, *54*(13), 663–668. https://doi.org/10.1016/j.ifacol.2021.10.527

Zhu, K., Zhang, Q., He, B., Huang, M., Lin, R., & Li, H. (2022). Immersive virtual reality-based cognitive intervention for the improvement of cognitive function, depression, and perceived stress in older adults with mild cognitive impairment and mild dementia: Pilot pre-post study. *JMIR Serious Games*, *10*(1), e32117. doi:10.2196/32117

13

Incorporating AI with a Multilingual Virtual Helper for Dementia Carers in Australia: A Case Study

Nalika Ulapane, Nilmini Wickramasinghe, Thu Ha Dang,
Antonia Thodis, and Bianca Brijnath

13.1 Introduction

Dementia has a global prevalence of 50 million, which is projected to triple by 2050 (Prince et al., 2016). Due to structural inequalities, exposure to obesogenic environments, and a paucity of culturally relevant preventive health interventions, rather than genetic factors per se, much of this increased prevalence will occur in low and middle-income countries and among ethnically diverse populations in high-income countries (The Lancet Regional Health-Western, 2022). Australia is no exception, experiencing a significant increase in the proportion of older Australians from diverse ethnic backgrounds, alongside a rising prevalence of dementia within these populations (Brijnath, 2014). A critical area thus becomes the need to support careers, often being family members of the person living with dementia. Hence, our study focuses on how we can use a digital health solution to address this key and growing need.

13.2 Literature Summary

There are numerous skill training and support programs available for family carers of people with dementia (hereafter "carers") (Cheng et al., 2020), yet, the availability of culturally appropriate and practical support is extremely limited in the low- and middle-income countries as well as for the ethnically diverse populations (Chowdhary et al., 2014), contributing to increased burden on family carers, especially women (Meyer et al., 2018; Temple & Dow,

DOI: 10.1201/9781003485681-13

2018). Studies indicate that carers from these backgrounds experience higher levels of psychological distress compared to those from the general populations (Meyer et al., 2018). Carer psychological distress is an indicator of elder abuse, deteriorating health outcomes, increased hospital admissions, hospitalizations, and institutionalization for care recipients (Coehlo et al., 2007; Stall et al., 2019). Moreover, many carers also faced a decrease in household productivity and income as a result of providing unpaid care (Prince et al., 2015). Therefore, providing high-quality, culturally appropriate support for carers to deliver care at home is a top priority for governments worldwide (WHO, 2017).

Digital media can potentially provide low-cost and sustainable non-pharmacological support to carers, such as communication, education, and services navigation (Abdel Haleem, 2022; Adamopoulou & Moussiades, 2020; Zheng et al., 2023). Apps, chatbots, virtual helpers, and other technologies have the potential to support carers by providing 24/7 education, offering instant and consistent answers, promoting engagement, and aiding in navigating services. Apart from that, they can overcome barriers of limited time, literacy, and geographic isolation (Thomas, 2019). Chatbots have been increasingly used for ageing and health over the past decade to provide information and social and emotional support in many areas (Piau et al., 2019; Portz et al., 2016), including dementia (Vedel et al., 2013; Zulman et al., 2013). However, there is no research on how to develop a multilingual chatbot that is culturally appropriate and usable for carers from ethnically diverse backgrounds (Ruggiano et al., 2021).

This study presents a case of a multilingual virtual helper for carers from an ethnic diverse background in Australia. The study is part of the Drawing Out Care project, aiming to develop and evaluate the DrawCare intervention, including six short-animated films, and six digital practical tip sheets, located on a website with a virtual helper, and available in ten languages: Arabic, Cantonese, Greek, Hindi, Italian, Mandarin, Spanish, Tamil, Vietnamese, and English (Thodis et al., 2023). Through this endeavor, we attempted to answer the following research question: How might we design and develop a virtual helper to support family carers of people with dementia from ethnically diverse backgrounds living in Australia?

13.3 Theoretical Background

Chatbots in general function as conversational agents, and they help in enhancing communication dynamics when designed thoughtfully (Zhou et al., 2023). Within healthcare, chatbots can be made to serve as decision support agents, enriching various decision-making processes (Suppadungsuk et al., 2023). As such, we propose a theoretical lens in this paper to group chatbots in healthcare. In our lens, we see chatbots as decision-support (conversational) agents, or essentially, decision support tools. Our lens is thus governed by two relevant dimensions: (1) Complexity of the human decision-making task(s) to which a chatbot assists; and (2) the intelligence-based capability of a chatbot.

Consider the first dimension. Human decision-making can be categorized into three fundamental types: structured, semi-structured, and unstructured (Ulapane & Wickramasinghe, 2021). Structured decisions entail clear procedures and well-defined problems, while semi-structured decisions involve a blend of structured frameworks and unstructured elements. Unstructured decisions, on the other hand, are characterized by ambiguity and subjective interpretation. We employ this classification of human decision-making in our theoretical lens.

For the second dimension, we draw inspiration from a categorization of clinical decision support systems (Ulapane & Wickramasinghe, 2022). Inspired by clinical decision support systems, we propose a nuanced three-fold classification for chatbots. Our proposed classification for chatbots includes: (1) Rule-based agents, semi-intelligent agents, and intelligent agents. Rule-based agents adhere strictly to predefined rules, semi-intelligent agents integrate rule-based algorithms with limited machine learning capabilities, and intelligent agents exhibit sophisticated Natural Language Processing (NLP) and decision-making prowess. We employ this

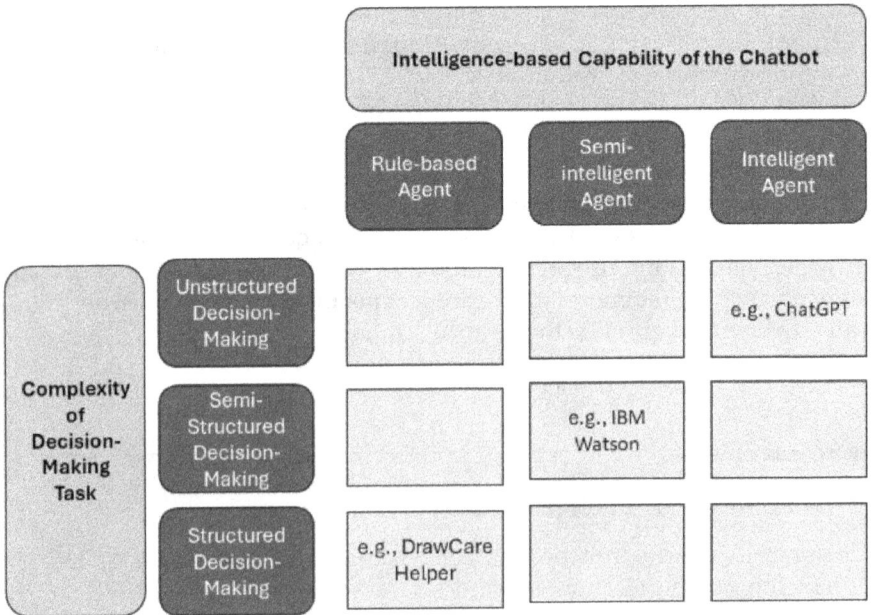

FIGURE 13.1
Proposed theoretical lens to group chatbots (or conversational agents).

interpretation and classification of chatbots (or conversational agents in general) too in our theoretical lens.

In healthcare contexts, where mostly unstructured decisions abound, chatbots prove invaluable aids. Therefore, we introduce a structured nine-celled matrix to classify chatbots tailored to assisting in health-related decision making, providing a comprehensive framework for understanding their roles and capabilities. Our matrix is bounded by the two dimensions discussed above. Some examples are thoughtfully embedded within some cells of the matrix to illuminate the distinct characteristics of each category. Our proposed theoretical lens for group chatbots is presented in Figure 13.1. In this context, the co-designed chatbot is referred to as the "DrawCare Helper" (Figure 13.1) and is focused on grouping and analyzing chatbots designed for healthcare. However, we envision broader applicability to group chatbots and other virtual or decision-support agents in healthcare and in other domains.

13.4 Research Method

This research adopted a single case study approach to develop a virtual supportive agent tailored to, and co-designed with ethnically diverse dementia carers in Australia. Robert Yin's case study methodology (Yin, 2013) was closely followed in the study design, and the design and validation of the virtual supportive agent were done closely following design science research principles (Vom Brocke et al., 2020).

The initial phase involved identifying the challenges encountered by carers, leading to the decision to develop a dedicated website called DrawCare, featuring a chatbot to assist carers. The website and chatbot aimed to provide videos and document resources to support carers, leveraging and modifying materials from the World Health Organization (WHO)'s iSupport Lite program (WHO, 2020).

Subsequently, the DrawCare website and chatbot were co-designed and developed across four stages. These stages encompassed: (1) Brainstorming and drafting the web layout and chatbot conversation flow; (2) Presenting prototypes to the research team for feedback; (3) Conducting six iterative co-design workshops with family and professional carers from diverse communities (Dang et al., 2023); and (4) Revising the website and chatbot based on co-design feedback.

Co-design workshops' participants were recruited nationally through convenience, purposeful and snowball sampling methods, utilizing existing national networks of carers, clinicians/service providers, and broader organizations. Participants were either family or professional carers of people with dementia, able to speak one of nine languages and English, and able to participate in an online workshop. Effort was made to recruit participants with diversity in age, gender, language, and educational background. The number of participants per workshop was between five and eight (excluding researchers).

After obtaining written informed consent, participants were given the iSupport Lite original poster, a draft script, and an animation storyboard related to the co-design theme, and access to the draft website before the workshop for review. Each two-hour online workshop was led by two researchers who were trained in qualitative research and had prior experience working with ethnically diverse participants on dementia-related topics. The workshop was recorded for transcription purposes. Notes were also taken by another researcher for data analysis. In the workshop, participants again reviewed the drafted film script, storyboard, and host website structure, and provided feedback and suggestions. The potential usefulness of an additional virtual assistant to help carers find resources was discussed.

Ethical clearance was obtained from the Human Research Ethics Committee (HREC) of Curtin University, Australia (HRE2022-0004), prior to commencing the study. A Stakeholder Advisory Group (SAG), comprising representatives from various organizations including the Australian government, ethno-specific aged care providers, and the World Health Organization (WHO), as well as three former carers, was assembled to guide the DrawCare project.

13.5 Findings

Main findings from stages 3 (co-design) and 4 (chatbot revision) of the study are reported in this paper. Twenty-one individuals participated in six online co-design workshops (mean age 57 years, 95% females) (Dang et al., 2023). Participant demographics are presented in Table 13.1.

The primary findings derived from feedback obtained from both the research team and participants engaged in the co-design phases (Dang et al., 2023) revealed several key insights. Notable feedback from workshop participants regarding the initial website and chatbot versions, along with subsequent adaptations, is detailed in Table 13.2.

Notably, it was suggested that the design of the website and chatbot should employ two contrasting colors to enhance aesthetics while maintaining clarity and minimizing clutter. Additionally, participants emphasized the importance of utilizing larger, easily readable text and employing clear language to enhance comprehension, while minimizing the overall text volume. These recommendations were duly considered during the refinement process, encompassing adjustments to the website, chatbot, text resources, and scripts for animated video resources.

TABLE 13.1

Demographics of Co-Design Workshop Participants

Characteristics		Participants (n = 22)
Sex	Male	1 (5%)
	Female	21 (95%)
Mean age	Years	57
Role	Family carer (FC)	5 (23%)
	Professional carer (PC)	14 (64%)
	Family and professional carer (dual role)	3 (13%)
Mean years as an FC		7.5
Mean years as a PC		10.5
Self-identified language group(s)	Chinese	3 (13%)
	English	3 (13%)
	Greek	4 (18%)
	Hindi	1 (5%)
	Italian	3 (13%)
	Spanish	1 (5%)
	Vietnamese	5 (23%)
	Chinese, Greek, Italian	1 (5%)
	Hindi, Tamil	1 (5%)

TABLE 13.2

Some Examples of the Feedback Received from Participants at the Co-Design Phase

Some Examples of Feedback Received	Corresponding Changes Made to the Website/Chatbot Design
Chatbot needed to be translated in all nine languages	Chatbot's content was translated into nine languages: Arabic, Cantonese, Greek, Hindi, Italian, Mandarin, Spanish, Tamil, and Vietnamese.
The current "chatbot" was more like an information box. "Chatbot" name sounds like it is going to be something that talks back to the user	The chatbot was renamed as "virtual helper."
The chatbot should function to help users navigating the website	The keywords or phrases from the short, animated films (videos) were used as a basis for creating a list of problem statements for users to select from, which then guided them to an appropriate film.
The chatbot prompts should be framed as carers' problems	The chatbot's prompt were developed in the way that when the user clicked on that, it took them to the specific film and tip sheet that deals with the problem.

13.6 Discussion

The challenges associated with caring for individuals with dementia are profound, underscoring the importance of culturally responsive support systems for carers. In response, we developed a website and virtual helper (i.e., DrawCare) specifically tailored to aid dementia carers from ethnically diverse communities in Australia, a demographic often underserved in healthcare.

This endeavor underwent iterative stages of co-design and development before transitioning into preliminary evaluation and then a clinical trial phase. Venturing into uncharted territory, we deliberated extensively on the design considerations for the website and chatbot within this unique context. Contemplating whether to pursue a fully fledged NLP-enabled chatbot, we opted for a gradual approach, starting with a simpler version to gather insights and evidence. Our theoretical lens in Figure 13.1 proved pivotal in shaping our design strategy. By conceptualizing decision-making for dementia carers in a structured manner, we could effectively leverage a rule-based chatbot to meet their needs. Co-design input from family carers helped us to collate a set of challenges that carers often face and which our films and other resources addressed. Thus, when carers sought the virtual helper, they were presented with short scenarios, could select options based on their need, and be directed to resources that matched that need. Such an approach lays the foundation for future advancements through delving into other domains in the matrix depicted in Figure 13.1.

Our contributions extend beyond practical tool development, encompassing theoretical advancements and broader implications for healthcare applications. The theoretical contribution includes a novel matrix for classifying conversational agents based on their role in assisting human decision-making, providing a valuable framework for analyzing such tools across various domains. Given the advancement in artificial intelligence (AI) (Wickramasinghe et al., 2024), it is only appropriate that these benefits are also incorporated into healthcare delivery in general and in dementia care specifically. Conversational agents that are tailored to specific healthcare contexts and issues will become of increasing importance given the current challenges facing healthcare delivery in a post-COVID environment. These challenges include: (i) escalating costs, (ii) aging population; (iii) longer life expectancy, (iv) need to provide more patient-centric care, (v) the need to provide high-quality care, (vi) the need to provide higher value care, and (vii) the impact of significant workforce shortages. Thus, bots and conversational agents fill a key and critical void. Not only can they be designed and developed (as exemplified in the present study) to be tailored to a specific context as well as support multi-lingual and multi-cultural needs, they also are available 24/7 365 days of the year and hence provide any time anywhere support. As more intelligence is incorporated into them, they will be able to provide even better precise and personalized support for any/all healthcare delivery issues. Thus, our developed framework, which serves to classify the key types of bots/conversational agents and thereby also enables an objective evaluation of them, serves as an important contribution as this area advances and develops. In practice, our multilingual website and chatbot serve to offer vital resources to ethnically diverse dementia carers, serving as a blueprint for similar initiatives in diverse healthcare contexts. Given the significant workforce shortages being experienced post COVID in both developed and developing countries coupled with the fact that it is never easy or simple to have an interpreter on the spot, this serves as a significant contribution to support superior healthcare delivery and support for CALD populations and thus also assists with ensuring a high quality of care can be received for all people irrespective of location, ethnicity, culture or language.

While our study is not without limitations, such as the rule-based nature of the chatbot and the small number of workshop participants per language, these constraints were balanced against feasibility and resource considerations. The modest sample sizes in the co-design phases were deemed adequate, although we acknowledge potential limitations in the scope of feedback obtained. To address this, we have initiated user-testing and a clinical trial (Thodis et al., 2023) with a larger sample size to gather more comprehensive insights.

13.7 Future Directions: Incorporating Advanced AI for Dementia Carers

As we look to the future, the integration of advanced AI technologies presents a promising avenue to further enhance support for dementia carers. Building on the foundation established by the DrawCare Virtual Helper, several key areas in AI can be identified to be helpful in enabling sophisticated AI-enabled care.

13.7.1 Natural Language Processing for Better Understanding

Enhanced Conversational Agents: By leveraging advanced NLP techniques, we can develop conversational agents that understand and respond to carers' queries with greater accuracy and empathy. These agents can handle more complex interactions, providing personalized advice and support tailored to the specific needs of each carer.

Multilingual and Multicultural Support: Next-generation advancements in NLP can improve a virtual helper's ability to understand

and generate responses in multiple languages and dialects along with cultural nuances, ensuring that carers from diverse backgrounds receive culturally and linguistically appropriate support.

13.7.2 Machine Learning and Predictive Analytics

Personalized Recommendations: Through the use of machine learning algorithms, a virtual helper can analyze patterns in carers' interactions and provide personalized recommendations for resources and support. This can help carers navigate the challenges of dementia care more effectively.

Predictive Insights: Predictive analytics can be incorporated to identify potential issues before they arise, offering proactive support to carers. For example, a virtual helper could alert carers to signs of caregiver burnout and suggest interventions to mitigate stress.

13.7.3 Integration with Wearable and IoT Devices

Real-Time Monitoring: Integrating a virtual helper with wearable devices and Internet of Things (IoT) sensors can provide real-time monitoring of both the carer and the person with dementia. This data can be used to offer timely advice and interventions, enhancing the overall care experience. It can also prevent accidents like falls, and incidents like dementia patients walking out of homes or care facilities unsupervised and getting lost.

Health Tracking: Wearable devices can be used to track vital signs and other health metrics, allowing a virtual helper to provide data-driven insights and recommendations for managing the health and well-being of both the carer and the care recipient.

13.7.4 Emotional and Mental Health Support

Sentiment Analysis: Advanced AI can be used to analyze the emotional tone of carers' interactions, offering empathetic responses and mental health support. This can help address the emotional challenges of caregiving and provide a source of comfort and reassurance. This can also help track and audit good care practice and incidence of things like elder abuse.

Mental Health Resources: A virtual helper can be equipped with resources and tools to support carers' mental health, such as mindfulness exercises, stress management techniques, and connections to professional counseling services, and AI can help provide resources personalized to a carer.

13.7.5 Continuous Learning and Improvement

Feedback Loops: Incorporating continuous feedback loops into AI-incorporated virtual helpers can ensure that a virtual helper evolves based on user interactions and feedback. This iterative improvement process can enhance the system's effectiveness and relevance over time.

Collaborative Learning: Engaging with a broader community of carers and healthcare professionals can provide valuable insights and data to refine and expand the capabilities of a virtual helper, and having AI-incorporated workflows can help in agile and evidence-based design of support tools.

Evidence Tracking: AI-incorporated helpers can be connected with edge, fog, or cloud networks to gather a lot of real-world care-related data, which will serve as evidence to facilitate continuous learning and improvement for future.

Through embracing such advanced AI capabilities, we can create a more robust and responsive support system for dementia carers. This not only addresses the immediate challenges faced by carers but also contributes to the broader goal of improving healthcare delivery and outcomes for individuals with dementia and their families. As we continue to explore these possibilities, our commitment to culturally responsive and empathetic care remains at the forefront of our efforts.

13.8 Conclusions

To address our research question regarding the development of a multilingual chatbot suitable for family carers of dementia patients from ethnically diverse backgrounds, we established a robust theoretical framework. By amalgamating decision-making principles with nuances from clinical decision support systems, as outlined in Figure 13.1, we provided a novel theoretical lens for this purpose, representing a significant theoretical contribution. Through our case study of the DrawCare Virtual Helper for ethnically diverse dementia family caregivers, we have outlined a practical roadmap for the design and development of such solutions, emphasizing their appropriateness and responsible design. Given the widespread adoption of chatbots across various domains and the growing prevalence of dementia, we anticipate that our findings will have broad-reaching implications. Our future research will delve more deeply into the proposed theoretical framework and analysis of our chatbot developments as well as investigate the possibility of including more AI capabilities.

Acknowledgment

The authors extend thanks and acknowledge all chief investigators and members of the Executive Committee of the Drawing-out Care project: Dr. Andrew Simon Gilbert, Prof. Briony Dow, Prof. Claudia Cooper, Ms. Danijela Hlis, A/Prof. Duncan Mortimer, Dr. Joanne Enticott, Dr. Josefine Antoniades, Prof. Lily Dongxia Xiao, Ms. Mary Gurgone, Prof. Mathew Varghese, Prof. Santosh Loganathan, and A/Prof. Tuan Nguyen. The authors also thank the co-design workshop participants for sharing their lived experiences in a cultural context to adapt the stories depicted in the animated films and information sheets. We acknowledge the expertise of our technical collaborators in translation, animation, and website design. The authors thank the following organizations for their financial or in-kind support to the project: the Department of Mental Health and Substance Use, World Health Organization (WHO), Dementia Australia, the Federation of Ethnic Communities Council of Australia (FECCA), Advance Care Planning Australia, and the National Ageing Research Institute (NARI).

Funding

The DrawCare study was funded by the Medical Research Future Fund (MRFF), Australian Government Department of Health [grant number APP2008065]. The study sponsor and funders do not have any role in the study's design, data collection, management, analysis, interpretation of data, or writing reports or publications.

References

Abdel Haleem, H. B. (2022). Global Media Ethics and the Digital Revolution, Noureddine Miladi (Ed.) (2022). *Journal of Arab & Muslim Media Research, 15*(2), 309–312. https://doi.org/10.1386/jammr_00052_5

Adamopoulou, E., & Moussiades, L. (2020). Chatbots: History, Technology, and Applications. *Machine Learning with Applications, 2.* https://doi.org/10.1016/j.mlwa.2020.100006

Brijnath, B. (2014). *Unforgotten: Love and the Culture of Dementia Care in India* (1 ed., Vol. 2). Berghahn Books.

Cheng, S.-T., Li, K.-K., Losada, A., Zhang, F., Au, A., Thompson, L. W., & Gallagher-Thompson, D. (2020). The Effectiveness of Nonpharmacological Interventions for Informal Dementia Caregivers: An Updated Systematic Review and Meta-Analysis. *Psychology and Aging, 35*(1), 55–77. https://doi.org/10.1037/pag0000401

Chowdhary, N., Jotheeswaran, A. T., Nadkarni, A., Hollon, S. D., King, M., Jordans, M. J. D., Rahman, A., Verdeli, H., Araya, R., & Patel, V. (2014). The Methods and Outcomes of Cultural Adaptations of Psychological Treatments for Depressive Disorders: A Systematic Review. *Psychological Medicine*, 44(6), 1131–1146. https://doi.org/10.1017/S0033291713001785

Coehlo, D. P., Hooker, K., & Bowman, S. (2007). Institutional Placement of Persons With Dementia: What Predicts Occurrence and Timing? *Journal of Family Nursing*, 13(2), 253–277. https://doi.org/10.1177/1074840707300947

Dang, T. H., Thodis, A., Ulapane, N., Antoniades, J., Gurgone, M., Nguyen, T. A., Gilbert, A., Wickramasinghe, N., Varghese, M., Loganathan, S., Enticott, J., Mortimer, D., Dow, B., Cooper, C., Xiao, L. D., & Brijnath, B. (2023). "It's Too Nice": Adapting iSupport Lite for Multicultural Family Carers of a Person with Dementia. *Clinical Gerontologist WCLI*. https://doi.org/10.1080/07317115.2023.2254296

Meyer, O. L., Liu, X., Nguyen, T. N., Hinton, L., & Tancredi, D. (2018). Psychological Distress of Ethnically Diverse Adult Caregivers in the California Health Interview Survey. *Journal of Immigrant & Minority Health*, 20(4), 784–791. https://doi.org/10.1007/s10903-017-0634-0

Piau, A., Crissey, R., Brechemier, D., Balardy, L., & Nourhashemi, F. (2019). A Smartphone Chatbot Application to Optimize Monitoring of Older Patients with Cancer [Research Support, Non-U.S. Gov't]. *International Journal of Medical Informatics*, 128, 18–23. https://doi.org/https://dx.doi.org/10.1016/j.ijmedinf.2019.05.013

Portz, J. D., Miller, A., Foster, B., & Laudeman, L. (2016). Persuasive Features in Health Information Technology Interventions for Older Adults with Chronic Diseases: A Systematic Review. *Health and Technology*, 6(2), 89–99. https://doi.org/10.1007/s12553-016-0130-x

Prince, M., Comas-Herrera, A., Knapp, M., Guerchet, M., & Karagiannidou, M. (2016). *World Alzheimer Report 2016: Improving Healthcare for People Living with Dementia: Coverage, Quality and Costs Now and in the Future*. A. s. D. International. https://www.alzint.org/u/WorldAlzheimerReport2016.pdf

Prince, M., Wimo, A., Guerchet, M., Ali, G., Wu, Y., & Prina, M. (2015). *World Alzheimer Report 2015*. A. s. D. International. https://www.alzint.org/resource/world-alzheimer-report-2015/

Ruggiano, N., Brown, E. L., Roberts, L., Framil Suarez, C. V., Luo, Y., Hao, Z., & Hristidis, V. (2021). Chatbots to Support People with Dementia and Their Caregivers: Systematic Review of Functions and Quality. *Journal of Medical Internet Research*, 23(6), e25006. https://doi.org/10.2196/25006

Stall, N. M., Kim, S. J., Hardacre, K. A., Shah, P. S., Straus, S. E., Bronskill, S. E., Lix, L. M., Bell, C. M., & Rochon, P. A. (2019). Association of Informal Caregiver Distress with Health Outcomes of Community-Dwelling Dementia Care Recipients: A Systematic Review. *Journal of the American Geriatrics Society*, 67(3), 609–617. https://doi.org/10.1111/jgs.15690

Suppadungsuk, S., Thongprayoon, C., Miao, J., Krisanapan, P., Qureshi, F., Kashani, K., & Cheungpasitporn, W. (2023). Exploring the Potential of Chatbots in Critical Care Nephrology. *Medicines*, 10(10), 58.

Temple, J. B., & Dow, B. (2018). The Unmet Support Needs of Carers of Older Australians: Prevalence and Mental Health. *International Psychogeriatrics*, 30(12), 1849–1860. https://doi.org/10.1017/S104161021800042X

The Lancet Regional Health-Western, P. (2022). Dementia in the Western Pacific Region: From Prevention to Care. *The Lancet Regional Health Western Pacific, 26,* 100607. https://doi.org/10.1016/j.lanwpc.2022.100607

Thodis, A., Dang, T.-H., Antoniades, J., Gilbert, A. S., Nguyen, T., Hlis, D., Gurgone, M., Dow, B., Cooper, C., Xiao, L.-D., Wickramasinghe, N., Ulapane, N., Varghese, M., Loganathan, S., Enticott, J., Mortimer, D., & Brijnath, B. (2023). Improving the Lives of Ethnically Diverse Family Carers and People Living with Dementia Using Digital Media Resources – Protocol for the Draw-Care Randomised Controlled Trial. *Digital Health, 9,* 20552076231205733. https://doi.org/10.1177/20552076231205733

Thomas, A., Ryan, C. P., Caspi, A., Liu, Z., Moffitt, T. E., Sugden, K., Zhou, J., Belsky, D. W. Pace of Biological Aging, and Risk of Dementia in the Framingham Heart Study, *Measuring Australia's Digital Divide: The Australian Digital Inclusion Index 2019.* https://doi.org/10.1002/ana.26900

Ulapane, N., & Wickramasinghe, N. (2021). Clinical Decision-Making as a Subset of Decision-Making: Leveraging the Concepts of Decision-Making and Knowledge Management to Characterize Clinical Decision-Making. In *Healthcare and Knowledge Management for Society 5.0* (pp. 47–62). CRC Press.

Ulapane, N., & Wickramasinghe, N. (2022). Scoping Mobile Clinical Decision Support Systems to Enhance Design and Recording of Usage Data Effectively: A Suggested Approach. In *Digital Disruption in Healthcare* (pp. 209–225). Springer.

Vedel, I., Akhlaghpour, S., Vaghefi, I., Bergman, H., & Lapointe, L. (2013). Health Information Technologies in Geriatrics and Gerontology: A Mixed Systematic Review. *Journal of the American Medical Informatics Association, 20*(6), 1109–1119. https://doi.org/10.1136/amiajnl-2013-001705

Vom Brocke, J., Hevner, A., & Maedche, A. (2020). Introduction to Design Science Research. *Design Science Research. Cases,* 1–13. https://www.researchgate.net/profile/Jan-Vom-Brocke/publication/345430098_Introduction_to_Design_Science_Research/links/5fc033bd299bf104cf8233a2/Introduction-to-Design-Science-Research.pdf

WHO. (2017). *Global Action Plan on the Public Health Response to Dementia 2017–2025.* WHO. file:///C:/Users/thuhadang/Downloads/9789241513487-eng.pdf

WHO. (2020). *WHO Launches iSupport Lite.* https://www.who.int/news/item/06-07-2020-who-launches-isupport-lite

Wickramasinghe, N., Kraus, M., & Bodendorf, F. (2024). *Analytics and AI for Healthcare.* CRC.

Yin, R. K. (2013). Validity and Generalization in Future Case Study Evaluations. *Evaluation, 19*(3), 321–332.

Zheng, J., Gresham, M., Phillipson, L., Hall, D., Jeon, Y.-H., Brodaty, H., & Low, L.-F. (2024). Exploring the Usability, User Experience and Usefulness of a Supportive Website for People with Dementia and Carers. *Disability and Rehabilitation: Assistive Technology, 19*(4), 1369–1381. https://doi.org/10.1080/17483107.2023.2180546

Zhou, Q., Li, B., Han, L., & Jou, M. (2023). Talking to a Bot or a Wall? How Chatbots vs. Human Agents Affect Anticipated Communication Quality. *Computers in Human Behavior, 143,* 107674.

Zulman, D. M., Piette, J. D., Jenchura, E. C., Asch, S. M., & Rosland, A. M. (2013). Facilitating Out-of-Home Caregiving through Health Information Technology: Survey of Informal Caregivers' Current Practices, Interests, and Perceived Barriers. *Journal of Medical Internet Research, 15*(7), e123. https://doi.org/10.2196/jmir.2472

14

Co-Design of Digital Health Interventions in Dementia

Ellen Gaffy, Frances Batchelor, Bobby Redman, and Anita Goh

14.1 Importance of Co-Designing Digital Health Interventions

Co-design involves bringing together people with professional and lived experience in design processes to collaboratively identify problems and develop solutions (Sanders & Stappers, 2008). Several key characteristics differentiate co-design from other participatory and design approaches. Co-design is a process, guided by underlying values and principles of inclusivity, diversity, equality and active involvement, and facilitated through practical skills, tools and methods (Blomkamp, 2018; McKercher, 2020). Co-design applies creative problem solving throughout an iterative process of continuous design improvement by ideating, testing and refining ideas (Sanders & Stappers, 2008, 2014). It is a way to meaningfully engage people with lived experience in development and design processes to ensure relevancy and applicability of design outcomes. To achieve this, designers use their visual thinking skills, making skills and communication skills along with a mindset of valuing lived experience and having curiosity and empathy towards the experiences of other people.

When applied in the design and development of digital health technology and interventions for dementia, co-design can enable a better understanding of people's experiences and their care requirements, leading to more innovative and creative solutions and interventions that are tailored to specific user requirements and preferences and can adapt to changing support needs. This results in more relevant products that are more likely to be adopted, used effectively and integrated into daily routines. Co-design processes may involve a combination of involvement methods to achieve the various aims of different project stages in the development, design and testing of the digital health intervention.

Involving historically marginalised or at-risk groups in co-design, including people living with dementia, requires critical reflection by co-design facilitators during co-design planning to ensure effective and

DOI: 10.1201/9781003485681-14

appropriate co-design methods and processes are used (Moll et al., 2020). Particularly when developing interventions intended for use by people living with dementia, and involving people living with dementia in the process of co-designing them, an inclusive approach is needed. This approach should consider how their experiences, history, any cognitive and physical impairments, and personal strengths affect comfortable, safe and supported involvement and contribution (Goh et al., 2022; Lord et al., 2022).

In this chapter, we discuss the critical success issues when co-designing digital health solutions with and for people impacted by dementia. This includes the people who are living with dementia, and also the people involved in their life such as family, friends, and carers. We reflect on the benefits, challenges and issues faced by designers and researchers when engaging with people impacted by dementia to develop digital health interventions, and how to address these to ensure successful co-design. We discuss considerations to ensure active and meaningful involvement of people living with dementia across the design process and various project stages, including establishing collaborative relationships and consideration of human rights, equity, safety and accessibility. We also discuss key considerations and challenges when implementing and evaluating co-designed interventions to ensure sustainability and integration into practice and daily use.

Author Bobby Redman is a retired psychologist and dementia advocate. Following her diagnosis of dementia, Bobby committed herself to advocacy – creating awareness, giving support and participating in dementia research. In addition to her contributions to the content of this chapter, quotes from Bobby are also included to highlight the topics in her own voice.

14.2 Benefits, Issues, and Challenges When Engaging People Impacted by Dementia in the Co-Design of Digital Health Interventions

14.2.1 Overview

Digital health interventions, such as mobile Health Applications (mHealth), wearable devices, assistive devices, digital therapeutic devices and communication support interventions have huge potential to improve quality of life, assist in self-management and provide support for those living with dementia and for those caring for people living with dementia. However, these beneficial health outcomes may not be achieved if people living with dementia and family carers are not involved in designing them, which can result in interventions that are of poor quality or irrelevant, and designs that are not useable, functional or accessible.

14.2.2 Issues and Challenges

It is important to include people with living experience of dementia *at all stages* of the co-design process, but especially in the initial problem identification stages to ensure useful and relevant designs that address the direct needs (including care and support) identified by people living with dementia themselves. However, this does not always happen in practice (Span et al., 2013) and presents the risk of technology developers and designers making incorrect assumptions about needs and preferences. In a systematic review of the involvement of people living with dementia in the development of supportive technologies, Suijkerbuijk et al. (2019) identified that people living with dementia were most often involved in the design and development of assistive technology in a passive, rather than active, capacity. Only 7 of the 49 studies (14%) included in the review involved people living with dementia as co-designers. In these seven studies, the label of co-designer was attributed if participants had been involved in multiple phases of development and were consulted iteratively throughout the design process. However, in most cases, people living with dementia were just informants, most often involved in only the generative or the evaluative design phases, and not in the problem identification stages. That is, people living with dementia were not continually involved throughout the design process; rather, they were involved in interviews to provide feedback or approval of a design or were only observed using an already-developed prototype solution. These points in the design process are often when meaningful changes are unable to be made or when developers or designers are unwilling to make changes.

Often, the focus of digital interventions is on addressing risk or safety issues, which are exacerbated by cognitive or physical impairments. Proxy informants, such as family carers, are often involved in providing input on behalf of people living with dementia. However, while carers also have important insights, preferences and priorities may differ between family carers and people living with dementia. For example, family carers may assign a higher priority to safety, monitoring and risk reduction than people living with dementia do (Hirt et al., 2019). People living with dementia indicate preferences for assistive technology and devices that can support health self-management, completing daily tasks and activities, shared care and collaborative care planning, social connection and participation in meaningful activities (Astell, 2019; Wilson et al., 2024). Design outputs that don't identify the needs and preferences of people living with dementia may unintentionally diminish rather than support personhood. For example, wearable GPS devices, while seen as helpful for carers in monitoring falls, changes in behaviour and limiting walking outside the home, may be viewed by people living with dementia as infringing on privacy and autonomy (Leorin et al., 2019).

It is natural for carers to worry about their loved ones, but at times this worry may result in taking away our right to dignity of risk, resulting in a loss of control of our own lives

Bobby Redman

The REAFF Framework (Responding, Enabling, Augmenting and Failure-free) (Astell, 2019) proposes four key principles to guide the development of digital solutions for people living with dementia. Key considerations include whether a particular digital solution is responsive to the needs of people living with dementia, whether it will enhance their life and not be disabling, whether it builds on retained skills and abilities of the person living with dementia who is using the digital intervention, and whether it is intuitive and accessible for people living with dementia (Astell, 2019). As technology and digital health interventions have a clear role in actively engaging and empowering people living with dementia, active involvement of people living with dementia in the design and development of this technology is critical.

Key fundamental underlying values of co-design include equality and inclusivity, which are achieved by sharing power and decision-making. Co-designing digital health technologies involves multi-disciplinary collaboration between various stakeholder groups, including people living with dementia, family carers, healthcare professionals, designers, technology developers and researchers. Working effectively with multiple different stakeholder groups requires active and continual reflection of the power dynamics between the different groups and awareness of the barriers to achieving shared power and equal contribution to decision-making. Co-design also requires designers and other stakeholders with professional expertise to have a mindset where different types of knowledge are equally valuable in order to avoid tokenistic involvement of people with lived experience. Often, the value of the expertise provided by people with a diagnosis of dementia is underestimated. Even when well-intentioned, researchers and people with technology expertise may still talk over or disregard input of those with living experience, assuming a lack of knowledge.

At times suggestions are met with patronising smiles, or responses that suggest that we are just being humoured, as is sometimes seen when adults interact with children.

Bobby Redman

Power dynamics to be aware of when developing dementia-related digital interventions may include the involvement of people with lived or living experience and those with professional experience, and the involvement of people living with dementia and people without dementia. It is important to know how best to support involvement, be aware of barriers to involvement and contribution, and how to optimise and support communication and involvement in conversations and discussions. Some stakeholder groups involved may be unfamiliar with certain technology or devices or may have limited digital literacy. Also, some people or groups may be unfamiliar with dementia or have not collaborated with people who have a diagnosis of dementia. For example, engineers or software developers may have had limited experience of, or exposure to, working with people living with dementia. Power differentials may also arise due to the focus on technology and use of technical language in discussions (Fox et al., 2022). Diverse stakeholder groups may also mean differing or conflicting priorities, potentially leading to difficulties in decision-making. Also, not all stakeholder groups will have delegated decision-making power, depending on project-specific requirements (Gaffy et al., 2022). Therefore, transparency around decision-making processes is essential to meaningful involvement and is also important to ensuring a sense of ownership over the final output or outcomes (Sakamoto et al., 2023). Finally, co-design is both a time and resource intensive process. It is often long, spanning multiple years and requiring thorough planning and lead-in time, particularly when involving people impacted by dementia to ensure involvement is accessible, supported, and ultimately meaningful. The following section outlines key considerations when engaging with people impacted by dementia to co-design digital interventions.

14.3 Co-Designing with People Impacted by Dementia to Develop Digital Health Interventions: Key Considerations

14.3.1 Overview

To actively and meaningfully engage people living with dementia and family carers in co-design, aspects of the co-design process may need to be adapted or modified to support involvement across the lifespan of the project. While general guidance for collaborating with people living with dementia is useful for a range of engagement methods and purposes (Dementia Australia, 2022; Dementia Enquirers, 2023), when developing digital health interventions, additional topic and output specific considerations are presented. The focus on digital devices, products and platforms, and likely need to interact with and use technology during the design process presents specific considerations around digital literacy, ensuring digital accessibility for people living with dementia and a greater focus on usability testing and ongoing product refinement and updates.

14.3.2 Considerations for Co-Designing Digital Health Interventions with People Impacted by Dementia

14.3.2.1 Developing Relationships

People living with dementia should be involved in the design process as early as possible. As previously discussed, early involvement is not only important in ensuring the right needs and priorities for a project are being identified, but it is also essential in developing trust, effective working relationships and genuine partnerships. When identifying and engaging people to be involved, ways to reduce the burden of involvement should be explored. Fox et al. (2022) connected with local dementia support groups to develop the MyMindCheck app to monitor cognitive change and variability. Workshops were held in the same venues to ensure a familiar environment and were scheduled to fit in with existing meetings. Later in the design process, support groups with a special interest in technology were engaged to enable continuity in ongoing usability testing (Fox et al., 2022). The purpose, aims, and involvement requirements of the project should be discussed early and transparently to develop clear shared goals and objectives. Being transparent about what can be achieved can help manage expectations and mitigate potential conflicts over priorities. Having role transparency, developing Terms of Reference together, and introducing people to each other according to the expertise they are contributing rather than their role can be ways to mitigate power differences and help to establish collaborative relationships (Metro North Health, 2024).

14.3.2.2 Accessibility

Whether it is intended that the co-design process will be conducted in-person, virtually or a combination of both, accessibility issues in the environment are a key consideration. In-person co-design needs to be dementia accessible. This involves reviewing the type and amount of travel required, the building facilities, signage, and other accessibility needs (Dementia Australia, 2022) and ensuring as-needed support is available. For example, way finding in large buildings with complex infrastructure can be challenging – the availability of someone to meet a person living with dementia and to support way finding should be considered. The application of co-design practice in virtual and online methods of delivery increased due to the COVID-19 pandemic, with co-design methods adaptable to use in virtual settings (Kennedy et al., 2021). Sakamoto et al. (2023) observed that while virtual co-design was beneficial in enabling their project to continue in pandemic restrictions (and is also useful in engaging people who live in rural or remote areas, or who may be unable to travel to in-person venues), not being able to have informal conversations and interactions with people living with dementia, in conjunction with managing the various types and platforms being used to facilitate the co-design, prevented connection and emotional and meaningful engagement.

Additional considerations when exploring the feasibility of virtual co-design may include needing time to become familiar with any technology that is being used to facilitate the co-design itself, i.e., workshops, meetings and in-between contact. For example, video conferencing platforms, online whiteboards used to facilitate virtual collaborative work, such as Mural and Miro, and the use of email. While many people living with dementia may be comfortable participating in video meetings, it is important to clarify beforehand (with all attendees, not just the people with dementia) that they are familiar with the specific video-conferencing platform being used and provide assistance if required. Platforms that are intuitive and simple to use should be used as much as possible (one often-used platform is Zoom). Online whiteboards, which are increasingly being used for co-design activities, can be useful for brainstorming, but the process is often fast-moving and can be a barrier to participation for people who need more time to process information or who are unfamiliar with using these types of collaboration tools. Arrangements should be offered for support to input responses for those unable to do so, either by regular check-ins with the person or by using telephone, chat or message functions to provide input depending on the individual's preference, or ensuring in-person support.

14.3.2.3 Family Carer Involvement

While the intended primary user of an intervention being designed may be the person living with dementia themselves, involvement of their family supporter/carer may also be an essential component of the co-design process. For example, digital interventions may be intended for use by the family carer as well as the person living with dementia such as digital interventions supporting shared care and decision-making. In addition, other digital health interventions are intended for use by family carers themselves, such as carer support, learning about dementia and how to support someone living with dementia. When people living with dementia and their family supporter are involved in design processes together, it is important to ensure that family carers do not speak on behalf of the person living with dementia, unless this has been discussed prior as their communication preference. It is also important that digital designs adapt to the progression of dementia, which may include capacity for integration of carer support if required and is desired by people living with dementia themselves (Wilson et al., 2024); otherwise, there is the risk of technology becoming unusable (Cheraghi-Sohi et al., 2023).

14.3.2.4 Communication

Understanding the communication strengths, needs and preferences of someone who has a diagnosis of dementia, and barriers they may face in group settings, is essential to creating a safe and comfortable environment in meetings, design sessions, workshops or consultations. Providing short, plain language summaries about the project and what involvement will require (including a breakdown of what is to be discussed during design sessions or meetings) is helpful for people to prepare and organise their thoughts. Some people may prefer video calls, telephone calls, or written instructions to refer to as memory prompts. Technical language and jargon should be avoided in any written materials (Dementia Australia, 2022). Overall, each person has different strengths, needs and preferences and it is important to ask each co-designer how best to communicate with them to optimise their input.

People living with dementia should be given the same respect as others in the team when planning meeting times and it should never be assumed that people living with dementia do not have any other time commitments. Reminders leading up to the meeting are useful (not only to people living with dementia) and the agenda and any necessary paperwork provided in advance, in the format requested by the person with dementia. People living with dementia may have sensory or physical issues that make it difficult to read from a screen, and some people may not have access to email or to a printer to print multipage colour documents. Following meetings or design sessions, notes or summaries should be provided as soon as possible in readable format for people living with dementia to review and add to (in whatever format they wish).

Participating in group discussions, answering questions that are addressed to a group and keeping track of conversations can be barriers for people living with dementia to participate in discussion-based co-design activities (Lord et al., 2022). Designers and discussion facilitators need to be mindful of including all co-designers in the discussion, particularly in fast moving and larger meetings. Flexibility, patience, and empathy are key. Allowing people living with dementia to set the pace of discussions can ensure adequate time and space are provided for all people to voice their suggestions (Dementia Australia, 2022). Assigning someone to monitor the discussion to ensure all co-designers are given opportunities to be heard is a useful approach. Small groups, short design sessions, ensuring questions are not confronting and are not asked in a way where someone may feel like they are being tested all create a comfortable environment (Lord et al., 2022; G. Wang et al., 2019).

Further, having a range of verbal and non-verbal methods is essential for ensuring the meaningful involvement of people with different communication needs. Having options for non-verbal participation, rather than just discussion-based involvement, can support the involvement of people with more progressed dementia (G. Wang et al., 2019). For example, using art-based tactile and sensory materials (Kenning, 2018; Winton & Rodgers, 2019) and playful activities and games (Branco et al., 2017) may be suitable ways to support a person living with dementia to communicate their needs, preferences, ideas and feedback other than through verbal means. Designers and facilitators should remain flexible in design sessions, workshops and meetings and across the entire design process to be able to adapt or change approaches to respond to changing support needs or people's capacity to be involved (Dementia Australia, 2022).

14.3.2.5 Co-Design Tools and Activities

People living with dementia have diverse and individual strengths and needs, and co-design processes should be representative and inclusive of people living with dementia at various stages of the condition. The key to co-designing digital health interventions is to recognise that people living with dementia may face different challenges, not just to people without dementia but also from each other. There are many different types of dementia, which may result in different symptoms. Additionally, people will be at different stages of the condition, meaning that capacity in different co-design situations can be extremely variable. Different methods of engagement should be considered to support the involvement of people at different stages of dementia progression (Winton & Rodgers, 2019).

Consulting with people prior to their involvement about individual support requirements is vital to ensure these needs are catered to, and that planned tools and activities can be modified or adapted to ensure equitable participation. Practical tools, activities and other methods applied throughout the co-design process may need to be adapted or modified to be suitable for people living with dementia to participate in, as people living with dementia have different communication, sensory and cognitive support needs (Hendriks et al., 2015b). Involvement in co-design can require those involved to process complex information, provide input and suggestions, and contribute to discussions. Typically, design activities, tools and methods are selected based on whether they align with the primary aims of the project stage (Hendricks, F. et al., 2015a). However, when involving people living with dementia, the needs and abilities of those involved should be the primary driver of tool and activity selection (Hendriks et al., 2015b).

Co-design tools or methods relevant for use in developing digital interventions include those that can facilitate the exploration of needs and preferences for support that can be provided by a digital device, and those that can ensure the user-friendliness of technology and devices (Astell et al., 2020). Methods and tools such as surveys, interviews, diaries, storytelling and photovoice can be used to obtain rich information about the experiences, needs, preferences and requirements of people living with dementia. As part of the MinD project, Niedderer et al. (2020) developed a suite of co-design data collection tools with and for people living with dementia, including visual cards to support conversation and diary probes to explore goals and needs to identify areas for intervention. Using co-created personas (a representation of a user group developed with people living with dementia) is also a suitable approach to exploring experiences and needs of people living with dementia. Presentation of personas can serve as memory and discussion prompts and can be useful in de-personalising involvement to help people feel more comfortable when critiquing issues or providing negative feedback (Neate et al., 2019). However, personas should not be used in place of the involvement of people living with dementia themselves (McKercher, 2020).

Prototyping, prioritisation activities and usability testing are commonly used in the ideation, testing and refinement stages of co-design. Prototyping helps to visualise design concepts and simulate use of the design to get feedback on usability and potential design issues, and preferencing and prioritisation activities (e.g., card sorting) aid and facilitate decision-making. Usability testing can be used to observe how people interact with the design and provide an opportunity to give real-time feedback on usability and function, rather than having to report back later. Prototypes may also be taken home for use to obtain feedback on how the intervention or device integrates with daily life. Prototyping can identify usability issues such as interface accessibility, interaction and navigation, points where instructions are required, interaction with the device (e.g., using swipes or clicks), font and button size, and suitable contrast and colours (Kerkhof et al., 2019), and the requirement of images or other multimedia, providing screen readers and use of overlay accessibility tools (Alzheimer's Society, 2022). Usability testing also requires other technology-specific considerations such as providing adequate time for people to familiarise themselves with any devices being used, e.g., using a smartphone/app/iPad/computer, or to become familiar with any relevant technical language. As technology development can also require significant hands-on involvement, activities will need to consider how people with any physical and cognitive support needs can be involved.

The TUNGSTEN approach to technology design (Tools for User Needs Gathering to Support Technology Engagement) provides a framework and practical tools to engage older people in technology development process and has been adapted to use with people living with dementia and family carers (Astell et al., 2020). In the development of "Data Day," an app to empower people with a diagnosis of dementia in the self-management of their daily tasks and activities, the tools were used to build confidence in people living with dementia in talking about and using technology, and to support involvement in all decision making related to usability, accessibility, functionality, interface design, navigation and interaction with the app. The activities involved people living with dementia and family carers initially interacting with existing technology to establish comfort in talking about and using technology, then demonstrating using existing technology their likes and dislikes, and finally exploring and providing feedback on emerging prototypes (Astell et al., 2020).

14.3.3 Summary

The adaptability and flexibility of co-design methods allow for ongoing and iterative adaptation, monitoring and evaluation to update digital interventions based on real-world use to ensure the designed intervention remains useable and workable for the proposed end-users. Sustainability of the digital health intervention requires consideration and planning for ongoing resourcing, implementation, scalability beyond initial pilot phases and maintaining stakeholder engagement (such as consumers, technology partners and healthcare providers). These issues will be discussed in the following section.

14.3.4 Resources

Alzheimer's Society Guide (includes Digital accessibility best practice guidelines): https://www.alzheimers.org.uk/sites/default/files/2022-05/alzheimers-society-co-creation-guide.pdf

Dementia Australia engagement guidelines – Half the story https://www.dementia.org.au/sites/default/files/2023-12/Half-the-story.pdf

14.4 Implementing and Embedding Digital Health Interventions: Key Considerations for Co-Design

Despite the increasing application of co-design with the dementia community, often resulting in innovative and successful interventions to improve health outcomes and well-being, there remains a persistent gap between research and real-world implementation. Even the most promising innovations derived from rigorous co-design can fail to deliver benefits if not effectively implemented.

To bridge this gap, co-design needs to go beyond the design of the innovation, and also focus on the collaborative co-design of the *implementation* plan – that is, for co-designers to also devote time to the "how" – how the strategies for putting an intervention or program will be put into practice. This ensures the specific environment or context where the intervention will be implemented is considered, and requires a deliberate effort to embed and integrate user needs, implementation of "real-world" realities, and research evidence, leading to more effective and sustainable interventions. In addition, to ensure both research and implementation considerations are addressed, implementation plans should be designed with validated implementation strategies and then robustly evaluated.

Implementation science is the science of translating research findings into real-world practice (Bauer et al., 2015). It furthers understanding of the factors that influence how well an intervention is adopted and delivered in real-world settings. By addressing implementation challenges (examples include user adoption, workflow integration, and fidelity to the intervention), implementation science can help ensure interventions are delivered as intended, ultimately maximising their effectiveness. Implementation science helps ensure that interventions with the potential to improve health and well-being are optimally translated into practice and reach the communities that would benefit most, in this instance, people living with dementia and those who care for them.

Co-design and implementation science approaches share a strong emphasis on collaboration, context, and user involvement. While co-design often focuses on the development of an intervention, implementation science specifically addresses the process of putting it into practice. That is, how can the intervention be effectively integrated into actual practice – for individuals, and for organisations? Both co-design and implementation science share the goal of ensuring successful adoption and use. Implementation science findings can (and should) inform the design of interventions from the beginning. By considering implementation factors early on, co-designers can design, test, and roll out interventions that are more likely to be successfully adopted and delivered in real-world settings.

By incorporating implementation science principles into the co-design process, it is possible to develop digital health interventions for dementia that are not only effective but also feasible, sustainable, and impactful. Digital interventions often face challenges in adoption and use and implementation science approaches can help to identify and address potential barriers to implementation (such as lack of training, resistance to change, or technical difficulties) and optimise sustainability and maintenance of the intervention over time.

14.4.1 Implementation Frameworks

There are numerous frameworks and theories in implementation science that are useful in co-designing digital health interventions for dementia. These can guide the co-design process, ensuring a focus on both translational research and implementation factors from the outset. Existing frameworks are grounded in diverse theoretical backgrounds or perspectives within implementation science, and are used across the various aspects of planning, implementation and evaluation of interventions. Using standardised methodologies and frameworks in the co-creation process of technology solutions can also support analysis and comparison in a field where there are currently large variations in methodology and approaches. While the field of implementation science is continually evolving, we have highlighted two frameworks, which can also be used to complement each other.

14.4.1.1 The RE-AIM Framework

The RE-AIM framework (Holtrop et al., 2021) is a validated and widely used framework for evaluating and planning interventions, particularly those focused on public health (including digital health). The RE-AIM framework focuses on five key dimensions for successful intervention uptake:

Reach: The co-designed intervention should reach the target population effectively.

Effectiveness: Co-designers should integrate evidence-based practices to maximise effectiveness and ensure the intervention achieves its intended outcomes.

Adoption: Consider the intervention's feasibility and acceptability within its intended setting. Will the end-users accept and integrate the intervention into their systems, workflow, and policies?

Implementation: This assesses how faithfully the intervention is delivered in real-world settings. Co-designing with providers can ensure the intervention fits seamlessly into existing workflows.

Maintenance: This dimension looks at whether the intervention can be sustained over time. Co-designing a plan for ongoing support and training can promote long-term use.

By considering all five RE-AIM dimensions during co-design and in the evaluation of the co-designed innovation, digital health interventions can be developed that are not only effective but also widely used, well-integrated, and sustainable.

There are examples of the RE-AIM framework being employed to guide the implementation and evaluation of dementia-related digital interventions, such as interventions aimed at supporting informal carers of older people (Dale et al., 2023), and supporting self-management (Lee et al., 2024), but there are very few studies relating to co-designed digital interventions for the dementia community.

14.4.1.2 Consolidated Framework for Implementation Research (CFIR)

The Consolidated Framework for Implementation Research (CFIR) (Damschroder et al., 2022) provides a validated implementation science framework, covering specific factors influencing implementation success. The CFIR can be combined with RE-AIM to provide a more comprehensive picture and a more nuanced understanding of an intervention's impact. Whereas RE-AIM can be used to support overall evaluation, the CFIR will help to identify specific implementation factors (e.g., intervention characteristics, immediate environment, broader context within the RE-AIM framework's "implementation" dimension.

The CFIR provides practical guidance for the systematic assessment of facilitators and barriers to implementation, supporting tailoring of implementation strategies and needed adaptations, and/or to explain outcomes. The CFIR promotes consistent use of constructs, systematic analysis, and organisation of findings related to implementation. This is particularly useful in co-designing dementia-related interventions as facilitators and barriers to implementation have been historically under-recognised or not taken into consideration.

The CFIR has most often been used within healthcare settings but has also been used across a diverse array of settings including low-income contexts. In co-design of digital interventions in the dementia field, the CFIR has been used in settings such as hospitals and long-term care. Guo et al. (2023) explored barriers and facilitators that impact healthcare staff participation in co-design activities for digital applications for dementia care. Three main themes were identified: (a) information sharing between projects and staff allowed for meaningful engagement, (b) a sense of accomplishment and satisfaction promoted commitment to continuity and (c) creativity and open-mindedness created access to collective resources. Hung and colleagues (2023) found CFIR useful when engaging stakeholders in project planning and team reflection for implementation, helping to overcome challenges and meet the needs of multiple organisations.

The CFIR has also been used in the process evaluation of large randomised controlled trials (e.g., Wilding et al., 2022) and in systematic reviews. For example, Gilliam et al. (2022) found that key factors in implementing eHealth assessment and decision-making for residents with dementia in long-term care related to the "inner setting" construct, such as providing a conducive learning climate, engaged leadership, and sufficient training and resources. These results support the need to adopt practical strategies to maximise implementation of digital health interventions to optimise uptake and drive improvements.

14.4.2 Summary

By using validated and reliable implementation frameworks, developers and designers can increase the likelihood of creating digital health interventions that meet the needs of the target population and are successfully implemented (and evaluated) in real-world settings. Allocating adequate and dedicated resources (including time, budget, personnel) to consider robust co-design, consideration of implementation factors, and the evaluation of both, is key.

14.4.3 Resource

RE-AIM framework: https://re-aim.org/

14.5 Evaluation of Co-Design of Digital Health Interventions in Dementia

14.5.1 Introduction

Despite the exponential increase in the use of co-design across a wide range of contexts, there is relatively little literature or information directly addressing the evaluation of co-design and even less relating to the evaluation of co-design and technology. For example, Bird et al. (2021) describe a co-design framework for health innovation which includes the stages of pre-design, co-design and post-design, yet does not include specific reference to evaluation. Evaluation of outcomes and participatory processes is particularly important to ensure that co-design has benefits for all involved (Malloy et al., 2023). In the context of co-design and dementia, this could be rephrased as: was a positive change achieved or a digital health intervention created that benefits people with dementia and/or those who care for them, and was a collaborative co-design process used that engaged people living with dementia and/or their carers? (Metro North Health, 2024).

Co-design evaluation frameworks that are more generic may be used to guide evaluation in the context of digital health interventions and dementia. For example, a framework for evaluating the *processes* involved in co-design could potentially be adapted for technology design contexts. As successful processes and outcomes are inextricably linked with successful implementation, implementation frameworks such as RE-AIM and CFIR discussed above are also useful tools for designing and undertaking evaluation. In line with the principles of co-design more broadly, evaluation (including planning the evaluation from the outset) needs to actively involve the most relevant stakeholders, in this instance, people living with dementia and those who support and/or care for them. Indeed, as the whole co-design process moves towards a monitoring and evaluation phase, it is important to consider how the co-designers can continue to have meaningful involvement (McKercher, 2020). Wang et al.'s (2022) literature review provides a recommended co-design evaluation framework, which could be adapted for dementia-related technology design contexts. The suggested steps include:

1. Planning the evaluation from the beginning of the co-design process
2. Setting the evaluation criteria and ensuring criteria for success are established from the start
3. Choosing appropriate evaluation methods relevant to approach, process and outcome
4. Critically interpreting the results
5. Communication of evaluation outcomes

With respect to digital health interventions, evaluation often focuses on the *outcome* of a co-designed intervention, rather than evaluation of the co-design process itself. For example, a systematic review focussing on co-design of digital health interventions for younger people described the evaluation approach used by 15 of the included studies, but only outcome measures related to user experience of the final digital health intervention were described (Malloy et al., 2023). Outcomes included measures of usability, acceptability, feasibility and end-user satisfaction. As outcomes and processes are inextricably linked in co-design, process evaluation is essential and evaluation of one without the other would not be desirable.

14.5.2 Considerations When Evaluating Co-Design

Key considerations when evaluating co-design include:

- The need to evaluate processes involved in co-design as well as the experiences of co-design participants and the outcomes achieved (Hyett et al., 2020).
- Understanding the impact of co-design on stakeholders (Malloy et al., 2023), that is, the process of being a co-designer.
- The need to adopt multiple methods including qualitative and quantitative process and outcome data to collect, analyse and interpret data to support the evaluation (Hyett et al., 2020). People living with dementia and those who care for them have a key role in identifying the most relevant process and outcome measures.
- Understanding the design criteria specified in the planning and development phases of co-design – as the design criteria will guide ongoing monitoring, evaluation and learning (McKercher, 2020).
- Inclusion of sustainability as a key evaluation component. This should incorporate an evaluation of the sustainability of the co-design activities (process), and the overall sustainability of the end product or digital health intervention and its impacts (outcome) (Hayward et al., 2017).

Overall, the outcomes of co-designing a digital health intervention need to be carefully considered, including specifying the most appropriate outcome measures. This also requires careful consideration of and collaboration with the intended end-user. A successful outcome from the perspective of a family member may not be seen as positive by the person living with dementia themselves. For example, remote monitoring of a person's movement may be seen as a positive outcome of the co-design of a digital health intervention in the case where family members are concerned about a person living with dementia walking outside of the home, but may be seen as intrusive by the person living with dementia.

14.5.3 Key Challenges in Evaluation of Co-Design for Digital Health Interventions in Dementia

The active and meaningful participation of people living with dementia in co-design requires strong processes in place to recognise and respond to the unique capacities, strengths and needs of individuals with potentially varying degrees and types of cognitive and/or physical impairment (see section above). The degree to which this has occurred also needs to be reflected in the evaluation. Evaluation therefore needs to consider:

- The degree to which the person living with dementia and/or their carer have been supported throughout all of the co-design activities (McKercher, 2020). Evaluation questions to address this factor could include:
  - How well were support needs of the person with dementia and/or their carer identified and addressed?
  - For the person providing support, were they provided with adequate training and resources to enable them to provide appropriate support?
  - What was the experience of support like for all co-designers?
- The degree to which the co-design process has been safe (McKercher, 2020) and beneficial for all stakeholders (Man et al., n.d.). Key evaluation questions include:
  - Was there a framework of safety developed?
  - Were there any adverse events/negative experiences?
  - How well were any disclosures managed?

The lack of relevant process and outcome data to support meaningful co-design evaluation can also be a significant challenge (Wang et al., 2022). The overall co-design process, particularly in the case of co-designing dementia-related digital technologies, may involve relatively small numbers of people, who may then decline or not be available to participate in an evaluation process. This is particularly relevant to people with dementia and their carers, who may be experiencing fatigue or burnout in everyday life (Takai et al., 2009) and not have the capacity or time to be able to contribute to evaluation beyond the co-design process itself.

Inherent in co-design is the principle that involving users in all aspects of the design process will result in a final product that is aligned with the co-designer's strengths, needs and preferences. This is especially important when creating digital health interventions for older adults, including people living with dementia and those who care for them, who are often left out of design decisions even though they may be the main users (Comincioli et al., 2022).

However, even when people living with dementia are included in the design process, implicit ageism and/or ableism, biases that can affect both designers and people living with dementia, can still negatively influence the processes and outcomes (Comincioli et al., 2022). These biases should be considered across all aspects of the co-design process, for example, in selecting co-designers, and also when developing, conducting, analysing and interpreting the evaluation.

14.5.4 Summary

The evaluation of co-design, particularly in the context of digital health interventions for dementia, is crucial yet underexplored. While frameworks like those proposed by Bird et al. (2021) and Wang et al. (2022) offer structured approaches, they often lack specific guidelines for evaluating the co-design process itself. Effective evaluation should encompass both the outcomes and the participatory processes to ensure that the benefits are realised for all stakeholders, including people living with dementia and those who care for them. This involves planning the evaluation from the outset, setting clear criteria for success, choosing appropriate methods, and critically interpreting and communicating the results. The involvement of people living with dementia and key stakeholders throughout the evaluation process is essential to maintaining the integrity and inclusivity of the co-design approach.

Key considerations for evaluating co-design include assessing the processes, experiences of co-designers, and the outcomes achieved. It is important to adopt multiple methods, both qualitative and quantitative, to gather comprehensive data. Evaluation should also consider the sustainability of both the co-design activities and the final product. Challenges such as the active participation of people living with dementia, managing implicit and explicit biases, and ensuring meaningful data collection must be addressed. Ultimately, the goal is to create digital health interventions that are aligned with the needs and preferences of people living with dementia and those who care for them, ensuring that the co-design process is safe, supportive, and beneficial for all involved.

14.5.5 Resources

Guide to Evaluating Co-design (Metro North Health, 2024)

Beyond Sticky Notes (McKercher, 2020)

Beyond Sticky Notes website https://www.beyondstickynotes.com/

Implementing and evaluating co-design: A step-by-step toolkit (Man et al., n.d.)

References

Alzheimer's Society. (2022). *Dementia and co-creation: A practical guide to designing products and services.* https://www.alzheimers.org.uk/sites/default/files/2022-05/alzheimers-society-co-creation-guide.pdf

Astell, A. (2019). Creating Technologies with People Who Have Dementia. In S. Sayago (Ed.), *Perspectives on Human-Computer Interaction Research with Older People* (pp. 21–36). Springer International Publishing. https://doi.org/10.1007/978-3-030-06076-3_2

Astell, A., Dove, E., Morland, C., & Donovan, S. (2020). Using the TUNGSTEN Approach to Co-Design DataDay: A Self-Management App for Dementia. In R. Brankaert & G. Kenning (Eds.), *HCI and Design in the Context of Dementia* (pp. 171–185). Springer International Publishing. https://doi.org/10.1007/978-3-030-32835-1_11

Bauer, M. S., Damschroder, L., Hagedorn, H., Smith, J., & Kilbourne, A. M. (2015). An Introduction to Implementation Science for the Non-Specialist. *BMC Psychology, 3*(1), 32. https://doi.org/10.1186/s40359-015-0089-9

Bird, M., McGillion, M., Chambers, E. M., Dix, J., Fajardo, C. J., Gilmour, M., Levesque, K., Lim, A., Mierdel, S., Ouellette, C., Polanski, A. N., Reaume, S. V., Whitmore, C., & Carter, N. (2021). A Generative Co-Design Framework for Healthcare Innovation: Development and Application of an End-User Engagement Framework. *Research Involvement and Engagement, 7*(1), 12. https://doi.org/10.1186/s40900-021-00252-7

Blomkamp, E. (2018). The Promise of Co-Design for Public Policy. *Australian Journal of Public Administration, 77*(4), 729–743. https://doi.org/10.1111/1467-8500.12310

Branco, R. M., Quental, J., & Ribeiro, Ó. (2017). Personalised Participation: An Approach to Involve People with Dementia and Their Families in a Participatory Design Project. *CoDesign, 13*(2), 127–143. https://doi.org/10.1080/15710882.2017.1310903

Cheraghi-Sohi, S., Davies, K., Gordon, L., Jones, H., Sanders, C., & Ong, B. N. (2023). A Study to Explore the Usefulness of a Mobile Health Application to Support People with Mild Cognitive and/or Communication Impairment Due to Dementia and Their Carers. *Digital Health, 9*, 205520762311735. https://doi.org/10.1177/20552076231173560

Comincioli, E., Hakoköngäs, E., & Masoodian, M. (2022). Identifying and Addressing Implicit Ageism in the Co-Design of Services for Aging People. *International Journal of Environmental Research and Public Health, 19*(13). https://doi.org/10.3390/ijerph19137667

Dale, J., Nanton, V., Day, T., Apenteng, P., Bernstein, C. J., Grason Smith, G., Strong, P., & Procter, R. (2023). Uptake and Use of Care Companion, a Web-Based Information Resource for Supporting Informal Carers of Older People: Mixed Methods Study. *JMIR Aging, 6*, e41185. https://doi.org/10.2196/41185

Damschroder, L. J., Reardon, C. M., Widerquist, M. A. O., & Lowery, J. (2022). The Updated Consolidated Framework for Implementation Research Based on User Feedback. *Implementation Science, 17*(1), 75. https://doi.org/10.1186/s13012-022-01245-0

Dementia Australia. (2022). *Half the Story – A guide to meaningful consultation with people living with dementia, families and carers.* https://www.dementia.org.au/sites/default/files/2023-12/Half-the-story.pdf

Dementia Enquirers. (2023). *The dementia enquirers gold standards for ethical research.* https://www.dementiavoices.org.uk/wp-content/uploads/2020/07/The-DEEP-Ethics-Gold-Standards-for-Dementia-Research.pdf

Fox, S., Brown, L. J. E., Antrobus, S., Brough, D., Drake, R. J., Jury, F., Leroi, I., Parry-Jones, A. R., & Machin, M. (2022). Co-Design of a Smartphone App for People Living with Dementia by Applying Agile, Iterative Co-Design Principles: Development and Usability Study. *JMIR mHealth and uHealth, 10*(1), e24483. https://doi.org/10.2196/24483

Gaffy, E., Brijnath, B., & Dow, B. (2022). Co-Producing Research with People Impacted by Dementia and Service Providers: Issues and Challenges. *Public Health Research & Practice, 32*(2). https://doi.org/10.17061/phrp3222216

Gillam, J., Davies, N., Aworinde, J., Yorganci, E., Anderson, J. E., & Evans, C. (2022). Implementation of eHealth to Support Assessment and Decision-Making for Residents with Dementia in Long-Term Care: Systematic Review. *Journal of Medical Internet Research, 24*(2), e29837. https://doi.org/10.2196/29837

Goh, A. M., Doyle, C., Gaffy, E., Batchelor, F., Polacsek, M., Savvas, S., Malta, S., Ames, D., Winbolt, M., Panayiotou, A., Loi, S. M., Cooper, C., Livingston, G., Low, L.-F., Fairhall, A., Burton, J., & Dow, B. (2022). Co-Designing a Dementia-Specific Education and Training Program for Home Care Workers: The "Promoting Independence through Quality Dementia Care at Home" Project. *Dementia, 21*(3), 899–917. https://doi.org/10.1177/14713012211065377

Guo, Y. P. (Ellen). (2023). *Co-designing a digital application for dementia care with health-care staff in hospital and long-term care.* https://doi.org/10.14288/1.0423804

Hayward, B., Hayward, P., & Walsh Dr, C. (2017). Increasing Sustainability in Co-Design Projects: A Qualitative Evaluation of a Co-Design Programme in New Zealand. *Patient Experience Journal, 4*(2), 44–52.

Hendriks, F., Kienhues, D., & Bromme, R. (2015a). Measuring Laypeople's Trust in Experts in a Digital Age: The Muenster Epistemic Trustworthiness Inventory (METI). https://doi.org/10.1371/journal.pone.0139309

Hendriks, N., Slegers, K., & Duysburgh, P. (2015b). Codesign with People Living with Cognitive or Sensory Impairments: A Case for Method Stories and Uniqueness. *CoDesign, 11*(1), 70–82. https://doi.org/10.1080/15710882.2015.1020316

Hirt, J., Burgstaller, M., Zeller, A., & Beer, T. (2019). Needs of People with Dementia and Their Informal Caregivers Concerning Assistive Technologies: A Scoping Review. *Pflege, 32*(6), 295–304. https://doi.org/10.1024/1012-5302/a000682

Holtrop, J. S., Estabrooks, P. A., Gaglio, B., Harden, S. M., Kessler, R. S., King, D. K., Kwan, B. M., Ory, M. G., Rabin, B. A., Shelton, R. C., & Glasgow, R. E. (2021). Understanding and Applying the RE-AIM Framework: Clarifications and Resources. *Journal of Clinical and Translational Science, 5*(1), e126. https://doi.org/10.1017/cts.2021.789

Hung, L., Mann, J., & Upreti, M. (2023). Using the Consolidated Framework for Implementation Research to Foster the Adoption of a New Dementia Education Game during the COVID-19 Pandemic. *The Gerontologist, 63*(3), 467–477. https://doi.org/10.1093/geront/gnac138

Hyett, N., Bagley, K., Iacono, T., McKinstry, C., Spong, J., & Landry, O. (2020). Evaluation of a Codesign Method Used to Support the Inclusion of Children with Disability in Mainstream Schools. *International Journal of Qualitative Methods, 19*, 160940692092498. https://doi.org/10.1177/1609406920924982

Kennedy, A., Cosgrave, C., Macdonald, J., Gunn, K., Dietrich, T., & Brumby, S. (2021). Translating Co-Design from Face-to-Face to Online: An Australian Primary Producer Project Conducted during COVID-19. *International Journal of Environmental Research and Public Health*, 18(8), 4147. https://doi.org/10.3390/ijerph18084147

Kenning, G. (2018). Reciprocal Design: Inclusive Design Approaches for People with Late Stage Dementia. *Design for Health*, 2(1), 142–162. https://doi.org/10.1080/24735132.2018.1453638

Kerkhof, Y., Pelgrum-Keurhorst, M., Mangiaracina, F., Bergsma, A., Vrauwdeunt, G., Graff, M., & Dröes, R.-M. (2019). User-Participatory Development of findMyApps; a Tool to Help People with Mild Dementia Find Supportive Apps for Self-Management and Meaningful Activities. *Digital Health*, 5, 205520761882294. https://doi.org/10.1177/2055207618822942

Lee, A. R., McDermott, O., & Orrell, M. (2024). Findings from the Promoting Independence in Dementia app (PRIDE-app) Study a Reach, Effectiveness, Adoption, Implementation, and Maintenance Framework Discussion. *Journal of Geriatric Psychiatry and Neurology*, 08919887241246237. https://doi.org/10.1177/08919887241246237

Leorin, C., Stella, E., Nugent, C., Cleland, I., & Paggetti, C. (2019). The Value of Including People with Dementia in the Co-Design of Personalized eHealth Technologies. *Dementia and Geriatric Cognitive Disorders*, 47(3), 164–175. https://doi.org/10.1159/000497804

Lord, K., Kelleher, D., Ogden, M., Mason, C., Rapaport, P., Burton, A., Leverton, M., Downs, M., Souris, H., Jackson, J., Lang, I., Manthorpe, J., & Cooper, C. (2022). Co-Designing Complex Interventions with People Living with Dementia and Their Supporters. *Dementia*, 21(2), 426–441. https://doi.org/10.1177/14713012211042466

Malloy, J., Partridge, S. R., Kemper, J. A., Braakhuis, A., & Roy, R. (2023). Co-Design of Digital Health Interventions with Young People: A Scoping Review. *Digital Health*, 9, 20552076231219117. https://doi.org/10.1177/20552076231219117

Man, M., Abrams, T., & McLeod, R. (n.d.). *Implementing and evaluating co-design*. https://www.thinknpc.org/wp-content/uploads/2019/07/Co-design-guidance-July-2019.pdf

McKercher, K. A. (2020). *Beyond sticky notes. Doing co-design for real: Mindsets, methods, and movements, 1st Edn.* Sydney, NSW: Beyond Sticky Notes.

Metro North Health. (2024). *Guide to evaluating co-design*. Queensland Government. https://metronorth.health.qld.gov.au/wp-content/uploads/2022/10/evaluation-guide-co-design.pdf

Moll, S., Wyndham-West, M., Mulvale, G., Park, S., Buettgen, A., Phoenix, M., Fleisig, R., & Bruce, E. (2020). Are You Really Doing "Codesign"? Critical Reflections When Working with Vulnerable Populations. *BMJ Open*, 10(11), e038339. https://doi.org/10.1136/bmjopen-2020-038339

Neate, T., Bourazeri, A., Roper, A., Stumpf, S., & Wilson, S. (2019). *Co-created personas: engaging and empowering users with diverse needs within the design process*. 650. https://dl.acm.org/doi/10.1145/3290605.3300880

Niedderer, K., Tournier, I., Coleston-Shields, D. M., Craven, M., Gosling, J., Garde, J., Salter, B., Bosse, M., & Griffioen, I. (2020). Designing with and for People with Dementia: Developing a Mindful Interdisciplinary Co-Design Methodology. In G. Muratovski & C. Vogel (Eds.), *Re:Research Volume 4: Design and Living Well* (pp. 147–168). Intellect.

Sakamoto, M., Guo, Y. P. E., Wong, K. L. Y., Mann, J., Berndt, A., Boger, J., Currie, L., Raber, C., Egeberg, E., Burke, C., Sood, G., Lim, A., Yao, S., Phinney, A., & Hung, L. (2023). Co-Design of a Digital App "WhatMatters" to Support Person-Centred Care: A Critical Reflection. *International Journal of Geriatric Psychiatry, 38*(10), e6014. https://doi.org/10.1002/gps.6014

Sanders, E. B.-N., & Stappers, P. J. (2008). Co-creation and the New Landscapes of Design. *CoDesign, 4*(1), 5–18. https://doi.org/10.1080/15710880701875068

Sanders, E. B.-N., & Stappers, P. J. (2014). Probes, Toolkits and Prototypes: Three Approaches to Making in Codesigning. *CoDesign, 10*(1), 5–14. https://doi.org/10.1080/15710882.2014.888183

Span, M., Hettinga, M., Vernooij-Dassen, M., Eefsting, J., & Smits, C. (2013). Involving People with Dementia in the Development of Supportive IT Applications: A Systematic Review. *Ageing Research Reviews, 12*(2), 535–551. https://doi.org/10.1016/j.arr.2013.01.002

Suijkerbuijk, S., Nap, H. H., Cornelisse, L., IJsselsteijn, W. A., De Kort, Y. A. W., & Minkman, M. M. N. (2019). Active Involvement of People with Dementia: A Systematic Review of Studies Developing Supportive Technologies. *Journal of Alzheimer's Disease, 69*(4), 1041–1065. https://doi.org/10.3233/JAD-190050

Takai, M., Takahashi, M., Iwamitsu, Y., Ando, N., Okazaki, S., Nakajima, K., Oishi, S., & Miyaoka, H. (2009). The Experience of Burnout among Home Caregivers of Patients with Dementia: Relations to Depression and Quality of Life. *Archives of Gerontology and Geriatrics, 49*(1), e1–e5. https://doi.org/10.1016/j.archger.2008.07.002

Wang, Z., Jiang, T., Huang, J., Tai, Y., & Trapani, P. M. (2022, June 16). *How might we evaluate co-design? A literature review on existing practices.* DRS2022: Bilbao. https://doi.org/10.21606/drs.2022.774

Wang, G., Marradi, C., Albayrak, A., & Van Der Cammen, T. J. M. (2019). Co-Designing with People with Dementia: A Scoping Review of Involving People with Dementia in Design Research. *Maturitas, 127*, 55–63. https://doi.org/10.1016/j.maturitas.2019.06.003

Wilding, C., Morgan, D., Greenhill, J., Perkins, D., O'Connell, M. E., Bauer, M., Farmer, J., Morley, C., & Blackberry, I. (2022). Web-Based Technologies to Support Carers of People Living with Dementia: Protocol for a Mixed Methods Stepped-Wedge Cluster Randomized Controlled Trial. *JMIR Research Protocols, 11*(5), e33023. https://doi.org/10.2196/33023

Wilson, M., Doyle, J., Turner, J., Nugent, C., & O'Sullivan, D. (2024). Designing Technology to Support Greater Participation of People Living with Dementia in Daily and Meaningful Activities. *Digital Health, 10*, 20552076231222427. https://doi.org/10.1177/20552076231222427

Winton, E., & Rodgers, P. A. (2019). Designed with Me: Empowering People Living with Dementia. *The Design Journal, 22*(sup1), 359–369. https://doi.org/10.1080/14606925.2019.1595425

15

The Potential of Digital Solutions for Caregivers of Individuals with Dementia

Sara J. Czaja and Laura N. Gitlin

15.1 Introduction

By 2030, 1 in 6 people in the world will be aged 60 years or over, and by 2050, the world's population of people aged 60 years and older will double (2.1 billion). Further, the number of persons aged 80 years or older is expected to triple between 2020 and 2050 to reach 426 million (World Health Organization, 2024). As age is the primary risk factor for Alzheimer's disease and related dementia (ADRD), the growth in the number of older people, especially those older than 85 years, has vast implications for society and the healthcare system and specifically dementia care. Figure 15.1 shows the number of people with ADRD in the United States (U.S.) according to age category, as shown incidence of ADRD is higher among the older cohorts. Currently, there are over 55 million people worldwide living with dementia in 2020. This number will almost double every 20 years, reaching 78 million in 2030 and 139 million in 2050 (Prince et al., 2015). Moreover, the number of people with ADRD will continue to increase in the upcoming decades (Fang et al., 2025).

Most older adults (~96%) with ADRD live at home in communities and rely on family members or friends to provide the care and support needed. Although estimates vary regarding the prevalence of caregivers, it is estimated to be about 11 million people in the U.S. adult population are providing unpaid care to someone with ADRD (Alzheimer's Association, 2024). Further, the prevalence of family members serving in a caregiving role is projected to increase in the upcoming years with the aging of the population, the projected shortage in geriatric healthcare workers, and increases in the cost of long-term care.

The roles of family caregivers are complex and range from assistance with daily activities and providing direct care to the care recipient to navigating complex healthcare and social services systems (Gitlin & Hodgson, in press). Specific caregiving tasks include assistance with household tasks, self-care tasks, and mobility; provision of emotional and social support; health and

DOI: 10.1201/9781003485681-15

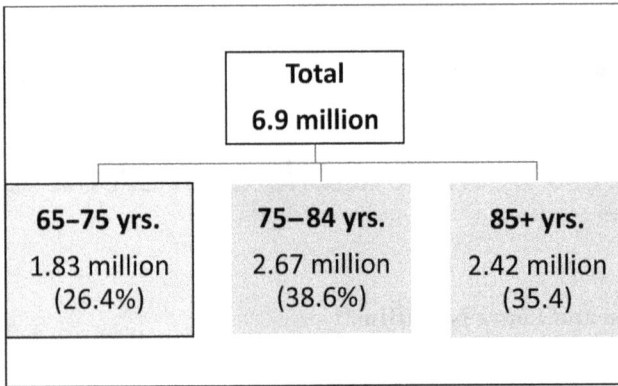

FIGURE 15.1
Number of adults with Alzheimer's disease or dementia by age. (Based on data from Rajan et al., 2021.)

medical care; advocacy and care coordination; and surrogacy (National Academies of Sciences, Engineering, and Medicine, 2016). Given the current movement toward more home-based (National Academies of Sciences, Engineering, and Medicine, 2011) as opposed to clinically based care for patients with a chronic illness such as ADRD, caregivers also frequently need to interact with complex medical technologies such as infusion pumps or feeding tubes when performing medical tasks. Importantly, few caregivers have received training or are prepared to perform these activities. As such, numerous studies have documented the negative consequences associated with dementia caregiving and a myriad of interventions have been developed to aid family caregivers and relieve caregiver burden and distress (e.g., Schulz et al., 2020). Additionally, unfortunately, for a variety of reasons, many caregivers do not avail themselves of existing services and programs. For example, barriers such as transportation problems, insufficient support from others, lack of knowledge among caregivers about available services, workforce limitations such as staff shortages and poor dementia training, and cultural beliefs often limit caregivers from participating in intervention programs. Further, very few evidence-based programs have been translated for and implemented in community and healthcare settings (e.g., Gitlin et al., 2015, 2020). An essential challenge in dementia care is closing the research to practice gap by disseminating, scaling, and sustaining impactful and proven supportive interventions for caregivers (Gitlin & Czaja, in press).

One approach to address this research to practice gap is the delivery of supportive approaches through technologies. Specifically, technologies such as digital tools have the potential to reach caregivers and provide on demand support. Currently, there are a variety of digital tools available that hold promise in terms of providing supportive approaches to caregivers, enhancing their ability to provide care, reducing their burden and stress, and enhancing the well-being of caregivers as well as dementia patients. For example, communication technologies may help caregivers overcome logistic barriers and access needed programs and services and facilitate communication with family and other caregivers and healthcare providers. Web-based platforms and apps can also be used to enhance access to health-related information or information about available community resources. Monitoring technologies may also allow caregivers to maintain a check on the status or activities of their loved one while they are at work or at a distant location. Developments in artificial intelligence (AI) also present opportunities for new digital solutions for caregivers such as virtual reality (VR). Examination of innovative strategies to support family caregivers is especially critical as many are long distance caregivers (live at least 1 hour away). Current estimates indicate that about 5 to 7 million caregivers are long distant caregivers, and this number is projected to increase (Ülgüt et al., 2023).

In this chapter, we discuss the potential role of technology in providing support for caregivers. We also discuss the potential benefits and challenges associated with these technologies, factors that affect adoption, successful use of these technologies, and examples from the literature. Finally, we provide some suggestions for needed research in this area. This chapter is not intended as an exhaustive review of the literature in this expansive area, but rather provides an overview of the state of the science in this area and the potentiality of technology solutions for caregivers.

For the chapter, we are adopting the definition of caregiving provided by Schulz and Martire (2004, p. 240), that caregiving involves "the provision of extraordinary care, exceeding the bounds of what is normative or usual in family relationships." We recognize that there are distinct groups of caregivers such as children with chronic illness and disability who are typically cared for by young adult parents; adult children suffering from conditions such as mental illness, intellectual or physical challenges who are cared for by middle-aged parents; and older individuals who are cared for by their spouses, heir middle-aged children or some other relative or friend. The nature of caregiving differs substantially for children vs. adults and the patient population. Thus, the focus of our discussion will be on caregivers of older adults with ADRD patients. However, we believe that much of the discussion can generalize to other caregiver populations.

15.2 Digital Technology Platforms

15.2.1 What Are Digital Technologies?

Digitization, the process of converting information into a computer readable format (Merriam-Webster, 2025) has resulted in a myriad of digital technologies which permeate most aspects of daily living and, in many cases, enhance our ability to perform daily tasks. Currently, many activities of daily living necessitate the use of electronic devices such as smartphones and laptops. Technology generally refers to the application of scientific knowledge to the practical domains of human life (The Britannica Dictionary, 2023) and includes machines, tools, or applications used to perform or aid in the performance of activities. Digital technologies include personal computers, mobile devices and apps, the Internet of Things (IOT), robotic devices, and extended reality (e.g., VR), as well as big data and real-time analytics. Generally, these technologies, technology applications can be used in a variety of ways: as vehicles to deliver information and access to support services (e.g., mHealth apps for providing therapeutic support); as data collection tools (e.g., wearables to track behaviors); and as data analytic tools (e.g., machine learning algorithms to predict behavior; Gitlin & Czaja, in press).

For example, mobile technologies such as smartphones and tablets can be used to send prompts and reminders to users via text, pop-up notifications, or audio/visual messages; to deliver educational and support programs and counseling; and as a way for healthcare providers to provide suggestions for behavior modifications based on real-time user information. Social media platforms, such as Facebook, allow the sharing of ideas and information through virtual networks and communities. There are also current and emerging developments in AI, which are technologies and applications that are programmed to think and act like humans; recognize objects, understand language, make decisions, solve problems, and perform functions. For example, VR systems provide an immersive experience that can provide users with a realistic impression of being present in a context such as a museum or a situation (e.g., classroom) outside their home, alone, or with others. Digital assistants such as Alexa and ChatGPT can process natural human language and generate a response. Smart Home technologies with embedded AI can help individuals achieve the goal of living independently and help to reduce reliance on formal and informal (e.g., family members) caregivers. Smart home technologies with embedded include applications in household appliances, home safety and security, the ambient environment, and entertainment, and offer a range of management, monitoring, support, and responsive services.

Specifically with respect to family caregivers these applications include interventions that focus on the health and well-being of caregivers; connect them to sources of information and resources, facilitate access to healthcare providers; foster access to sources of support; help prepare the caregiver for caregiving tasks (e.g., tutorials on how to perform personal tasks) or health with care management activities. Other applications are designed to improve the safety, security, and well-being of care recipients, which in turn can help alleviate caregiver burden and distress (Lindeman et al., 2020). For example, the IOT and Smart Home devices can alert caregivers as well as providers to changes in a patient's activity patterns, health status, or an adverse event such as a fall. Below we provide examples of technology applications that support family caregivers. This is just a snapshot of applications as there are numerous technologies available and more on the horizon. Also, note that there is an overlap across the functionality of applications and devices. For example, both websites and digital assistants can facilitate access to information, and mobile apps and digital assistants can be used to schedule reminders.

BOX 15.1   EXAMPLES OF TECHNOLOGY APPLICATIONS FOR FAMILY CAREGIVERS

Telehealth Applications

- Virtual visits with providers
- Appointment scheduling
- Access to electronic health records
- Enhanced access to specialty care
- Prescription management

Information and Educational Applications

- Informational websites
- YouTube channels

Communication Applications (e.g., Videoconferencing, Text, Email)

- Communication with providers
- Online support groups with other caregivers
- Access to other family members (e.g., long distant)

Care Management Applications

- Transportation apps
- Online shopping and delivery apps
- Assistive technologies
- Reminder and scheduling apps

Online Caregiver Intervention Programs (Delivery of Interventions via Tech)

- Websites
- Interactive real-time programs

Digital Assistants (e.g., Alexa, ChatGPT)

- Reminders
- Appliance control
- Access to information

Internet of Things/Smart Devices

- Appliance management
- Location tracking
- Sensing and monitoring – safety, health indicators, activity patterns

Wearables

- Health and activity monitoring
- Location tracking

Virtual Reality Applications

- Skill building
- Respite (e.g., travel; cultural events)
- Rehabilitation

15.2.2 Use of Digital Technologies by Caregivers

Generally, the literature though limited indicates that caregivers are receptive to and are using various forms of technology to support their caregiving role. Early data from the Pew Research Center, which surveyed a representative sample of family caregivers in the U.S., found that caregivers frequently used the internet to engage in activities such as searching for health information and to find information about medications, available resources, and peers in similar situations as a source of support (Fox et al., 2013).

A more recent study by the American Association of Retired Persons (Keenan, 2022) interviewed 1,003 adults aged 18 or older currently providing unpaid care for an adult loved one to gather information about how caregivers use technologies to help them in their caregiving role. The findings indicated that caregivers use their phones and the internet to search for support services, food deliveries, and prescription refills, among other items, and use technology and software for making home modifications and keeping track of health and financial records. Additionally, although overall caregivers expressed interest in and comfort using technology, there were age group differences such that caregivers under the age of 50 expressed more comfort with and greater use of technology than older caregivers.

Lee and colleagues (Lee et al., 2024) conducted a web-based survey about technology use among unpaid caregivers of older adults (N = 486) who were recruited through a Qualtrics panel. The survey differentiated between technology devices and technology functions. The respondents were asked whether they used each of the seven devices (e.g., cell phone, smartphone, tablet, computer, e-reader, voice-activated assistant, and wearable or smartwatch for activity tracking) and eight functions (e.g., communication, ridesharing, online shopping, online banking, navigation, online entertainment, medication alerts or tracking, and physical activity tracking). Generally, the findings indicated that caregivers used all examined technologies, except for the medication alerts or tracking functions. The most frequently used devices were smartphones, tablets, and computers, and the most frequently used functions were communication, navigation to websites, online banking, and shopping. Like the findings by Keenan (2022), younger age, higher income, and education were associated with more technology use. Generally, technology is more likely to be adopted if it is accessible, usable, useful, and affordable.

Noteworthy, available data indicate that technology support tools are used by caregivers and that caregivers are comfortable using technology to support them in their caregiving role. However, the available data is U.S. centric, somewhat dated, and general. What is needed is a more current, comprehensive database on the types of technology tools used by caregivers, the frequency of use of these tools, perceived benefits of these tools, barriers to adoption, and caregiver preferences. Data are also needed on the cost-effectiveness of using technology to provide caregiver support.

15.2.3 The Promise of and Challenges of Digital Platforms for Caregivers

15.2.3.1 Technology Support Applications

As noted earlier in this chapter, there are multiple ways that technology can support family caregivers. Clearly, technologies such as the Internet and mobile devices can aid caregivers by enhancing their access to information about caregiving, ADRD, and available resources. A requisite to providing quality care is having the necessary knowledge about a care recipient's illness or disability, how to provide care, and how to access and utilize available services. However, obtaining knowledge and skills in these areas remains challenging for most caregivers. There are a vast number of websites available that can provide caregivers with information on illnesses/diseases, medications and treatments, healthcare providers, and health resources. These applications can also enhance direct access to experts and professional organizations, which can also facilitate decision-making by the caregiver. Box 15.2 provides a sample of websites that may be beneficial to caregivers.

Networks can also link caregivers to other family members or long distant caregivers to the person for whom they are providing care. The Internet is increasingly being used as a forum for individuals to exchange information about health difficulties, needs, and strategies for managing health challenges. As discussed earlier, data from the Pew Research Center indicates that caregivers frequently use the internet to search for information about health and available resources and to access support (Fox et al., 2013).

BOX 15.2 EXAMPLES OF WEBSITES FOR CAREGIVERS

American Association of Retired Persons (AARP): https://www.aarp.org/caregiving

Alzheimer's Disease International: https://www.alzint.org

Alzheimer's Association: https://act.alz.org

Embracing Carers: https://www.embracingcarers.com/us-en-resources-for-carers-around-the-world/

Family Caregiving Alliance: https://www.caregiveraction.org

National Alliance for Family Caregiving: https://www.caregiving.org

National Institute on Aging: https://www.nia.nih.gov/health/caregiving

World Health Organization: https://www.who.int/news-room/fact-sheets/detail/dementia

Technology applications can also be used as a vehicle to deliver interventions (e.g., mHealth apps for providing therapeutic support). Although this is a common use of technology applications for caregivers it became more prevalent during the COVID-19 pandemic. Generally, the literature suggests that using technology to deliver interventions is feasible, acceptable to caregivers, and results in beneficial caregiver outcomes.

In one study, Czaja and colleagues collaborated with a community agency (Finkel et al., 2007) and used a computer-telephone system (CTIS) designed for family caregivers of patients with ADRD to deliver a multicomponent psychosocial intervention to family caregivers. We found that caregivers with high levels of depressive symptoms that used the system exhibited statistically significant decreases in depression at follow-up. Caregivers also reported increased confidence in their skills as caregivers and in their ability to deal with difficult caregiving challenges.

In another study, Czaja and colleagues (2010) evaluated the efficacy and feasibility of a videophone-based psychosocial intervention aimed at reducing stress and burden and enhancing quality of life of minority family caregivers of patients with dementia. The intervention was modeled after the REACH II caregiver intervention (Belle et al., 2006) and was compared to an information only control and wellness contact control conditions. The videophone was installed in the homes of minority caregivers (Haitian, Hispanic, African American) of dementia patients and included text and voice information features (e.g., a resource guide and information/tips) and allowed for face-to-face communication between the caregivers and their interventionist and facilitated support groups. The videophone was preprogrammed so that the information was available in the preferred language of the caregivers – Creole, Spanish, and English. The findings indicated that the intervention alleviated caregiver distress and increased perceived social support. In addition, the caregivers were able to use the videophone system, and the majority indicated that the videophone was understandable and easy to use. The caregivers in this sample were generally of lower socio-economic status and had limited experience with technology prior to this study.

More recently, this team evaluated a computer-based intervention, Caring for the Caregiver Network, among family caregivers of Alzheimer's patients. The intervention was multicomponent and designed to provide education, skills training, and support and reduce stress. During the intervention period, participants completed individual skill-building sessions with a trained interventionist, participated in videoconferencing support groups, and had access to skill building and expert videos and a resource guide. The results indicate that the intervention was beneficial to the caregivers and resulted in reduced burden and depressive symptoms, and enhanced caregiver preparedness. Further, the caregivers found the intervention to be beneficial and the technology easy to use. They also found participation in the online support groups helpful as it increased their knowledge of caregiving and feelings of emotional support (Czaja et al., in preparation).

Noel and colleagues (2022) evaluated whether a virtual caregiver education program changes caregiver confidence, self-efficacy, and burden. The findings indicated that the virtual caregiver education program was effective in improving caregiver confidence and self-efficacy and participants' self-reported impact was equivalent to those who had taken previous courses in person. Xie et al. (2024) analyzed the impact of an internet-based caregiver skill training program on behavioral and psychological symptoms of dementia in patients and explored how the training impacted caregiver abilities and burden among family caregivers of patients with dementia. The findings indicated that the intervention reduced behavioral symptoms among the patients with dementia and alleviated caregiver burden on caregivers, and enhanced caregiver knowledge and skills.

Recently, there have been reviews of online interventions for family caregivers. For example, Irani and colleagues (Irani et al., 2020) conducted a systematic review to synthesize the study design features as well as the attributes and outcomes of technology-based health interventions targeting chronically ill adults and their family caregivers. Interventions either aimed to support patient self-management and improve patient outcomes or enhance shared illness management and improve patient and caregiver outcomes. The interventions included educational, behavioral, and support components and were delivered via various technologies ranging from text messaging to Internet use. Overall, patients and caregivers expressed improvements in self-management outcomes (or support) and quality of life. However, the authors noted that most of the included studies had some methodological limitations that might have influenced the findings and that some caregivers experienced technological challenges. They stressed that future research should test technology-based interventions in larger samples using robust study designs.

Pleasant et al. (2020) conducted a systematic review of online dementia-based training programs for formal and informal caregivers. They found that overall, the interventions improved caregiver outcomes and preparedness of caregivers. However, they underscore that future evaluations should consider study designs with multiple time points, control groups, and content that is personalized and interactive.

De-Moraes-Ribeiro and colleagues (2024) also conducted a systematic review of the effectiveness of internet-based or mobile app interventions for family caregivers of older adults with dementia. The interventions were classified into three main types of interventions: psychoeducational, psychotherapeutic, and multicomponent. Overall, the results indicated that the interventions were efficacious in improving caregiver knowledge and outcomes such as burden and distress. Zhai et al. (2023) conducted a system review of interventions using digital health tools to support family caregivers. The interventions included a variety of technology applications such as text messaging, internet resources (static and interactive), mHealth applications, wearables, and videoconferencing. The general purposes of the interventions included provision of education, data collection and monitoring, psychotherapy, and connection and support. The review revealed that digitally enhanced health interventions were effective at providing high-quality assistance and support to caregivers and improved caregiver psychological health, self-efficacy, caregiving skills, quality of life, social support, and problem-coping abilities. The authors concluded that Future research should include more marginalized caregivers from diverse backgrounds, improve the accessibility and usability of the technology tools, and tailor the intervention to be more culturally and linguistically sensitive.

Atefi et al. (2024) conducted a meta-analysis and systematic review to examine adherence to online interventions among family caregivers of dementia patients. The review was based on 18 studies and involved 1215 caregivers. The overall pooled drop-out rate was 18.5% which is comparable to that seen in other caregiver interventions, including those that are in person. The findings also showed that interactive social support, personalization strategies, and co-design of the intervention enhanced adherence. The authors underscored the importance of exploring factors that influence adherence in intervention studies.

In addition to technology-based interventions, computer networks, social media applications, and videoconferencing applications (e.g., Zoom) can also link caregivers to other family members or long distant caregivers to the person for whom they are providing care. (Fox et al., 2013). Other applications include sensing and monitoring systems, digital assistants, robotic applications, and VR applications (see Box 15.1).

Monitoring and tracking could, for example, help to identify potential health problems, emergencies, or safety situations. Various monitoring systems for older adults and their caregivers are already on the market, and many more are being developed. These include systems such as fall detection and prevention systems, wearable activity monitors, non-wearable embedded sensor activity monitors, medication compliance systems, and safety monitors such as smoke and temperature monitors. Developments in AI are increasing the power of *smart home* applications, which involve integrated networks of sensors – which may include a combination of safety, health, and wellness, and social connectedness technologies – installed into homes to continuously monitor environmental conditions, daily activity patterns, vital signs, sleep patterns, etc. over the long term. The goal is to capture physical and cognitive behavioral patterns and develop algorithms to detect deviations from normal patterns in the hopes of early detection of health problems and prevention of health declines.

Gaugler and colleagues (2022) assessed whether remote monitoring activity (RAM), used to track and alert users such as caregivers to behaviors and challenging events that may presage more adverse health outcomes such as hospitalizations or nursing home admissions among persons with Alzheimer's disease or a related dementia over an 18-month period in a randomized controlled trial. The results showed that reported emergency room visits and falls were significantly lower for care recipients in the intervention arm compared with the control arm in the months preceding the 18-month survey interval. In addition, the odds of experiencing a higher frequency of falls (i.e., being in a higher response category) versus a lower frequency of falls were lower for those in the intervention group compared with controls.

Web applications are also a promising approach as they are scalable and can reach caregivers who have broadband and either a smartphone, tablet, or computer. For example, Gitlin and colleagues have developed a web-app, the WeCareAdvisor, that is designed for family caregivers to learn about nonpharmacological strategies to implement in order to prevent, minimize, or resolve common dementia-related behavioral symptoms such as agitation, aggression, apathy, and more (Gitlin et al., 2021). It is the first application that operationalizes the describe, investigate, create, evaluate (DICE) approach (Kales et al., 2019). DICE is a systematic process that involves four steps: describe the behavioral symptom, investigate possible underlying contributors (e.g., medication change, infection, sleep deprivation, noisy or overstimulating), create a WeCareAdvisor Prescription that provides strategies tailored to descriptive and investigative factors, and then evaluate whether strategies worked. A pilot randomized trial involving 57 family caregivers showed that use of the WeCareAdvisor resulted in less caregiver distress with behavioral symptoms, and there was a trend toward reduced behavioral disturbances (Kales et al., 2018). A larger randomized trial of 261 caregivers across the United States is in process with initial emerging results suggesting high usage of the app, generation of WeCareAdvisor Prescriptions for all 14 behavioral symptoms represented and important positive benefits for both caregivers and persons with dementia.

Plans4Care™ is another web-app for dementia caregivers to provide dementia education and actionable strategies for common care challenges. It consists of over 80 common dementia-related care challenges (e.g., behavioral symptoms, care coordination, respite needs, and more) and over 2,000 nonpharmacological strategies. Caregivers select a care challenge they seek help with, respond to brief statements about the functional abilities of the person for whom they care using a novel scale (Everyday Function Scale, EFS), and then generate an Action Plan that explains the functional capacity of the person with dementia (e.g., what the person is able to do and what may be problematic or unsafe for them to do), why the care challenge may occur and specific nonpharmacological strategies personalized to the EFS score. Plans4Care also has other features including a Resource Library consisting of blogs, videos to instruct in use of key nonpharmacologic strategies, tracking stress levels as well as telephone access to a care advisor who can address questions, help caregivers use the strategies, and more (Jutkowitz et al., 2024). Plans4Care has been shown to be feasible and acceptable, and a randomized trial will now test whether its use can reduce hospitalizations among people with dementia and enhance caregiver well-being. Plans4Care has been designed with the end-user (caregivers and providers) testing each of its components as part of a user-design iterative evaluative process.

Other web applications specifically for family caregivers of people living with dementia are in varying stages of development and testing. These apps provide caregivers with a range of supportive approaches from addressing depression, providing meditation guidance (Jain et al., 2022; Madarasmi et al., 2024), or helping caregivers link to and coordinate with providers (Cajavilca et al., 2024).

Digital voice assistants such as Alexa or Google Assistant can also prove to be beneficial as they can provide reminders for medication, appointments, and other everyday tasks such as control of appliances or other smart home features. Findings from recent qualitative studies (Salai et al., 2022), that examined the use of digital voice that aimed to explore the expectations of family caregivers and professionals who use voice assistants to support people with a cognitive impairment at home, and to identify the barriers to using voice assistants by family carers of people with dementia and professionals. The results indicated that caregivers and professionals use voice assistants for home automation, prompts and reminders, behavior and environment monitoring, and for leisure and social interaction support. The findings also show that family carers encountered specific challenges that need to be overcome for them to realize the full benefits of voice assistants such as connectivity issues, cost, lack of familiarity with and complexity of the technology, and potential anxiety on the part of the dementia patient due to hearing unfamiliar voices.

As noted, technological solutions may also provide benefits to care recipients, which may in turn be beneficial to caregivers. For example, Czaja et al. (2024) developed a computer-based functional skills assessment and training program that included computer-based simulations of everyday technology-based tasks. The tasks include using an automatic teller machine (ATM), online banking and shopping, prescription refill, medication management, and using a ticket kiosk. The simulations are based on actual real-world systems. Each task includes a series of subtasks that progress from simple to complex. A fixed difficulty assessment without training feedback precedes training. During training, instructional feedback is provided following any error. The first error results in a repetition of the instructions. The next two errors lead to increasingly detailed instruction and the fourth error leads to the program demonstrating the correct response, followed by progression to the next subtask. Participants who do not master a subtask during training are returned to that subtask at their next training session.

The program was designed using a user-centered design approach, which included usability testing with representative trainees. The system was evaluated in two field trials with non-cognitively impaired older adults and older adults with mild cognitive impairment (MCI). In the initial field trial, the training was guided by an instructor and took place in senior centers (Czaja et al., 2020). In the second field trial, the training took place unguided in the participants' homes (Czaja et al., 2024). In both studies, performance of all six tasks improved significantly from baseline with training for both non-impaired and MCI participants. There were also significant increases in performance for trained and untrained everyday functional activities associated with the FUNSAT™ training across both samples. Further, participants who completed training reported, on average, 95% confidence that they could perform the tasks in the real world. Although the training in this study was focused on non-impaired and MCI older adults, gains in the abilities of these populations can reduce the care burden of caregivers and enhance the independence of those with a cognitive impairment as well as their feelings of mastery.

In summary, there are a variety of current and emerging digital technology applications that can provide support to caregivers of dementia patients, enhance their ability to provide care and their quality of life and that of the patient. Digital technology can also aid intervention researchers by offering new forms of data collection and analytic tools. Recently, there has also been an increased emphasis on using Ecological Momentary Assessment (EMA) techniques as a data collection tool. EMA involves repeated sampling of a person's emotions, thoughts, or behaviors in real-time via a prompt on a smartphone or other mobile device.

Recently, Kiselica and colleagues (2024) provided a useful framework (CARES) to describe the pathways by which technology might be deployed to aid caregivers of dementia patients. These pathways include cognitive offloading, offloading of tasks or activities such as remembering medication schedules and protocols; automated task management, e.g., online delivery services, remote monitoring and interventions; provision of emotional social support and symptom treatment (Table 15.1). They also provide potential outcome measures for these pathways.

TABLE 15.1

Cares Framework: Pathways Linking Technology Support to Caregivers (adapted from Kiselica et al., 2024)

Technology Pathway	Technology Examples	Examples of Potential Outcomes Measures
Cognitive Offloading of Tasks and Activities	Digital Assistant Reminders (e.g., medications, appointments)	Medication Adherence Caregiver Burden Usability metrics Acceptability metrics
Automated Task Management (perform tasks more efficiently)	Online Shopping and Delivery Autopay	Caregiver Burden Time spent on caregiving activities Usability metrics Acceptability metrics
Remote Monitoring	Sensors Wearables	Safety Measures (e.g. falls) Care Recipient Health Measures Caregiver Burden Usability metrics Acceptability metrics
Emotional/Social Support	Online Support Groups Social Virtual Reality Applications	Caregiver Burden Caregiver Depression Caregiver and Care Recipient Quality of Life Usability metrics Acceptability metrics
Symptom Management	Caregiver websites Sensors	Care Recipient Health Measures Caregiver Burden Usability metrics Acceptability metrics

15.2.3.2 Benefits and Challenges of Digital Technology Applications

Digital technology tools offer important advantages such as increased ability to deliver and access information on demand, asynchronously and over long distances; increased access to health professionals and social support; enhanced opportunities to monitor and track health indicators and activity patterns; and enhanced ability to manage daily activities and help address environmental safety concerns. Technology also affords the opportunity to present information in a wide variety of formats to suit the needs of the user population. For example, multimedia offers the potential of providing information in text with narration and animation. Developments in extended reality, such as VR, also offer the opportunity for immersive experiences. Further, technology-based interventions can extend the reach of support to more caregivers such as those in rural locations. Computer or mobile devices can also be an efficient means for delivering health risk assessments and health promotion material. Technology-based data collection tools also enable researchers to gather objective measures of behavior in real time. Additionally, developments in AI allow for prediction of behavioral patterns and precise tailoring of interventions and support materials (Box 15.3).

Technology, however, is not a panacea. There are challenges with technology solutions. Despite the increased uptake of technology by most sectors of the population, challenges accessing technology and internet connectivity persist and this is especially the case for some segments of the population such as older cohorts, those in rural locations, or of lower socio-economic status (DiMaria-Ghalili et al., 2021). Currently, in the United States, only 64% of those aged 65 and older indicate that they have home broadband and access to home broadband is lower among minorities. With respect to other technologies, 61% of people ages 65 and older own a smartphone and only about 45% of those 65 and older reported using social media (Faverio, 2022). Findings based on data from the United States Health and Retirement Survey (Choi et al., 2022) also indicate that those living in rural locations had lower internet access rates, used communication, financial, and media technology applications less, and had more unfavorable perceptions of technology than those living in more urban areas. Cost is another barrier to the use of technology by many caregivers.

Other potential challenges associated with technology include the lack of available training and technical support for the use of technology devices and the complexity of many applications and systems. Many technology applications are not designed using a user-centered design approach, and the needs, capabilities, and preferences of user groups such as caregivers are ignored in the design process (Czaja et al., 2019). There are also issues associated with privacy and security. For example, with respect to monitoring technologies, concerns related to adoption relate to what type of information is recorded, how it is recorded, and with whom it is shared. A national web-based survey of 1,518 disabled and non-disabled baby boomers (age 45–64) and older adults (65+), found variation in attitudes across these variables (Beach et al., 2009, 2010) according to what type of information was being recorded (e.g., vital signs, moving about the home, taking medications, toileting), methods of recording (video with sound, video without sound, sensors) and the target recipient of the information (self, family, doctor, researchers, insurance companies, government). The results showed that potential users were less accepting of the use of video cameras, either with or without sound, than of sensors, less acceptance of sharing information about toileting behavior, and, to a lesser extent, driving behavior, and insurance companies and the government as the least acceptable potential recipients of health information, while family members and doctors are most acceptable. The other major finding of the study was that both baby boomers and older adults reporting higher levels of disability were more accepting of having information recorded and shared than those with lower levels or no disability.

There are also other potentially negative consequences associated with digital technologies. For example, technology use may result in decreased activity engagement. Technology use may also have a negative impact on social engagement (Box 15.3). Overall, there needs to be a stronger evidence base regarding the benefits and challenges of technology solutions among family caregivers. This requires well-designed, systematic longitudinal trials with large and diverse samples of caregivers across the caregiver trajectory. Additionally, data gathered from these trials must expand beyond positive outcomes and include metrics of negative consequences and cost effectiveness.

BOX 15.3   SUMMARY OF THE POTENTIAL BENEFITS AND CHALLENGES OF DIGITAL TECHNOLOGIES

Benefits

- Broader reach of interventions to target populations
- Flexibility in information delivery modes (e.g., audio, text, graphic)
- Ability to access information on demand (e.g., any time or place)
- Ability to access interventions anonymously
- Enhanced ability to personalize information or interventions
- Enhanced ability to communicate with healthcare providers
- Enhanced access to resources and social support
- Enhances ability to perform tasks (e.g., reminders, appliance control)
- Enhanced ability to monitor and track health metrics and activity patterns

Challenges

- Connectivity issues
- Technology access
- Cost and access to stable broadband
- Lack of attention to user-centered design and integrating caregiver or end user input at each developmental stage of the technology
- Complex technologies and interfaces that are constantly changing
- Lack of available training and instructional support
- Privacy and security concerns
- Lack of information about potential negative consequences associated with use
  - Decreased physical activity
  - Decreased social engagement
- Unreliable systems
- Lack of knowledge and access

Exemplars
FUNSAT™

15.2.4 Summary and Future Research Directions

While digital technologies hold the promise of improving the quality of life for caregivers and care recipients, there are a number of issues that must be addressed before the full benefits of these technologies can be realized for these populations. For example, there are a number of existing barriers to widespread adoption for current cohorts of caregivers and care recipients including: large and diverse user groups with varying needs and abilities, lack of knowledge about the potential benefits of technology; low technology self-efficacy and anxiety; cost and accessibility; training opportunities; and system design characteristics.

Much more research is needed regarding the relative advantages of more advanced technologies, such as multimedia and smart mobile devices, relative to simpler technologies needs to be understood. There is also a great deal that needs to be examined with monitoring devices related to preferred formats for monitoring, privacy issues, and data integration, management, and sharing issues. There exist numerous usability issues associated with interface design that are particularly important for caregivers as they are already faced with many demands and do not need to be burdened with complex or cumbersome technologies. Clearly, it is also essential to investigate sources of potential harm inherent in some technologies such as privacy intrusions, false perceptions about the capabilities and safety of technology systems, the proliferation of too much and inappropriate information and miscommunications between caregivers, patients, and healthcare providers. Strategies need to be developed for minimizing these types of consequences.

Much more work also needs to be done in user need analyses from the perspective of caregivers, patients, and other healthcare providers. System designers need to adopt a user-centered design approach where family caregivers, care recipients, and healthcare providers are actively involved in the design process. People who receive and those who provide care are very diverse and possess variable skills, resources, knowledge, and experiences. They also differ on a number of other characteristics such as age, cultural and ethnic backgrounds, education, health status, and living arrangements. Thus, when considering the design and implementation of digital technologies for these user groups it is important to remember that "one size does not necessarily fit all."

It is also important to note that caregiving is not static and that the demands of caregiving may change over the course of a caregiver's career. For example, in the early stage of a patient's illness, a caregiver may need information about the disease and available resources, whereas in the later stages, they may need assistance with the treatment of behavioral or emotional problems. Thus, designers of technologies need to be aware of the trajectories and changing needs of caregiving when designing caregiver support systems.

Optimal strategies for combining technology with other types of interventions and healthcare interactions need to be identified. There is also very limited work examining the impact of combining caregiver and care recipient technology-based interventions. Research is also needed to identify strategies for training caregivers to use information technologies and to help caregivers maintain technology systems. More rigorous studies are also needed to evaluate the effectiveness of technology-based interventions with large and diverse caregiver populations. Data are also needed on the cost effectiveness of technological interventions.

Finally, there is great potential for digital approaches to reach more caregivers and provide on demand support and mobile apps and use of other digital platforms is proliferation. Still, developing platforms do not always include the user perspective or engagement in the development process. Digital approaches may reach more caregivers than other, more clinically intensive face-to-face psychosocial and supportive interventions. Yet, there remain the issues of dissemination, implementation, scaling, and commercialization that need to be addressed. Unknown, are the best practices and proven strategies for implementation and dissemination of technology-oriented approaches (Gitlin & Czaja, in press). Furthermore, prior to commercialization, more rigorous testing using randomized trial methodologies is an imperative, along with examining a broad range of health and psychosocial outcomes of these approaches. Another important direction for these types of interventions is understanding the mechanisms of action or why caregivers engage and improve from utilization.

References

Alzheimer's disease facts and figures. (2024). *Alzheimer's & Dementia 20*(5), 3708–3821. https://www.alz.org/alzheimers-dementia/facts-figures

Atefi, G. L., Koh, W. Q., Kohl, G., Seydavi, M., Swift, J. K., Akbari, M., & de Vugt, M. E. (2024). Adherence to online interventions for family caregivers of people with dementia: a meta-analysis and systematic review. *The American Journal of Geriatric Psychiatry: Official Journal of the American Association for Geriatric Psychiatry, 32*(10), 1271–1291.

Beach, S., Schulz, R., Downs, J., et al. (2010). Monitoring and privacy issues in quality of life technology applications. *Gerontechnology, 9*, 78–79.

Beach, S. R., Schulz, R., Downs, J., Matthews, J., Barron, B., & Seelman, K. (2009). Disability, age, and informational privacy attitudes in quality of life technology applications: results from a national web survey. *Transactions on Accessible Computing (TACCESS), Special Issue on Aging and Information Technologies ACCESS), Special Issue on Aging and Information Technologies, 2*(1), Article 5.

Belle, S. H., Burgio, L., Burns, R., et al. (2006). Enhancing the quality of life of dementia caregivers from different ethnic or racial groups: a randomized, controlled trial. *Annals of Internal Medicine, 145*, 727–738.

Choi, E. Y., Kanthawala, S., Kim, Y. S., & Lee, H. Y. (2022). Urban/rural digital divide exists in older adults: does it vary by racial/ethnic groups? *Journal of Applied Gerontology, 41*(5), 1348–1356. https://doi.org/10.1177/07334648211073605

Czaja, S. J., Boot, W. R., Charness, N., & Rogers, W. A. (2019). *Designing for Older Adults: Principles and Creative Human Factors Approaches* (3rd ed.). Boca Raton, FL: CRC Press.

Czaja, S. J., Kallestrup, P., & Harvey, P. D. (2020). Evaluation of a novel technology-based program designed to assess and train everyday skills in older adults. *Innovation in Aging, 4*(6), igaa052. https://doi.org/10.1093/geroni/igaa052

Czaja, S. J., Kallestrup, P., & Harvey, P. D. (2024). The efficacy of a home-based functional skills training program for older adults with and without a cognitive impairment. *Innovation in Aging, 8*(7), igae065. https://doi.org/10.1093/geroni/igae065

de-Moraes-Ribeiro, F. E., Moreno-Cámara, S., da-Silva-Domingues, H., Palomino-Moral, P. Á., & Del-Pino-Casado, R. (2024). Effectiveness of internet-based or mobile app interventions for family caregivers of older adults with dementia: a systematic review. *Healthcare (Basel, Switzerland), 12*(15), 1494.

DiMaria-Ghalili, R., Foreshaw Rouse, A., Coates, M., Hathaway, Z., Hirsch, J., Wetzel, S., Park, Y., Johnston-Walsh, B., Clark, K., & Gitlin, L. N. (2021). Disrupting Disparities in Pennsylvania: Retooling for Geographic, Racial and Ethnic Growth [White paper]. AARP Pennsylvania. https://aldianews.com/en/leadership/advocacy/barriers-healthcare-pa

Fang, M., Hu, J., Weiss, J., et al. (2025). Lifetime risk and projected burden of dementia. *Nature Medicine*. https://doi.org/10.1038/s41591-024-03340-9

Faverio, M. (2022, January 13). *Share of those 65 and older who are tech users has grown in the past decade*. Pew Research Center. https://www.pewsr.ch/3HZd2ao

Cajavilca, M. F., Zheng, A., Bamidele-Sanni, K., & Sadarangani, T. (2024). Exploring family caregivers' likelihood of adopting a novel app that connects care teams of persons living with dementia: a mixed-methods study. *Gerontology and Geriatric Medicine*, 10. doi:10.1177/23337214241275638

Finkel, S. I., Czaja, S. J., Schulz, R., Martinovich, Z., Harris, C., & Pezzuto, D. (2007). E-care: a telecommunications technology intervention for family Caregivers of dementia patients. *Am J Geriatric Psychiatry*, 15, 443–448.

Fox, S., Duggan, M., & Purcell, K. (2013). Caregivers are wired for health. Pew Research Center. Available online https://www.pewresearch.org/internet/2013/06/20/family-caregivers-are-wired-for-health.

Gaugler, J. E., Rosebush, C. A., Zmora, R., & Albers, E. A. (2022). Outcomes of remote activity monitoring for persons living with dementia over an 18-month period. *Journal of the American Geriatrics Society*, 70(8), 2439–2442. https://doi.org/10.1111/jgs.17839

Gitlin, L. N., Baier, R. R., Jutkowitz, E., Baker, Z. G., Gustavson, A. M., Sefcik, J. S., Hodgson, N. A., Koeuth, S., & Gaugler, J. E. (2020). Dissemination and implementation of evidence-based dementia care using embedded pragmatic trials. *Journal of the American Geriatrics Society*, 68 Suppl 2(Suppl 2), S28–S36.

Gitlin, L. N., Bouranis, N., Kern, V., Koeuth, S., Marx, K. A., McClure, L. A., Lyketsos, C. G., & Kales, H. C. (2021). WeCareAdvisor, an online platform to help family caregivers manage dementia-related behavioral symptoms: an efficacy trial in the time of COVID-19. *Journal of Technology in Behavioral Science*. doi:10.1007/s41347-021-00204-8

Gitlin, L. N., & Czaja, S. J. (2025). *Handbook of Intervention Science: From Design to Implementation*. Academic Press.

Gitlin, L. N., Cigliana, J., Cigliana, K., & Pappa, K. (2017). Supporting family caregivers of persons with dementia in the community: Description of the 'Memory Care Home Solutions' Program and its impacts. *Innovations in Aging*, 1(1), igx013. doi:10.1093/geroni/igx013

Gitlin, L. N., Winter, L., & Stanley, I. H. (2015). Compensatory strategies: prevalence of use and relationship to physical function and well-being. *Journal of Applied Gerontology*. doi:0733464815581479

Irani, E., Niyomyart, A., & Hickman, R. L., Jr (2020). Systematic review of technology-based interventions targeting chronically ill adults and their caregivers. *Western Journal of Nursing Research*, 42(11), 974–992. https://doi.org/10. 1177/0193945919897011

Jain, F., Okereke, O. I., Gitlin, L. N., Pedrelli, P., Onnela, J. P., Nyer, M., Ramirez Gomez, L. A., Pittman, M., Sikder, A., Ursal, D., & Mischoulon, D. (2022). Mentalizing imagery therapy for family dementia caregivers: protocol for mobile application with digital phenotyping. *Contemporary Clinical Trials*, 116, 106737. doi:10.1016/j.cct.2022.106737

Jutkowitz, E., Piersol, C. V., Koeuth, S., & Gitlin, L. N. (2024, November 16). *Plans4Care: Translating evidence from in-person caregiver interventions to a digital platform* [Conference presentation]. Gerontological Society of America Annual Meeting, Seattle, WA.

Kales, H. K., Gitlin, L. N., & Lyketsos, C. G. (January 2019). *The DICE Approach: Guiding the Caregiver in Managing the Behavioral Symptoms of Dementia*. Michigan Publishing.

Kales, H. C., Gitlin, L. N., Stanislawski, B., Myra Kim, H., Marx, K., Turnwald, M., Chiang, C., & Lyketsos, C. G. (2018). Effect of the WeCareAdvisor™ on family caregiver outcomes in dementia: a pilot randomized controlled trial. *BMC Geriatrics, 18*(113). doi:10.1186/s12877-018-0801-8

Kiselica, A. M., Hermann, G. E., Scullin, M. K., & Benge, J. F. (2024). Technology that CARES: enhancing dementia care through everyday technologies. *Alzheimer's & Dementia: The Journal of the Alzheimer's Association, 20*(12), 8969–8978. https://doi.org/10.1002/alz.14192

Lee, S., Ory, M. G., Vollmer Dahlke, D., & Smith, M. L. (2024). Technology use among older adults and their caregivers: cross-sectional survey study. *JMIR Aging, 7*, e50759. https://doi.org/10.2196/50759

Lindeman, D. A., Kim, K. K., Gladstone, C., & Apesoa-Varano, E. C. (2020). Technology and caregiving: emerging interventions and directions for research. *The Gerontologist, 60*(Suppl 1), S41–S49. https://doi.org/10.1093/geront/gnz178

Madarasmi, S., Gutierrez-Ramirez, P., Barsoum, N., Banerjee, S., Ramirez Gomez, L., Melero-Dominguez, M., Gitlin, L. N., Pederson, A., Liu, R. T., & Jain, F. A. (2024). Family dementia caregivers with suicidal ideation improve with mentalizing imagery therapy: results from a pilot study. *Journal of Affective Disorders Reports, 16*(100721). doi:10.1016/j.jadr.2024.100721

Merriam-Webster. (2025). https://www.merriam-webster.com/dictionary/digitization.

National Academies of Sciences, Engineering, and Medicine. (2011). *Health Care Comes Home: The Human Factors*. The National Academies Press.

National Academies of Sciences, Engineering, and Medicine. (2016). *Families Caring for an Aging America*. Washington, DC: The National Academies Press. https://doi.org/10.17226/23606.

Noel, M. A., Lackey, E., Labi, V., & Bouldin, E. D. (2022). Efficacy of a virtual education program for family caregivers of persons living with dementia. *Journal of Alzheimer's Disease: JAD, 86*(4), 1667–1678. https://doi.org/10.3233/JAD-215359

Pleasant, M., Molinari, V., Dobbs, D., Meng, H., & Hyer, K. (2020). Effectiveness of online dementia caregivers training programs: a systematic review. *Geriatric Nursing (New York, N.Y.), 41*(6), 921–935. https://doi.org/10.1016/j.gerinurse.2020.07.004

Prince, M., Wimo, A., Guerchet, M., Ali, G.-C., Wu, Y.-T., & Prina, M. (2015). World Alzheimer Report 2015. The Global Impact of Dementia. An Analysis of Prevalence, Incidence, Cost and Trends. https://www.alzint.org/u/WorldAlzheimerReport2015.pdf

Salai, A. M., Kirton, A., Cook, G., & Holmquist, L. E. (2022). Views and experiences on the use of voice assistants by family and professionals supporting people with cognitive impairments. *Frontiers in Dementia, 1*, 1049464. https://doi.org/10.3389/frdem.2022.1049464

Schulz, R., Beach, S. R., Czaja, S. J., Martire, L. M., & Monin, J. K. (2020). Family caregiving for older adults. *Annual Review of Psychology, 71*, 635–659. https://doi.org/10.1146/annurev-psych-010419-050754

Schulz, R., & Martire, L. M. (2004). Family caregiving of persons with dementia: prevalence, health effects, and support strategies. *American Journal of Geriatric Psychiatry, 12*(3), 240–249.

The Britannica Dictionary. (2023). *Technology.* https://www.britannica.com/dictionary/technology#:~:text=Britannica%20Dictionary%20definition%20of%20TECHNOLOGY,things%20or%20to%20solve%20problems

Ülgüt, R., Stiel, S., & Herbst, F. A. (2023). Experiences and support needs of informal long-distance caregivers at the end of life: a scoping review. *BMJ Open, 13*, e068175. doi:10.1136/bmjopen-2022-068175

World Health Organization. (2024). Aging and Health, Available online at: https://www.who.int/news-room/fact-sheets/detail/ageing-and-health.

Xie, Y., Shen, S., Liu, C., Hong, H., Guan, H., Zhang, J., & Yu, W. (2024). Internet-based supportive interventions for family caregivers of people with dementia: randomized controlled trial. *JMIR Aging, 7,* e50847. doi:10.2196/50847

Zhai, S., Chu, F., Tan, M., Chi, N.-C., Ward, T., & Yuwen, W. (2023). Digital health interventions to support family caregivers: an updated systematic review. *Digital Health, 9.* doi:10.1177/20552076231171967

16

Dementia Empowerment with Heart Health Intervention and LLM-based Health AI Research Assistant

Luuk P.A. Simons, Pradeep K. Murukannaiah, and Mark A. Neerincx

This research was (partly) funded by the https://www.hybrid-intelligence-centre.nl/ a 10-year programme funded the Dutch Ministry of Education, Culture and Science through the Netherlands Organisation for Scientific Research, grant number 024.004.022 and by EU H2020 ICT48 project "Humane AI Net" under contract $\# $952026.

16.1 Introduction

Dementia is one of the largest health problems in the world. It is the most expensive disease in most of the industrialized world (Sherzai & Sherzai, 2019), and it places a very large emotional load on caregivers. It is estimated that 15 billion hours of unpaid care are provided yearly to Alzheimer's patients in the USA alone (Alzheimer's Association, 2022). Moreover, it is one of the fasted growing diseases in the world (Sherzai & Sherzai, 2019).

There is a common misconception that dementia cannot be avoided (Hudson, Pollux, Mistry & Hobson, 2012; Cahill, Pierce, Werner, Darley et al., 2015). However, it is largely preventable. For example, the risk scoring system of (Kivipelto, Ngandu, Laatikainen, Winblad et al., 2006) indicates that males of 50 years old can have a factor of 50 times (!!) increase in Alzheimer's risk, depending on lifestyle-related risk factors. In any case, dementia is much better avoidable than treatable (De la Torre, 2010). The summary of that literature is that promoting heart health also promotes brain health (Singh-Manoux, Kivimaki, Glymour, Elbaz et al., 2012). More details follow in Section 16.2, Theory.

Another misconception, or at least a dominant bias from Big Hospital and Big Pharma (Cummings, Lee, Nahed, Kambar, et al., 2022), appears to be the idea that the best one can hope for in dementia care is alleviation of some of its symptoms, using drugs (Ayton & Bush, 2021). However, biologically, we know that dementia is not a drug deficiency disease, but a cardiovascular-health-related condition (Barnes & Yaffe, 2011; Sabbagh, Perez, Holland, Boustani et al., 2022), building up in our bodies for many decades (Braak & Braak, 1997). There are more than 100,000 recent papers on Alzheimer's (Greger, 2023) and a huge number of them revolve around (pharmaceutical) interventions targeting amyloid plaques. This strategy has been strikingly unsuccessful, with an abysmal 99.6% drug failure rate, the worst of any therapeutic area (Torres-Acosta, O'Keefe, O'Keefe, Isaacson et al., 2020), and some authors labelled this approach as "a congregation of the church of the holy plaque" (Joseph, Shukitt-Hale, Denisova, Martin et al., 2001). This label follows from scientific discussions that it may well be that amyloid plaques and tau tangles are a byproduct of dementia and part of the brain's defence mechanisms, instead of a causal factor (Ayton & Bush, 2021). For a more extensive review, we refer the reader to Greger (2023), chapter "Preserving your mind."

At the same time, interventions that foster brain health, which can improve mental functioning (Barnard, Bush, Ceccarelli, Cooper et al., 2014), dementia biomarkers (Bredesen, 2017; Bredesen et al., 2018), and symptoms of cognitive decline (Williamson, 2019) remain largely unknown and under-utilized. See also our previous work on this underused potential (Simons, 2020, 2023). (There may be a third misconception at work here, namely the assumption that (senior) people will hardly improve their health behaviours (Verweij, Coffeng, van Mechelen & Proper, 2011). An assumption we will refute in Section 16.2, Theory, and Section 16.5, Discussion.)

Given the importance of healthy lifestyle and dementia prevention, an important question becomes *how to empower patients, caregivers, and their day-to-day health professionals* (physiotherapists, nurses, dieticians, physician assistants) *to effectively reduce dementia risk and progression.* As discussed elsewhere (Simons, 2023), the "pill-paradigm" tends to disempower patients, whereas a "self-healing paradigm" is more empowering and biologically better suited for lifestyle-related conditions like dementia. In this chapter, we combine an innovation or design perspective (in which we argue for using "heart health" intervention experiences and a Heart Health AI self-management support (SMS) tool for treating early-stage dementia and cognitive decline) with an empirical element: conducting a user evaluation of the added value of such a Health AI tool with participants who had recent experience with intensive self-management health improvements.

So as a first contribution of this chapter, from an *innovation and design perspective*, we propose *two empowerment opportunities*. To start with, based on literature, in Section 16.2, we will propose why and how a daily blood pressure intervention is a cheap, effective, and attractive SMS option for early-stage treatment of dementia and cognitive decline. Secondly, we argue (more details in Section 16.2) that it is becoming increasingly difficult to keep up with the scientific literature on effective health behaviours for dementia prevention (since there are simply too many new research papers published each year), and that a Health AI Research Assistant may be helpful for health SMS.

Within our design perspective, the empowerment mantra of "Heart health = Brain health" will lead the way, not only because it is biologically relevant and easy to measure daily blood pressure improvements as a proxy for effective dementia prevention, but also since there is so much more intervention experience in the heart health than in the dementia domain, on which we can build. Similarly,

As a second contribution of this chapter, the empirical element is a user evaluation of the added value of a Health AI Research Assistant concept (hereafter also called "Health AI") with n = 8 participants who had just completed a successful heart health intervention, using various information sources. Hence, the focus of the *user evaluation* in this chapter is: *For users with hypertension health self-management experience, what are perceived usefulness and intention to use for a Health AI, compared to their other health information sources?*

The Research Questions for the user evaluation are:

1. *In users' solution space, what are their information needs and priorities? What would they most want to ask the Health AI tool?*

2. *How do they use and value other information sources (besides the Health AI)?*

3. *What is their "Technology Acceptance" evaluation and intention to use the Health AI?*

16.2 Theory

In this section we address three topics. Firstly, how heart-healthy behaviours and hypertension management can reduce dementia and cognitive decline risks. Secondly, the power of health SMS and daily social microlearning to achieve large blood pressure improvements through healthier behaviours (thus also reducing dementia risk). Thirdly, we address the design of a Health AI to add value for patients, caregivers, and their health professionals. And we discuss related work on large language models (LLMs) and claims analysis approaches for developing a Health AI.

16.2.1 Improving Blood Pressure and Cardiovascular Health for Dementia

The most common forms of dementia are Alzheimer's disease and cardiovascular dementia. Dementia incidence varies widely worldwide, with patterns very similar to those of heart disease, and with risk levels depending largely on the same health behaviours (Barnes & Yaffe, 2011).

Like in heart disease, consumption of saturated fats (Okereke, Rosner, Kim, Kang et al., 2012; Cao, Li, Han, Tayie et al., 2019), cholesterol (Barnard, 2018), and other foods that worsen atherosclerosis (Roher, Tyas, Maarouf, Daugs et al., 2011) are known risk factors for dementia and cognitive decline, just like blood cholesterol levels are a dementia risk factor (Corsinovi, Biasi, Poli, Leonarduzzi et al., 2011). There is extensive research explaining how pro-atherosclerotic behaviours and pathogenesis promote dementia, which is out of scope of this chapter (Roher, Tyas, Maarouf, Daugs et al., 2011). As is a broader review of the dementia preventive effects of anti-inflammatory, anti-oxidant, and anti-aging foods and lifestyle. Extensive reviews can be found in (Greger & Stone, 2016) and (Greger, 2023).

In this section we focus on the biological benefits of blood pressure reduction for dementia treatment, while at the same time acknowledging that most food and lifestyle choices that lower blood pressure will also lower serum cholesterol levels, systemic inflammation, oxidative stress and other know cardiac- and brain aging risk factors (Bredesen, 2017, Bredesen et al., 2018, Li, 2019, Greger, 2023).

Illustrating heart health relevance for early-stage dementia treatment, Professor Dean Ornish and coworkers have recently shown that their heart health intervention (Ornish, Scherwitz, Billings, Gould, et al., 1998, Ornish, Magbanua, Weidner, Weinberg et al., 2008, Lippman, Stump, Veazey, Guimarães et al., 2024) is surprisingly effective for improving cognitive function in those early-stage Alzheimer's participants that implemented the largest health behaviour improvements (Ornish, Madison, Kivipelto, Kemp et al., 2024).

Blood pressure and vascular function (= elasticity as well as protective and regulative properties of our arteries) are important for brain health, since elastic artery walls function as shock absorbers. As our arteries stiffen, the pressure pulses caused by the pumping of our heart can damage the small vessels in our brain (Pase, Herbert, Grima, Pipingas et al., 2012). This causes three times as many "brain microbleeds" in people with high blood pressure (Henskens, Van Oostenbrugge, Kroon, De Leeuw et al., 2008) and more lacunar infarcts (Kovacic & Fuster, 2012). These lacunar infarcts are small, silent brain infarcts associated with cognitive decline and a double dementia risk (Vermeer, Longstreth & Koudstaal, 2007).

Besides, high blood pressure is linked to brain shrinking, specifically in the memory centre (Beauchet, Celle, Roche, Bartha, et al., 2013). In general, hypertension in midlife is more strongly associated with risks of cognitive decline and dementia at later age than having the APOE Alzheimer's gene (Peila, White, Petrovich, Masaki et al., 2001). In summary of research reviews on the topic: "Fourteen of fifteen cross-sectional studies correlated increased arterial stiffness with impaired cognitive performance, and six of the seven longitudinal studies found that arterial stiffness appeared predictive of cognitive decline" (Singer, Trollor, Baune, Sachdev et al., 2014). Eleven randomized controlled trials (RCTs) show that reducing sodium intake is one effective way to reduce blood pressure (Filippini, Malavolti, Whelton, Naska et al., 2021), as well as artery stiffness (D'Elia, Galletti, La Fata, Sabino, et al., 2018). And salt is now recognized as a dementia risk factor, independent of its blood pressure effects, caused by the fact that salt impairs artery function (Santisteban & Iadecola, 2018).

One of the largest interventions to show cognitive improvement with blood pressure treatment was published in 2019 (Williamson, Pajewski, Auchus, Bryan et al., 2019). More than 9,000 participants (avg. 68 years old) were randomized to lower their systolic blood pressure to either under 140 or under 120 in the SPRINT trial (Cushman, Ringer, Rodriguez, Evans, et al., 2022). The trial was meant to last six years, but was stopped halfway, since the more intensive drug regimen saved so many more lives, lowering mortality by 27% (unfortunately at the cost of negative side effects like kidney failure etc (Wright, 2015); achieving these results with healthy lifestyle would have been better and would have created positive side effects, instead of negative ones). In terms of neurological outcomes, the 17% reduction in dementia was not statistically significant, but the 19% lower risk of developing mild cognitive impairment was (Williamson, Pajewski, Auchus, Bryan et al., 2019).

16.2.2 Empowerment through Intensive Health Self-Management Support with Daily Blood Pressure Measurements and Social Microlearning

There are many challenges in creating successful health interventions (Simons & Hampe, 2010, Simons, Hampe & Guldemond, 2013, 2014, Simons, Heuvel & Jonker, 2019), and some of the key lessons are (besides the fact that it is indeed not sufficient to just tell people to "eat healthier" Simons, Gerritsen, Wielaard & Neerincx, 2023), also confirmed in the field of health SMS (Jonkman, Schuurmans, Jaarsma, Shortridge-Baggett et al., 2016, Dineen-Griffin, Garcia-Cardenas, Williams, & Benrimoj, 2019). This is because participants have diverse questions and individual support needs. For example, questions about health beliefs and what is healthy, about goal setting and -achievement, about all the automatic daily health choices (what to do for eating/drinking/being physically active, or what not to do, with over 200 "mindless" decision moments per day (Wansink, 2011)); about dealing with potentially unhealthy situations such as social events, including mental preparation- and coping strategies (Simons, Heuvel & Jonker, 2018, 2019, 2020)

Because of these health intervention challenges (see details in Jonkman, Schuurmans, Jaarsma, Shortridge-Baggett et al., 2016, Dineen-Griffin, Garcia-Cardenas, Williams, & Benrimoj, 2019, Simons, Gerritsen, Wielaard & Neerincx, 2024):

a. SMS must be customized, very regular, and very specific.

b. Success experiences and progress confirmation must occur as soon as possible, preferably multiple times per day.

c. It is crucial to coach participants for ownership and experimentation.

d. Patients and caregivers must be guided from "short-term abstinence or willpower strategies" (which are a true pitfall for long-term success (ref Baumeister) to behaviour that fits their (long term) preferences and fosters intrinsic motivations.

In other words: SMS interventions must be attractive for the individual, but also showing biological effectiveness on a relatively short notice. Thus paradoxically, ambitious and high-intensity interventions which use daily experiment-and-measurement feedback cycles to create both biological and psychological successes can be relatively effective and attractive, due to the large benefits that participants experience in a matter of days or weeks (Simons, Pijl, Verhoef, Lamb et al., 2016, 2017, 2022, Simons, Gerritsen, Wielaard & Neerincx, 2024). Blood pressure challenges, with daily self-measurement and achieving −20 to −30 points lower systolic pressure in two weeks on average, are examples of such an approach (Simons, Gerritsen, Wielaard & Neerincx, 2023, 2024).

Given our interventional desire for rapid progress feedback, for dementia and its biologically slow processes, a quicker proxy measurement is needed. Thus, we propose blood pressure challenges as a potentially suitable approach for preventing dementia or treating early-stage cognitive decline.[1] This would have the following benefits for participants: (a) getting a daily biological proxy for biological progress, (b) supporting their ownership and engagement via experiment-and-feedback cycles: which new health behaviours are sufficiently attractive additions to my life as well as biologically effective?

More details on blood pressure challenges are given elsewhere (Simons, Gerritsen, Wielaard & Neerincx, 2023, 2024), but in summary, it is a hybrid eHealth intervention with ***twice-daily blood pressure biofeedback*** consisting of:

- Telephone intake and instructions for BP home measurements
- Start—and final group sessions (two weeks apart, face-to-face)
- Daily MS Teams eCoaching in week 1
- Twice-daily BP measurements and logging email
- Feedback on group progress after first week
- Healthy recipe suggestions
- Content (portal and/or email) on health, BP, and behaviour strategies
- Light weight follow-up support, group sessions in week 5 or 6 and 9 or 10

16.2.3 Health AI Research Assistant for Personalized "Health Hacks" Mining

As stated in our introduction, there are simply too many new health research papers published every year for a human brain to digest. Even if we limit ourselves to "cardiovascular health," more than 6,000,000 studies can be found in Google Scholar. In the years 2023 and 2022, the number of scientific publications on this topic referenced by Google Scholar is 249,000 and 307,000, respectively, per year. Hence, we are looking at artificial intelligence (AI) tools for assistance.

In line with the biology of Sections 16.2.1 and 16.2.2, and to limit our scope in the first phase of our health AI design, we initially focus the AI on cardiovascular health. The AI Research Assistant tool is meant to add value by enabling patients, caregivers, and their everyday healthcare professionals (like physiotherapists, dieticians, nurse practitioners, family doctors, or physician assistants) to self-source the most effective lifestyle choices and the best available medical evidence. For most of these individual optimization questions, the generic and "watered down" suggestions of our main health institutions are not specific enough (Simons, Neerincx & Jonker, 2021, 2022, Simons, Gerritsen, Wielaard & Neerincx, 2023, 2024). As described elsewhere (Simons, Bodegom, Dumaij & Jonker, 2015, Simons, Foerster, Bruck, Motiwalla et al., 2015, Simons, Heuvel & Jonker, 2018, 2019) people face a wide variety of health choices and gain most health benefits and competences when it is not a coach telling them what to do (Simons, 2020), but when they develop their own health patterns which best suite their personal preferences, home situation, social context, etc.

The recent advances in generative AI, LLMs conversing in natural language, and automation in analyzing health claims, open interesting new opportunities for health AI Research Assistant tools. So, as a final step in this section, we summarize related work on (1) LLMs for health, (2) claims analysis in AI (Guo, Schlichtkrull & Vlachos, 2022), and (3) the role of competing tools or information sources when designing and evaluating the added value of new information tools.

In recent years, multiple papers have been published on using *LLMs for healthcare*. Some using a review on opportunities and risks from mostly editorials (Sallam, 2023) or testing several use cases with health professionals (Cascella, Montomoli, Bellini & Bignami, 2023) or interviewing health professionals versus surveying the general public on their ChatGPT use in health (Raina, Mishra & Kumar, 2024). Some of the benefits that are relevant to our research question and generally mentioned in these papers are: utility in health research and benefits for healthcare practice (improving health literacy and efficiency in reviewing the literature). Risks that are often mentioned are: lack of transparency, risk of bias, incorrect citations, and risk of hallucinations. Other papers focusing more on the technology address privacy, security, and data architecture issues (Montagna, Ferretti, Klopfenstein,

Florio et al., 2023) or training and evaluating specialized LLMs to increase natural language qualities like perceived helpfulness, logic, and empathic phrasing (Lai, Shi, Du, Wu et al., 2023). Overall, given that LLMs can be described as "probable-word generators" (Shah, 2023), it is not so surprising that healthcare professionals describe their capabilities as lacking depth and argumentation in health expertise and lacking understanding of complex relationships between personal-, health- and behaviour-aspects (Raina, Mishra & Kumar, 2024).

However, we hold the view that from a design perspective it is not enough to explicate risks of misinformation or lack of transparency of health claims. We must also think about the next steps forward: How to design and enhance generative AI tools such that these risks can be better managed? For instance, when dealing with conflicting claims, mere transparency is insufficient. Metadata and additional tools are necessary to help users weigh different sources and claims. Human domain experts can provide valuable interpretations, creating a "hybrid intelligence" that combines the strengths of artificial and human intelligence (Simons, Neerincx & Jonker, 2021, 2022, Simons, Murukannaiah & Neerincx, 2024). The field of food and health is particularly challenging due to conflicting claims and interests. So, an important question is how to use metadata, information characteristics, and assessment criteria to help evaluate claims.

The task of analyzing claims is studied under the umbrella of *automated fact checking* (Guo, Schlichtkrull & Vlachos, 2022) in the AI (specifically, Natural Language Processing) literature. Automated fact checking typically involves four subtasks: (1) Claim detection involves identifying claims for verification. An important aspect here is identifying claims that are check-worthy (i.e., claims whose truthfulness the public is interested in); (2) Evidence retrieval involves retrieving information which can be used to evaluate the veracity of the claim; (3) Verdict prediction involves determining the veracity of the claim by synthesizing the pieces of evidence retrieved; and (4) Justification production involves generating a justification for why a certain claim was ruled true or not true (or somewhere in between). This is an important and challenging task, considering the black-box nature of the AI tools. The main challenge for us is to formulate these tasks for the domain of our interest in a systematic manner.

Finally, we must borrow some *value evaluation* principles from the field of new product design. This chapter reports on a user evaluation of a Health AI concept (see its description in Section 16.3, Methods and Materials). Besides the general frameworks of Technology Acceptance Model (TAM, Venkatesh & Davis, 2000) and Unified Theory of Acceptance and Use of Technology (UTAUT, Venkatesh, Morris, Davis & Davis, 2003), looking at concepts like perceived usefulness and ease of use, product design aims to specify and design these qualities in detail (Rondini, Pezzotta, Pirola, Rossi et al., 2016). Moreover, the added value of those new qualities should also be considered in comparison to competing alternatives (Herzwurm & Schockert, 2003, Rondini, Pezzotta, Pirola, Rossi et al., 2016). Hence, in our user evaluation, besides asking feedback on perceived usefulness of various Health AI functions, we will also ask which other information sources are used and/or preferred.

16.3 Methods and Materials

16.3.1 Research Design

Employing a design research approach (Vaishnavi & Kuechler, 2004, Verschuren & Hartog, 2005), we developed a high-level Health AI concept (described below) and gathered feedback from n = 8 participants with recent experience in a hypertension-reduction intervention (see Section 16.4, Results). We utilized a mixed-methods approach, combining quantified surveys, open-ended questions, and action research (during the intervention and user evaluation) to gain in-depth user insights and design suggestions while actively assisting participants[2] in navigating the complexities of health information. The user evaluations revealed a strong need for support in interpreting often ambiguous claims. In Section 16.5, Discussion, we propose several AI tool options to address these user requirements.

16.3.2 Participants

In early February 2024, we collected feedback from n = 8 Dutch participants who had begun an intensive hypertension-reduction intervention on January 15. All participants provided informed consent, and details of the intervention are available elsewhere (Simons, Gerritsen, Wielaard & Neerincx, 2022, 2023, 2024). Consistent with previous findings, average blood pressures were successfully reduced from 140/87 to 122/77 within 12 days through dietary and lifestyle modifications. The participants, all university employees, included two scientists and six support staff. Half were male, half female, with an average age of 45 (ranging from 29 to 58). All participants had experience with LLMs, with two having limited experience, three having average, and three having extensive experience. During the hypertension challenge, they utilized multiple information sources.

16.3.3 The Health AI Concept

- **Initial Scope:** Focussed on food and blood pressure.
- **Training Data:** Includes over 100,000 recent scientific publications in the domain.
- Specific Details are yet to be determined, but the foundation is:
- **User Interface:** Like ChatGPT, Copilot, and Gemini, with added capabilities for interpreting recent health studies.

TABLE 16.1

User Evaluation Topics

Topics Information Use and Health AI Added Value
1. Information usefulness, in general
2. "Voice of the user" Health AI preferences
3. Use of other information sources (during self-management)
4. "Technology acceptance" aspects for the Health AI

- **Language:** Operates in Dutch, allowing users to ask questions and receive answers in plain language.
- **Interactivity:** Supports follow-up questions and provides references to source publications used for answers.

16.3.4 User Evaluation & Data Analysis

When navigating health improvement iterations, participants often cycle through three design spaces: "problem," "solution," and "evaluation" (Simons, 2023). This chapter's user evaluation focuses on information usage within the "solution space" (identifying the most effective and appealing health behaviour options) and the potential benefits of the Health AI. Table 16.1 outlines the evaluation topics.

As discussed in Section 16.2, Theory, we sought insights into participants' general information preferences (topic 1), their desired functionalities and support from the Health AI (topic 2), their use of information sources during lifestyle changes (topic 3), and their technology acceptance feedback (topic 4). For the latter, we employed TAM (Venkatesh & Davis, 2000) and UTAUT (Venkatesh, Morris, Davis & Davis, 2003) to assess user evaluation concepts (perceived usefulness, ease-of-use, ability, trust, feeling, support, intention to use), focusing on individual usage preferences rather than UTAUT's organizational technology adoption processes (Carlsson, Carlsson, Hyvonen, Puhakainen et al., 2006).

Regarding data collection and analysis, we used questionnaire items for quantified evaluation of each topic. Additionally, we encouraged users to provide further input on their values and preferences, aligning with our design evaluation focus.

16.4 Results from the User Evaluation on the Health AI Tool Concept

We begin our results section by presenting the Research Questions (RQs) along with the Tables that summarize the user evaluations:

1. *In users' solution space, what are their information needs and priorities? What would they most want to ask the Health AI tool?* (Table 16.2, *scores* and Table 16.3, *open answers*)

2. *How do they use and value other information sources (besides the Health AI)?* (Table 16.4)

3. *What is their "Technology Acceptance" evaluation and intention to use the Health AI?* (Table 16.5)

In Table 16.2, we address the first Research Question by listing user responses on the usefulness of information, rated on a 7-point Likert scale. The table is divided into two parts: the first part covers general information and opinions, while the second part focuses on the usefulness of the Health AI tool. To highlight user preferences, we marked the top three highest scores in green for each question set.

For general information usefulness, the top three responses indicate that participants prioritize learning which health behaviours are most beneficial for health and hypertension, and how to make those changes easily. Notably, Question 1 received the maximum scores from all participants.

The second part of Table 16.2 reveals the most useful applications of the Health AI tool, according to participants. The top three scores are for understanding the effects of blood pressure and broader health impacts of food, along with practical tips on avoiding unhealthy foods. Just below the top

TABLE 16.2

Information Use and Health AI Preferences (7-Point (Dis)agree, n = 8, Avg = Average)

I Find the Following (General) Information Useful:	Avg Score
1. Connections between blood pressure, health, and behaviour	7.0
2. Most effective behaviour changes for hypertension	6.4
3. Knowing blood pressure effect sizes of behaviour changes	6.0
4. Tips for making behaviour changes *easy*	6.6
5. Tips for making behaviour changes *successful*	6.1
The Health AI Tool Would Be Useful for:	
1. Comparing blood pressure effects of foods	5.9
2. Getting health feedback on a specific (supermarket) product	5.8
3. Learning the optimum dosage of a food product	5.0
4. Learning the broader health effects of a food	6.0
5. Comparing effect sizes of foods with other health behaviours	4.9
6. Practical tips on how to increase daily intake of health foods	5.8
7. Tips on how to replace or avoid unhealthy foods	6.1
8. Tips on how to deal with pitfalls/difficult moments	5.8

TABLE 16.3

Information Use and Health AI Preferences (Open Answers)

Other Useful Information Sources Mentioned:

The conversations with the coach were most useful. I would hope the AI could have a similar conversation with us.

The context given during the Challenge in relation to healthy choices was very useful, like for example, "how sugar- and saturated-fat-spikes heighten artery systemic inflammation."

During the Challenge workshops, we heard many things that you would never think of yourself, like, for example, the blood pressure lowering effect of seeds like flaxseeds.

I was happy to hear about the updated hypertension guidelines from the AHA (American Heart Association), this is new for the Dutch context, and I will include this in my conversations with my family physician.

It's nice to see food intervention studies and effect sizes on hypertension.

Other Health AI Usefulness Mentioned:

It would be nice if the Health AI could filter information based on aspects like gender, age, weight, sports background, vegetarianism, etc., to increase relevance for my own situation.

I would like to input my existing breakfast, etc. (which I like) and ask for health improvement suggestions.

If certain foods are useful for my blood pressure, please show me the links to the original studies, so I can read them for myself (See also Table 16.5).

If the blood pressure food advice is distinct from the advice from my dietitian or weight watchers, can the Health AI explain why this may be so?

I want to ask questions on other topics like aspirin or sauna: do they also influence my blood pressure?

three, three items scored 5.8, all with a practical focus: daily eating patterns to increase healthy foods, strategies for dealing with pitfalls and difficult moments, and tips for making healthy choices when shopping.

Interestingly, opinions varied on practical advice items. Some participants preferred receiving practical tips from other participants, including context on usage and adoption. As one participant noted: *"By interacting with others about what works and why, our conversations become part of our usage intention. The goal is to apply these insights ourselves, making the* **conversation a part of our behaviour change** *rather than just information gathering."*

However, others preferred the AI tool for practical advice, while favouring the coach for understanding the broader health picture and its relevant connections. In Table 16.3, we list the main open answer inputs given in the user evaluation, regarding (1) the information sources that were found useful, and (2) other Health AI usefulness ideas and preferences.

In response to Research Question 2, Table 16.4 details the extent to which participants used various information sources during the two-week Challenge period. These sources can be seen as alternatives potentially competing with the Health AI we plan to introduce. All participants reported regular use of coach inputs, and all but one found inputs from other participants useful. The third most utilized source was official health institutes. Regarding the fourth source, personal networks, most participants indicated

TABLE 16.4

Use of Other Information Sources (Number of Times, n = 8, Avg Nr = Average Number of Times)

Number of Times during Challenge (of 2 Weeks)	Avg Nr
1. My personal network (family, friends, etc.)[3]	1.7
2. My physician or other health professionals	0.4
3. Sites/info from official health institutes	2.3
4. Other Internet sources	0.5
5. Google Scholar, PubMed, or similar	0.3
6. Individual scientific papers	0.9
7. Inputs/remarks from other Challenge participants	5.8
8. Inputs from Challenge coach	7.6

that these were more about sharing information rather than receiving it, although they did receive practical advice on implementing healthy lifestyle behaviours. Other Internet sources were often described as containing too much confusing or low-quality information.

When asked which information was most useful (open question), all participants cited the **Challenge workshops as the most beneficial.** This included materials, PowerPoints, references, an online portal with health information, and the explanations provided. *Reasons given included: providing a good summary, the value of practical tips, reflecting on their own behaviours, specific links and literature for focused follow-up, saving time, and not feeling the need to conduct their own research because the provided information was sufficient.*

Regarding Research Question 3, Table 16.5 presents responses to various aspects of Technology Acceptance. Since three of the highest-scoring items

TABLE 16.5

Technology Acceptance Factors (7-Point (Dis)Agree, n = 8, Avg = Average)

The Health AI Tool..:	Avg Score
1. is interesting	6.1
2. is useful for insights on improving my health	5.5
3. is easy to use for asking questions	6.0
4. is easy to interpret when presenting conflicting articles	4.9
5. will gain my trust, following the degree of clarity of its sources	6.1
6. I find it useful to discuss its outputs with other Challenge participants	5.5
7. I find it useful to discuss its outputs with the Challenge coach	6.5
8. I find it useful to practice its use in Challenge workshops	5.8
9. I would certainly use the Health AI	6.1

received the same score (6.1), we highlighted the top four in green. These responses indicate that participants find the Health AI interesting and intend to use it. However, it was also clear (from items 2, 4, and 6, as well as from open responses) that all participants were cautious about the risk of receiving unreliable answers from LLM tools like the Health AI. This concern is reflected in two of the top four items in Table 16.5: 5. ("it will gain my trust, following the degree of clarity of its sources") and 7. ("I find it useful to discuss the Health AI outputs with the coach").

Participants valued the ability to critically assess and interpret Health AI responses, especially when guided by human experts. They viewed this "hybrid intelligence" approach as a beneficial way to utilize the technology. However, they found interpretations from less knowledgeable participants to be less helpful.

Regarding *future Health AI use*, preferences varied ((in line with the variation in Table 16.2 answers). Some desired introductory training on how to use (or not use) the technology effectively, while others preferred a more hands-on approach. Similarly, some wanted to ask a wide range of health, food, and blood pressure questions, while others focused on scientific research or practical daily health tips. Additionally, some expressed interest in discussing potential Health AI suggestions with other participants during workshop sessions.

16.5 Discussion

16.5.1 Empowerment of Patients, Caregivers, and Health Professionals

In this chapter, we proposed two empowerment strategies for patients, caregivers, and healthcare professionals. Firstly, we showed how the successes in cardiac health, which have motivated senior citizens to make significant lifestyle changes, can be applied to the treatment of early-stage dementia and cognitive decline. This approach leverages the biological link between blood pressure, cardiovascular health, and dementia outcomes. Practically, it provides daily feedback on progress, empowering patients in their health improvement efforts. Secondly, we introduced and tested an AI Health Research Assistant designed to extract the most relevant lifestyle findings from the vast amount of new health literature published each year, ensuring that patients and professionals stay informed with the latest research.

Regarding the first point of lifestyle changes and despite the behaviour change challenges we discussed in Section 16.2, over the years we have seen many examples of large enthusiasm and satisfaction (even one or more years later, Simons, Bodegom, Dumaij & Jonker, 2015, Simons, Foerster, Bruck, Motiwalla et al., 2015, Simons, Pijl, Verhoef, Lamb et al., 2017, Simons, Pijl,

Verhoef, Lamb et al., 2022), based on the fact that participants were challenged to make large health behaviour improvements. This fostered empowerment, engagement, and satisfaction because of the short- and long-term health benefits that participants achieved. Results are very motivating. Especially when the health behaviours that one chooses fit well with one's preferences, personal life, and health ambitions (Simons, Hampe & Guldemond, 2014, Simons, Heuvel & Jonker 2019, Simons, 2023).

Whereas the large results in the blood pressure challenge we previously published were mostly realized in (busy) working populations (Simons, Gerritsen, Wielaard & Neerincx, 2023, 2024), these results were recently replicated in older, community-participant groups, see Figure 16.1. These results have yet to be more extensively analyzed and published, but this gives a preliminary idea of the large average systolic pressure drop in the most recent elderly community group (n = 7, avg age of 75 years old) over the course of 9 weeks (2 weeks intensive + 7 weeks light weight follow up), with average recommendation and satisfaction scores of 8.6 and 8.8 (out of 10).

In relation to the Health AI, participant evaluations were surprisingly positive, but also nuanced. This response fits well with previous other health content and tool evaluations in the context of intensive lifestyle interventions. Even though not every tool is equally valued by each participant, most participants appreciate and use at least several of the tools and content sources, since they feel that it helps them forward (Simons, Pijl, Verhoef, Lamb et al., 2016, 2017, Simons, Heuvel & Jonker, 2019, 2020, Simons, Pijl, Verhoef, Lamb et al., 2022).

When discussing the limitations of the empirical user evaluation of this chapter, a first limitation is its explorative nature, with only n = 8 participants. Still, for reaching input saturation at this design stage this appears sufficient; sometimes even five, six, or seven users are enough (Faulkner, 2003). Second,

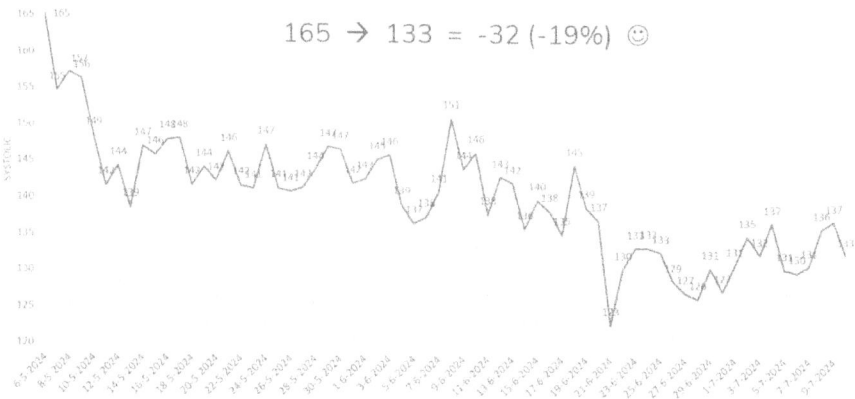

FIGURE 16.1
Average systolic pressure improvements (n = 7, avg. 75 yrs).

TABLE 16.6

Claims Evaluation Criteria

Evaluation Criteria and Interpretation Examples from Literature:

1. *Time Evolution of Claims:* Tools that track changes in health claims over time can be valuable. Dr. Neal Barnard (2018) highlights how claims about the cardiac health of eggs have evolved, often inaccurately becoming more positive in recent decades. This shift is attributed to the overwhelming negative evidence from earlier research, which led to a decline in serious investigation into the topic. This void was subsequently exploited by the egg industry to promote studies with questionable claims.

2. *Consistency of Claims:* A prime example of consistent scientific evidence is the established health benefits of fruits and vegetables. Despite this overwhelming consensus, some individuals, including intervention participants, online sources, and occasionally even dietitians, advise against consuming more than two servings of fruit per day due to concerns about their sugar content. While refined sugars may pose health risks, the consistent positive findings from numerous studies regarding the overall health benefits of fruits are clear and should prevail.

3. *Body of Evidence:* As a leading expert in health behaviours and risks highlights (Willett, 2012), it's crucial to evaluate the strength of scientific evidence. For over a century, a vast body of research, including animal studies, large-scale human migration studies, and randomized controlled trials, has consistently demonstrated a causal link between saturated fats, blood cholesterol, and cardiovascular disease.

4. *Burden of Proof:* Occasionally, new claims challenge prevailing scientific consensus. This can either represent a groundbreaking discovery or an error. A notorious example of the latter is the tobacco industry's claim that smoking is beneficial because it reduces the risk of Parkinson's disease (Greger & Stone, 2016, p.265). While it's true that tobacco and tomato plants contain substances with potential neuroprotective properties, this alone is insufficient. The burden of proof dictates that when overwhelming evidence points in one direction (smoking is harmful), extraordinary evidence is required to support the opposite claim (smoking is beneficial).

5. *Explicit Arguments and Proof for Conflicting Claims:* When introducing a claim that contradicts existing *body of evidence*, the *burden of proof* lies with the proponent to provide compelling arguments and/or evidence supporting the new claim, despite conflicting data. The health effects of soy consumption in humans are a case in point. While early animal studies suggested a potential link between high soy intake and cancer risk, this conflicted with the observed health of Asian populations with a high soy diet. Subsequent research revealed that rodents metabolize soy differently than humans, resolving this apparent contradiction (Setchell, Brown, Zhao, Lindley et al., 2011).

6. *Weighing Claims for Type of Study:* The soy example highlights a crucial principle in health research: large-scale, double-blind randomized controlled trials in humans provide significantly stronger evidence than animal studies or observational studies. While this may be evident to some, a Health AI can clarify and effectively utilize this distinction.

7. *Claimer and Industry Affiliation Analysis:* The prevalence of industry affiliations and conflicts of interest among scientists in the food sciences is alarming. Even the US Dietary Guidelines Advisory Committee, where objectivity should be paramount, has been found to have 19 out of 20 members with industry ties (Mialon, Serodio, Crosbie, Teicholz et al., 2022). To assess claim validity, a metadata analysis examining the identity of claimers and their industry affiliations can provide valuable insights.

the Health AI is only evaluated in concept. The next step in our research is to test a real prototype. Still, also on a concept level, their user inputs are useful, especially given their recent experience in dealing with ambiguous or conflicting claims from food and hypertension literature.

16.5.2 Health AI: Evaluation and Metadata Criteria for Ambiguous Claims

For a Health AI, besides analyzing and summarizing claims in scientific literature, there are other metadata that can be used to help evaluate the reliability of claims. In our health AI user evaluation, we heard several concerns regarding reliability and transparency of the answers. As a possible interpretation aid for users, Table 16.6 lists several criteria against which (possibly contradicting) claims can be evaluated. This is still early-stage design thinking, but we think these types of criteria are important for future AI transparency and usefulness.

16.5.3 Hybrid Intelligence for Ambiguity "Rationale capturing"

To summarize and conclude the user evaluation, it confirmed the importance of information quality and of scientific evidence for healthy lifestyle choices. Participants expressed particular concern regarding ambiguous or conflicting claims and emphasized the value of human expert support for interpreting such information. Based on their feedback, we believe this finding likely extends to other health domains, including cognition and dementia research.

Regarding the "hybrid intelligence" approach, providing expert explanations for confusing claims was deemed valuable. This addresses users' key questions of "How to interpret claims?" and "Is there an underlying reason for the ambiguity?" A hybrid solution, combining AI tools with expert human guidance, appears to be effective. In this model, the AI assists experts, while the final advice is grounded in human expertise, addressing users' primary concerns about claim confusion in the food and health domain.

16.6 Conclusion

Dementia is one of the most feared diagnoses in medicine (Greger, 2023). The aim of this chapter was to help empower patients, caregivers, and health professionals in becoming proactive in reducing future burdens of dementia and cognitive decline. For this purpose, we use biological causality: significantly reducing hypertension and improving cardiovascular health offers important potential to improve future dementia outcomes. We have attempted to illustrate how a specific form of intensive hypertension SMS, with daily blood pressure measurements, social learning, large health behaviour changes, and multiple microlearning moments per day, helps motivate people and can lead to large improvements in cardiovascular health, even within several weeks. Moreover, it is a type of intervention which has been shown to raise health self-management competencies and which leads to high satisfaction and recommendation scores, even in the long run.

In an empowerment approach like this, participants regularly take on a lot of ownership and they want to self-source information about their options regarding health choices. For this purpose, a Health AI Research Assistant can be valuable to help mine the vast amount of new health findings published every year. User evaluations have shown that experienced lifestyle participants have positive but nuanced expectations of such a Health AI, including risks of AI hallucinations, information in-transparency, or conflicting messages. To help with transparency and information evaluation, we have proposed several metadata criteria to be used by future versions of Health AI Research Assistant tools.

Notes

1 Moreover, since there are about 30% of misdiagnoses of Alzheimer's (Viña & Sanz-Ros, 2018), caused by other underlying issues like sleep problems, depression, or side effects of (ironically) cardiovascular or sleep medications causing cognitive impairment. In our experience, blood pressure challenges also help people tackle issues like sleep problems, depressive symptoms, or overmedication. Thus we can help solve cognitive impairment via the "positive side effects" of healthy lifestyle.
2 By supporting individuals during hypertension lifestyle interventions, as well as providing six months of healthy lifestyle coaching (Simons & Hampe, 2010, 2017) for literally thousands of participants and caregivers in these domains, over the course of the past ten years.
3 One of the participants was an outlier with score 15, hence excluded from this item average. Moreover, all participants said it was more about sharing information than receiving information, except for practical tips/discussions on how to implement health behaviours.

References

Alzheimer's Association. (2022). Alzheimer's disease facts and figures. Special Report More than normal aging. https://www.alz.org/media/Documents/alzheimers-facts-and-figures.pdf. Alzheimer's Association. Accessed January 8, 2003.

Ayton, S., & Bush, A. I. (2021). β-amyloid: the known unknowns. *Ageing Research Reviews, 65*, 101212.

Barnard, R. J. (2018). How the Egg Industry Skews Science. YouTube, accessed 26-2-2024: https://www.youtube.com/watch?v=FyG8wr0gWIA.

Barnard, N. D., Bush, A. I., Ceccarelli, A., Cooper, J., de Jager, C. A., Erickson, K. I., ... & Squitti, R. (2014). Dietary and lifestyle guidelines for the prevention of Alzheimer's disease. *Neurobiology of Aging, 35*, S74–S78.

Barnes, D. E., & Yaffe, K. (2011). The projected effect of risk factor reduction on Alzheimer's disease prevalence. *The Lancet Neurology, 10*(9), 819–828.

Beauchet, O., Celle, S., Roche, F., Bartha, R., Montero-Odasso, M., Allali, G., & Annweiler, C. (2013). Blood pressure levels and brain volume reduction: a systematic review and meta-analysis. *Journal of Hypertension, 31*(8), 1502–1516.

Braak, H., & Braak, E. (1997). Frequency of stages of Alzheimer-related lesions in different age categories. *Neurobiology of Aging, 18*(4), 351–357.

Cahill, S., Pierce, M., Werner, P., Darley, A., & Bobersky, A. (2015). A systematic review of the public's knowledge and understanding of Alzheimer's disease and dementia. *Alzheimer Disease & Associated Disorders, 29*(3), 255–275.

Cao, G. Y., Li, M., Han, L., Tayie, F., Yao, S. S., Huang, Z., ... & Xu, B. (2019). Dietary fat intake and cognitive function among older populations: a systematic review and meta-analysis. *The Journal of Prevention of Alzheimer's Disease, 6*, 204–211.

Carlsson, C., Carlsson, J., Hyvonen, K., Puhakainen, J., & Walden, P. (2006). Adoption of mobile devices/services—searching for answers with the UTAUT. In *System Sciences, 2006. HICSS'06. Proceedings of the 39th Annual Hawaii International Conference on* (Vol. 6, pp. 132a–133a). IEEE.

Cascella, M., Montomoli, J., Bellini, V., & Bignami, E. (2023). Evaluating the feasibility of ChatGPT in healthcare: an analysis of multiple clinical and research scenarios. *Journal of Medical Systems, 47*(1), 33.

Corsinovi, L., Biasi, F., Poli, G., Leonarduzzi, G., & Isaia, G. (2011). Dietary lipids and their oxidized products in Alzheimer's disease. *Molecular Nutrition & Food Research, 55*(S2), S161–SS172.

Cummings, J., Lee, G., Nahed, P., Kambar, M. E. Z. N., Zhong, K., Fonseca, J., & Taghva, K. (2022). Alzheimer's disease drug development pipeline: 2022. *Alzheimer's & Dementia: Translational Research & Clinical Interventions, 8*(1), e12295.

Cushman, W. C., Ringer, R. J., Rodriguez, C. J., Evans, G. W., Bates, J. T., & Cutler, J. A., ... & SPRINT Research Group. (2022). Blood pressure intervention and control in SPRINT. *Hypertension, 79*(9), 2071–2080.

D'Elia, L., Galletti, F., La Fata, E., Sabino, P., & Strazzullo, P. (2018). Effect of dietary sodium restriction on arterial stiffness: systematic review and meta-analysis of the randomized controlled trials. *Journal of Hypertension, 36*(4), 734–743.

De la Torre, J. C. (2010). Alzheimer's disease is incurable but preventable. *Journal of Alzheimer's Disease, 20*(3), 861–870.

Dineen-Griffin, S., Garcia-Cardenas, V., Williams, K., & Benrimoj, S. I. (2019). Helping patients help themselves: a systematic review of self-management support strategies in primary health care practice. *PLoS One, 14*(8), e0220116.

Faulkner, L. (2003). Beyond the five-user assumption: benefits of increased sample sizes in usability testing. *Behavior Research Methods, Instruments, & Computers, 35*, 379–383.

Filippini, T., Malavolti, M., Whelton, P. K., Naska, A., Orsini, N., & Vinceti, M. (2021). Blood pressure effects of sodium reduction: dose–response meta-analysis of experimental studies. *Circulation, 143*(16), 1542–1567.

Greger, M. (2023). *How not to age: the scientific approach to getting healthier as you get older.* Flatiron Books, New York.

Greger, M., & Stone, G. (2016). *How not to die: discover the foods scientifically proven to prevent and reverse disease.* Pan Macmillan, New York City.

Guo, Z., Schlichtkrull, M., & Vlachos, A. (2022). A survey on automated fact-checking. *Transactions of the Association for Computational Linguistics, 10,* 178–206.

Henskens, L. H., Van Oostenbrugge, R. J., Kroon, A. A., De Leeuw, P. W., & Lodder, J. (2008). Brain microbleeds are associated with ambulatory blood pressure levels in a hypertensive population. *Hypertension, 51*(1), 62–68.

Herzwurm, G., & Schockert, S. (2003). The leading edge in QFD for software and electronic business. *International Journal of Quality & Reliability Management, 20*(1), 36–55.

Hudson, J. M., Pollux, P. M., Mistry, B., & Hobson, S. (2012). Beliefs about Alzheimer's disease in Britain. *Aging & Mental Health, 16*(7), 828–835.

Jonkman, N. H., Schuurmans, M. J., Jaarsma, T., Shortridge-Baggett, L. M., Hoes, A. W., & Trappenburg, J. C. (2016). Self-management interventions: proposal and validation of a new operational definition. *Journal of Clinical Epidemiology, 80*(12), 34–42.

Joseph, J., Shukitt-Hale, B., Denisova, N. A., Martin, A., Perry, G., & Smith, M. A. (2001). Copernicus revisited: amyloid beta in Alzheimer's disease. *Neurobiology of Aging, 22*(1), 131–146.

Kivipelto, M., Ngandu, T., Laatikainen, T., Winblad, B., Soininen, H., & Tuomilehto, J. (2006). Risk score for the prediction of dementia risk in 20 years among middle aged people: a longitudinal, population-based study. *The Lancet Neurology, 5*(9), 735–741.

Kovacic, J. C., & Fuster, V. (2012). Atherosclerotic risk factors, vascular cognitive impairment, and Alzheimer disease. *Mount Sinai Journal of Medicine: A Journal of Translational and Personalized Medicine, 79*(6), 664–673.

Lai, T., Shi, Y., Du, Z., Wu, J., Fu, K., Dou, Y., & Wang, Z. (2023). Psy-LLM: Scaling up global mental health psychological services with AI-based large language models. *arXiv preprint arXiv:2307.11991.*

Li, W. W. (2019). *Eat to beat disease: the new science of how your body can heal itself.* Hachette UK.

Lippman, D., Stump, M., Veazey, E., Guimarães, S. T., Rosenfeld, R., Kelly, J. H., … & Katz, D. L. (2024). Foundations of lifestyle medicine and its evolution. *Mayo Clinic Proceedings: Innovations, Quality & Outcomes, 8*(1), 97–111.

Mialon, M., Serodio, P., Crosbie, E., Teicholz, N., Naik, A., & Carriedo, A. (2022). Conflicts of interest for members of the US 2020 Dietary Guidelines Advisory Committee. *Public Health Nutrition, 27*(1), 1–28.

Montagna, S., Ferretti, S., Klopfenstein, L. C., Florio, A., & Pengo, M. F. (2023). Data decentralisation of LLM-based chatbot systems in chronic disease self-management. In *Proceedings of the 2023 ACM Conference on Information Technology for Social Good, Lisbon, Portugal, Sept 6 2023 to Sept 8 2023,* (pp. 205–212).

Okereke, O. I., Rosner, B. A., Kim, D. H., Kang, J. H., Cook, N. R., Manson, J. E., … & Grodstein, F. (2012). Dietary fat types and 4-year cognitive change in community-dwelling older women. *Annals of Neurology, 72*(1), 124–134.

Ornish, D., Madison, C., Kivipelto, M., Kemp, C., McCulloch, C. E., Galasko, D., … & Arnold, S. E. (2024). Effects of intensive lifestyle changes on the progression of mild cognitive impairment or early dementia due to Alzheimer's disease: a randomized, controlled clinical trial. *Alzheimer's Research & Therapy, 16*(1), 122.

Ornish, D., Magbanua, M. J. M., Weidner, G., Weinberg, V., Kemp, C., Green, C., … & Carroll, P. R. (2008). Changes in prostate gene expression in men undergoing an intensive nutrition and lifestyle intervention. *Proceedings of the National Academy of Sciences, 105*(24), 8369–8374.

Ornish, D., Scherwitz, L. W., Billings, J. H., Gould, K. L., Merritt, T. A., Sparler, S., … & Brand, R. J. (1998). Intensive lifestyle changes for reversal of coronary heart disease. *JAMA, 280*(23), 2001–2007.

Pase, M. P., Herbert, A., Grima, N. A., Pipingas, A., & O'Rourke, M. F. (2012). Arterial stiffness as a cause of cognitive decline and dementia: a systematic review and meta-analysis. *Internal Medicine Journal, 42*(7), 808–815.

Peila, R., White, L. R., Petrovich, H., Masaki, K., Ross, G. W., Havlik, R. J., & Launer, L. J. (2001). Joint effect of the APOE gene and midlife systolic blood pressure on late-life cognitive impairment: the Honolulu-Asia aging study. *Stroke, 32*(12), 2882–2889.

Raina, A., Mishra, P., & Kumar, D. (2024). AI as a Medical Ally: Evaluating ChatGPT's Usage and Impact in Indian Healthcare. *arXiv preprint arXiv:2401.15605.*

Roher, A. E., Tyas, S. L., Maarouf, C. L., Daugs, I. D., Kokjohn, T. A., Emmerling, M. R., … & Beach, T. G. (2011). Intracranial atherosclerosis as a contributing factor to Alzheimer's disease dementia. *Alzheimer's & Dementia, 7*(4), 436–444.

Rondini, A., Pezzotta, G., Pirola, F., Rossi, M., & Pina, P. (2016). How to design and evaluate early PSS concepts: the product service concept tree. *Procedia CIRP, 50*, 366–371.

Sabbagh, M. N., Perez, A., Holland, T. M., Boustani, M., Peabody, S. R., Yaffe, K., … & Tanzi, R. E. (2022). Primary prevention recommendations to reduce the risk of cognitive decline. *Alzheimer's & Dementia, 18*(8), 1569–1579.

Sallam, M. (2023). ChatGPT utility in healthcare education, research, and practice: systematic review on the promising perspectives and valid concerns. *Healthcare MDPI, 11*(6), 887.

Santisteban, M. M., & Iadecola, C. (2018). Hypertension, dietary salt and cognitive impairment. *Journal of Cerebral Blood Flow & Metabolism, 38*(12), 2112–2128.

Setchell, K. D., Brown, N. M., Zhao, X., Lindley, S. L., Heubi, J. E., King, E. C., & Messina, M. J. (2011). Soy isoflavone phase II metabolism differs between rodents and humans: implications for the effect on breast cancer risk. *The American Journal of Clinical Nutrition, 94*(5), 1284–1294.

Sherzai, D., & Sherzai, A. (2019). Preventing Alzheimer's: our most urgent health care priority. *American Journal of Lifestyle Medicine, 13*(5), 451–461.

Simons, L. P. A., (2020). Health 2050: Bioinformatics for Rapid Self-Repair; A Design Analysis for Future Quantified Self, pp. 247–261, *33rd Bled eConference*. June 28–29, Bled, Slovenia, Proceedings retrieval from www.bledconference.org. ISBN-13: 978-961-286-362-3. https://doi.org/10.18690/978-961-286-362-3.17.

Simons, L. P. A., (2023). Health 2050: faster cure via bioinformatics & quantified self; A design analysis. *International Journal of Networking and Virtual Organisations, 28*(1), 36–52. https://doi.org/10.1504/IJNVO.2023.130957

Simons, L. P. A., Bodegom, D., Dumaij, A., & Jonker, C. M. (2015a). Design Lessons from an RCT to Test Efficacy of a Hybrid eHealth Solution for Work Site Health. Paper *presented at the 28th Bled eConference*. Bled, Slovenia, from www.bledconference.org.

Simons, L. P. A., Foerster, F., Bruck, P. A., Motiwalla, L., & Jonker, C. M. (2015b). Microlearning mApp raises health competence: hybrid service design. *Health and Technology, 5*, 35–43. doi:10.1007/s12553-015-0095-1

Simons, L. P. A., Gerritsen, B., Wielaard, B., & Neerincx, M. A. (2023). Hypertension Self-Management Success in 2 weeks; 3 Pilot Studies, pp. 19–34, *36th Bled eConference*. June 25–28, Bled, Slovenia, Proceedings retrieval www.bled conference.org. ISBN-13: 978-961-286-751-5. https://research.tudelft.nl/en/pub-lications/hypertension-self-management-success-in-2-weeks-3-pilot-studies/

Simons, L. P. A., & Hampe, J. F. (2010). Service Experience Design for Healthy Living Support; Comparing an In-House with an eHealth Solution. *The 23rd Bled eConference*, pp. 423–440. Retrieved from www.bledconference.org

Simons, L. P. A., Hampe, J. F., & Guldemond, N. A. (2013). Designing healthy living support: mobile applications added to hybrid (e)Coach solution. *Health and Technology, 3*(1), 85–95. doi:10.1007/s12553-013-0052-9

Simons, L. P. A., Hampe, J. F., & Guldemond, N. A. (2014). ICT supported healthy lifestyle interventions: design lessons. *Electronic Markets, 24*, 179–192. doi:10.1007/s12525-014-0157-7

Simons, L. P. A., Heuvel, AC van den, & Jonker, C. M. (2018). eHealth WhatsApp Group for Social Support; Preliminary Results, pp. 225–237, *Presented at the 31st Bled eConference*. Bled, Slovenia, Proceedings retrieval from www.bledconference. org. ISBN-13: 978-961-286-170-4. https://doi.org/10.18690/978-961-286-170-4

Simons, L. P. A., Heuvel, AC van den, & Jonker, C. M. (2020). eHealth WhatsApp for social support: design lessons. *International Journal of Networking and Virtual Organisations, 23*(2), 112–127. https://doi.org/10.1504/IJNVO.2020.108857

Simons, L. P. A., Gerritsen, B., Wielaard, B., & Neerincx, M. A. (2024). Employee hypertension self-management support with microlearning and social learning. *International Journal of Networking and Virtual Organisations, 30*(4), 350–365.

Simons, L. P. A., Murukannaiah, P. K., & Neerincx, M. A. (2024). Designing and Evaluating an LLM-based Health AI Research Assistant for Hypertension Self-Management; Using Health Claims Metadata Criteria, pp. 283–298, *37th Bled eConference*. June 9–12, Bled, Slovenia, Proceedings. ISBN-13: 978-961-286-871-0. doi:10.18690/um.fov.4.2024

Simons, L. P. A., Neerincx, M. A., & Jonker, C. M. (2021). Health Literature Hybrid AI for Health Improvement; A Design Analysis for Diabetes & Hypertension, pp. 184–197, *34th Bled eConference*. June 27–30, Bled, Slovenia, Proceedings retrieval from www. bledconference.org. ISBN-13: 978-961-286-385-9. https://aisel.aisnet.org/bled2021/5

Simons, L. P. A., Pijl, M., Verhoef, J., Lamb, H. J., van Ommen, B., Gerritsen, B., Bizino, M. B., Snel, M., Feenstra, R., & Jonker, C. M. (2016). Intensive Lifestyle (e)Support to Reverse Diabetes-2. Paper *presented at the 29th Bled eConference*. Bled, Slovenia, from www.bledconference.org. and http://aisel.aisnet.org/cgi/viewcontent. cgi?article=1023&context=bled2016

Simons, L. P. A., Pijl, H., Verhoef, J., Lamb, H. J., van Ommen, B., Gerritsen, B., Bizino, M. B., Snel, M., Feenstra, R., & Jonker, C. M. (2017). Diabetes Lifestyle (e)Coaching 50 Weeks Follow Up; Technology Acceptance & e-Relationships, pp. 545–560, *presented at the 30th Bled eConference*. Bled, Slovenia, Proceedings retrieval from www.bledconference.org. ISBN 978-961-286-043-1. https://doi. org/10.18690/978-961-286-043-1

Simons, L. P. A., Neerincx, M. A., & Jonker, C. M. (2022). Is Google making us smart? Health self-management for high performance employees & organisations.

International Journal of Networking and Virtual Organisations, 27(3), 200–216. doi:10.1504/IJNVO.2022.10053605

Simons, L. P. A., Gerritsen, B., Wielaard, B., & Neerincx, M. A. (2022). Health Self-Management Support with Microlearning to Improve Hypertension, pp. 511–524, *35th Bled eConference*. June 26–29, Bled, Slovenia, Proceedings retrieval from www.bledconference.org. ISBN-13: 978-961-286-616-7. doi:10.18690/um/fov.4. 2022

Simons, L. P. A., Pijl, H., Verhoef, J., Lamb, H. J., van Ommen, B., Gerritsen, B., Bizino, M. B., Snel, M., Feenstra, R., & Jonker, C. M. (2022). E-health diabetes; 50 weeks evaluation. *International Journal of Biomedical Engineering and Technology*, 38(1), 81–98.

Simons, L. P. A., van den Heuvel, W. A., & Jonker, C. M. (2019). WhatsApp Peer Coaching Lessons for eHealth. In *Handbook of research on optimizing healthcare management techniques* (pp. 16–32). IGI Global, ISBN 9781799813712.

Singer, J., Trollor, J. N., Baune, B. T., Sachdev, P. S., & Smith, E. (2014). Arterial stiffness, the brain and cognition: a systematic review. *Ageing Research Reviews*, 15, 16–27.

Singh-Manoux, A., Kivimaki, M., Glymour, M. M., Elbaz, A., Berr, C., Ebmeier, K. P., ... & Dugravot, A. (2012). Timing of onset of cognitive decline: results from Whitehall II prospective cohort study. *BMJ*, 344, 1–8.

Torres-Acosta, N., O'Keefe, J. H., O'Keefe, E. L., Isaacson, R., & Small, G. (2020). Therapeutic potential of TNF-α inhibition for Alzheimer's disease prevention. *Journal of Alzheimer's Disease*, 78(2), 619–626.

Vaishnavi, V., & Kuechler, W. (2004). Design Research in Information Systems. Last updated August 16, 2009, from https://scholar.google.com/citations?user=2AUiwBoAAAAJ&hl=en

Venkatesh, V., & Davis, F. D. (2000). A theoretical extension of the technology acceptance model: four longitudinal field studies. *Management Science*, 46, 186–204.

Venkatesh, V., Morris, M. G., Davis, G. B., & Davis, F. D. (2003). User acceptance of information technology: toward a unified view. *MIS Quarterly*, 27(3), 425–478.

Vermeer, S. E., Longstreth, W. T., & Koudstaal, P. J. (2007). Silent brain infarcts: a systematic review. *The Lancet Neurology*, 6(7), 611–619.

Verschuren, P., & Hartog, R. (2005). Evaluation in design-oriented research. *Quality and Quantity*, 39, 733–762.

Verweij, L. M., Coffeng, J., van Mechelen, W., & Proper, K. I. (2011). Meta-analyses of workplace physical activity and dietary behaviour interventions on weight outcomes. *Obesity Reviews*, 12, 406–429.

Viña, J., & Sanz-Ros, J. (2018). Alzheimer's disease: only prevention makes sense. *European Journal of Clinical Investigation*, 48(10), e13005.

Wansink, B. (2011). *Mindless eating*. Hay House UK Limited, London.

Willett, W. C. (2012). Dietary fats and coronary heart disease. *Journal of Internal Medicine*, 272(1), 13–24.

Williamson, J. D., Pajewski, N. M., Auchus, A. P., Bryan, R. N., Chelune, G., & Cheung, A. K., ... & Sprint Mind Investigators for the SPRINT Research Group. (2019). Effect of intensive vs standard blood pressure control on probable dementia: a randomized clinical trial. *JAMA*, 321(6), 553–561.

17

Digital Twins of Dementia Patients for Clinical Decision Support

Nilmini Wickramasinghe and Nalika Ulapane

17.1 Introduction

17.1.1 Dementia

Dementia is a growing health challenge worldwide. It is marked by decline in cognitive functions such as memory, reasoning, and communication. This condition significantly interferes with the daily life and independence of patients. That makes dementia one of the most serious public health issues worldwide. According to certain reports, approximately 57 million people were living with dementia worldwide in 2021 [1]. Nearly 10 million new cases emerge each year [1]. This number is expected to almost double every 20 years. That means, the number reaching 78 million in 2030 and 139 million by 2050 [2]. Most of these cases are in low and middle-income countries. In these countries, the healthcare systems are often less equipped to handle the burden of dementia [1].

The economic impact of dementia is staggering. In 2019, the worldwide cost of dementia was estimated at $1.3 trillion [2]. This figure is projected to rise to $2.8 trillion by 2030 [2]. These costs include different aspects such as direct medical expenses, social services, and the significant unpaid care provided by family members (i.e., family carers). In the United States alone, the economic burden of dementia is expected to reach $781 billion by 2025 [3]. This includes not only healthcare costs; this also includes the hidden financial impacts such as lost income and the emotional toll on caregivers [3].

The aging population is a critical factor that drives the increase in dementia cases. As people live longer due to advances in modern healthcare, the proportion of older adults in the population rises. Dementia primarily affects older individuals. The risk increases significantly with age. For instance, about one-third of people over the age of 85 have some form of dementia [4]. The aging trend is particularly pronounced in regions like China, India, and other South Asian and Western Pacific countries. These regions are

DOI: 10.1201/9781003485681-17

experiencing the fastest growth in their elderly populations [2]. This demographic shift highlights the urgent need for effective approaches to dementia care. These include strategies and support systems to manage this growing burden.

The combination of an aging population and the high costs associated with dementia care presents a challenge for healthcare systems worldwide. Addressing this issue requires comprehensive approaches that include early diagnosis, improved care models, and support for caregivers. As the prevalence of dementia continues to rise, so too does the need to develop innovative solutions to mitigate its impact on individuals, families, and societies at large.

17.1.2 Complexities in Dementia Care

Dementia care is inherently complex. It requires a multifaceted approach to address the diverse needs of individuals. The progression of dementia varies greatly among patients. This necessitates personalized care plans that adapt to changing cognitive and physical abilities. This complexity is compounded by the need for specialized training. This includes training for caregivers to manage behavioral and psychological symptoms, such as aggression, depression, and anxiety. Additionally, the coordination of care across various healthcare providers, including primary care physicians, neurologists, social workers, family carers, and more, adds to the complexity.

Family carers bear a significant burden in dementia care [5, 6]. They often provide extensive support. These include support with daily activities, medical appointments, emotional support, and more. This role can be physically and emotionally exhausting. It can lead to high levels of stress, burnout, and even health issues among caregivers. The financial strain is also considerable. Many family carers may need to reduce their working hours or leave their jobs entirely to provide care. This results in lost income and increases financial pressure. The hidden costs of caregiving, such as out-of-pocket expenses for medical supplies and home modifications, can further exacerbate this burden.

Globalization and immigration have created a multicultural and multilingual world. This presents unique challenges in dementia care. Immigrant families often face language barriers and cultural differences. These can hinder access to appropriate care and support services. In many cases, healthcare systems are not adequately equipped to provide culturally sensitive care [5, 6]. This can lead to misunderstanding, misdiagnosis, or delayed diagnosis of various health conditions including dementia, especially among minority groups. This lack of culturally and linguistically appropriate services can result in social isolation and inadequate support for dementia cases in minority communities.

The modern world of increased cost of living and other expenses adds another layer of difficulty. Dementia care can incur high costs, including residential care and specialized medical treatments. Many families are forced to make difficult financial decisions. This might include compromising other living expenses to balance out the costs of dementia care. This financial strain can lead to significant stress and impact the overall well-being of all involved, including the caregiver and the person with dementia and the whole family.

The complexities of dementia care are thus vast and multifaceted. They affect not only the individuals with dementia but also their families and caregivers. The challenges are further amplified in a multicultural and multilingual world. Minority groups may face additional barriers to accessing appropriate care and support. Addressing these complexities requires comprehensive and culturally sensitive approaches.

17.1.3 Precision in Personalization of Care

Precision medicine [7], sometimes also known as personalized medicine, is a novel concept and an innovative approach to healthcare. This attempts to tailor interventions to the individual characteristics of each patient. In different health contexts, this approach considers factors such as genetics, environment, and lifestyle to develop more effective and targeted interventions. Unlike the traditional "one-size-fits-all" model, precision medicine aims to provide the right treatment to the right patient at the right time. Thereby, the expectation is to enhance the efficacy of interventions while minimizing adverse effects.

Like in many other diseases, when it comes to dementia also, precision medicine holds promise. Dementia encompasses a range of conditions, including Alzheimer's disease, vascular dementia, and Lewy body dementia, each with distinct underlying causes and progression patterns. By leveraging precision and personalization of interventions, personalized care plans can be developed to address the specific needs of each patient based on their unique profiles. Moreover, precision medicine can inform non-pharmacological interventions as well, which are especially relevant for dementia. These include lifestyle modifications and cognitive therapies, tailored to the individual's specific risk factors and characteristics. For example, a patient with a predisposition to Alzheimer's disease, such as family background and early symptoms of mild cognitive impairment, might benefit from personalized exercises and diet designed to mitigate their risk.

17.1.4 Digital Twins (DTs) in Healthcare

DTs are virtual replicas of physical objects, systems, or processes [8]. They are used to simulate, predict, and optimize their real-world counterparts. DTs get continuously updated, often with real-time data. This allows for dynamic and accurate representations of their physical counterparts. The concept of DTs has evolved significantly since its inception. Applications of DTs span various industries, such as manufacturing and automation, construction and planning, supply chain and logistics, and healthcare.

In healthcare, DTs are often targeted at enabling precision and personalization of care [9]. By integrating data from various sources, including genetic information, medical records, real-time sensor data, and environmental factors, and more, DTs create comprehensive and dynamic models of patients' and other required healthcare-related processes. These models are used to simulate different scenarios, predict disease progression, and tailor interventions to the specific needs of each patient.

For example, DTs can be used to create personalized treatment plans for patients with chronic conditions such as cardiovascular disease or cancer [10]. By simulating how different treatments will affect a patient's condition, healthcare providers can select the most effective interventions and minimize adverse effects. This approach reduces the trial-and-error process often associated with medical interventions, leading to superior outcomes and improved patient satisfaction.

17.1.5 Research Question

Drawing synergy between the complexities and challenges in dementia care and the potential of delivering precision medicine and DTs, this chapter aims to address the following research question: **How might the concept of DTs be used to enhance precision and personalization of dementia care?**

As discussed earlier, the increasing prevalence of dementia, driven by an aging population worldwide, presents significant challenges for modern healthcare systems. Traditional approaches to dementia care often struggle to meet the unique and evolving needs of individual patients. This leads to suboptimal outcomes and increased burdens on families and caregivers. The integration of precision medicine offers a promising pathway to address these challenges by enabling interventions to be tailored to specific characteristics of each patient.

DTs, as virtual replicas of physical entities, provide a powerful tool to implement precise and personalized interventions in dementia care. By creating dynamic and comprehensive models of patients' profiles, DTs of dementia patients can be used to predict likely disease progression and design personalized care plans. This approach not only enhances the effectiveness of care but also allows for continuous monitoring and real-time adjustments to care.

Furthermore, DTs can help bridge the gaps in care for minority groups and immigrant populations. As discussed earlier, these groups often face barriers to accessing culturally and linguistically appropriate services. By incorporating diverse data inputs, DTs can ensure that care plans are sensitive to the unique needs of these communities. This also promotes fairness in healthcare delivery.

In this chapter, we present a simple DT construct for dementia care only using a few elements of data. Through this we aim to demonstrate how DTs can support more precise, personalized, and effective dementia care. By addressing our target research question, we hope to highlight the ways in which DTs can improve the quality of life for individuals with dementia and alleviate the broader societal and economic burdens associated with dementia.

17.2 Proposed Solution

The proposed DT solution is intended to function as a web-based application that can be accessed through desktop and mobile devices to assist with shared decision-making. The shared decision-making can be performed by clinicians in consultation with patients and/or carers, and also carers themselves. The idea is to take several data elements about a present dementia patient as input as described in Section 2.1. Then a cohort matching (i.e., finding cohorts of past patients that best match the present patient as per some statistical criteria) is performed as described in Section 2.2. Then, precision and personalization are achieved through matching the trend of the present patient's cognitive decline (based on the Mini-Mental State Examination (MMSE) score) to those of the past patients within the cohort. Finally, as outputs from the system, the clinicians and/or carers can have the likely trajectory of cognitive decline for the present patient, and recommended activities to maximize and prolong the quality of life of the present patient.

17.2.1 Inputs to the Solution

The proposed DT solution intakes a set of data about the present dementia patient. This data is used to create a personalized virtual model of the patient. At this preliminary stage, the following data elements are considered.

- **Patient's Age:** The patient's age is an important factor. It helps us understand the progression of dementia and it also helps us tailor interventions accordingly.
- **Patient's Sex:** Gender-specific differences are also notable in dementia prevalence and progression. Therefore, the patient's sex is also considered an important point of data.
- **Patient's Ethnicity:** The ethnicity of a patient is an important marker that succinctly summarizes a patient's genetic profile, and a lot of other factors that are culturally specific. These could include risk

factors, progression of dementia, and perhaps culturally specific nuances and practices of care and mitigation of dementia. This makes the patient's ethnicity an important variable to design personalized care.

- **Origin of Symptoms:** This is the rough date (i.e., year, month, and the exact date if possible). Information about the initial onset and the nature of dementia symptoms is helpful to plan appropriate interventions.

- **MMSE Scores:** The MMSE scores [11] provide a quantitative measure of cognitive function over time. These scores, recorded at different dates, are crucial for tracking the patient's cognitive decline and matching it with similar cases within past patients. These scores are recorded as follows: (Date1, Score1), (Date2, Score2), ...

There are of course a lot of other variables that can be considered. However, at this preliminary stage, we intended to keep our solution simple and small in scale. Therefore, we decided to go with the data elements mentioned above.

By integrating these data elements, the DT solution can create a model of the patient's condition. This model then serves as the foundation for cohort matching and the subsequent precision and personalization of dementia care.

17.2.2 Cohort Matching

Cohort matching is a critical step in the proposed DT solution. It enables identifying a group of past patients whose characteristics closely resemble those of the present patient. This process ensures that the recommendations and predictions generated by the DT solution are based on relevant and comparable cases. The following criteria are used for cohort matching:

- **Patient's Age (+/− 5 Years):** The age of the present patient is matched with past patients within a five-year age range. This criterion accounts for age-related differences in the progression and management of dementia and also the required elements of care.

- **Patient's Sex:** The sex of the present patient is matched with past patients. This ensures that gender-specific factors that influence dementia are considered.

- **Patient's Ethnicity:** The ethnicity of the present patient is matched with past patients. The cohort is selected to match the same ethnicity or the ethnicity that is as close as possible to the present patient. This criterion helps address cultural and genetic factors that may affect dementia, and also the culturally nuanced mitigation strategies and elements of care.

- **Origin of Symptoms:** Date (+/− 1 year). The onset date of dementia symptoms in the present patient is matched with past patients. Patients whose symptoms began within one year of the present patient's onset date are considered as a matching cohort. This ensures that the cohort includes patients at a similar stage of the disease.

By applying the aforesaid matching criteria, the DT solution can identify a cohort of past patients whose demographics closely align with those of the present patient. This cohort serves as a reference group for predicting the likely trajectory of cognitive decline of the present patient, and also as an assistive cohort to derive recommendations on personalized interventions.

17.2.3 Acquiring Precision and Personalization

To achieve precision and personalization, the proposed solution uses indicators of cognitive decline as indicated by the MMSE scores. Other scores can also be used or designed. However, for this analysis, we chose the MMSE scores. We expect these scores will be recorded on different dates, perhaps several months apart, to provide a quantitative measure of cognitive decline over time. The process involves the following steps:

- Data Collection: The MMSE scores of the present patient are collected, for example:

  (Date1, Score1)

  (Date2, Score2)

  (Date3, Score3)

  ...

- **Linear Interpolation:** Using the collected MMSE scores, we perform linear interpolation between the score coordinates to generate a piecewise continuous line graph. This graph visually represents the cognitive decline of the present patient over time. The interpolation ensures that the cognitive trajectory is depicted smoothly, capturing the progression between recorded scores.

- **Graph Comparison:** The piecewise continuous line graph of the present patient is then compared with similarly generated graphs of past patients within the matched cohort. Each past patient's MMSE scores are used to create their own piecewise continuous line graph, representing their cognitive decline trajectory.

- **Statistical Matching:** To identify the best matches, we employ statistical measures such as mean absolute error (MAE) or mean square error (MSE). These measures quantify the differences between the present patient's graph and each past patient's graph. The patients with the lowest MAE or MSE values are considered the best matches, as their cognitive decline trajectories closely resemble that of the present patient.

The selected cohorts are then used to derive personalized insights and recommendations for shared decision-making and planning care for the present patient.

17.2.4 Outcomes of the Solution

Based on the cohort matching through MMSE scores, the proposed DT solution can provide insights and recommendations to enhance the care of present dementia patients. The key outcomes of the solution include the following.

- **Likely Trajectory of Cognitive Decline:** By comparing the present patient's cognitive decline trajectory with those of past patients in the matched cohort, the DT solution can predict the likely future progression of the present patient's dementia. This prediction includes estimates of future MMSE scores and the expected rate of cognitive decline. Such information is crucial for clinicians and carers to anticipate changes in the patient's condition and plan appropriate interventions.

- **Recommended Activities:** The DT solution can suggest personalized activities and interventions designed to maximize and prolong the quality of life for the present patient drawing synergies from past patients in the matched cohort. In other words, these recommendations are based on the experiences and outcomes of past patients with similar cognitive decline trajectories. Activities may include cognitive exercises, physical activities, social engagement, and dietary modifications that have been shown to benefit individuals with dementia. These can be culturally sensitive too as the ethnicity of the present dementia patient is considered at the cohort matching stage. By tailoring these recommendations to the specific needs of the patient, the DT solution helps optimize their overall well-being.

- **Care Plan Adjustments:** Accompanying the DT solution with continuous monitoring and real-time data integration capabilities allows for dynamic adjustments to the care plan. As the patient's condition evolves, the DT system can update its predictions and recommendations, ensuring that the care plan remains relevant and effective. This adaptive approach helps address the changing needs of the patient and provides ongoing support to caregivers.

- **Enhanced Decision-Making:** The DT solution facilitates shared decision-making between clinicians, patients, and carers. By providing personalized information about the patient's condition and potential interventions, the DT system empowers all stakeholders to make informed decisions about the care plan. This collaborative approach enhances the overall quality of care. It also ensures that the patient's preferences and needs are prioritized.

The outcomes of the proposed DT solution as such, include the prediction of the patient's cognitive decline trajectory, personalized activity recommendations, facility for dynamic care plan adjustments, and support for enhanced and shared decision-making. These outcomes contribute to more precise and personalized dementia care. This ultimately aims at improving the quality of life for individuals with dementia and reducing the burden on carers and healthcare systems.

17.2.5 Continuous Learning

To further enhance the proposed DT solution, it can be integrated with a cloud-based system for continuous learning and outcome reporting. This integration allows for the collection and analysis of real-time data from various sources and sensors. This thereby provides a robust evidence-gathering tool that supports ongoing improvements in dementia care. Some of the key elements that can be captured are listed below.

- **Carer-Reported Outcomes:** Family (or other) carers play a crucial role in the daily management of dementia patients. By incorporating carer-reported outcomes into the cloud-based system, the DT solution can gather valuable insights into the patient's condition and the effectiveness of recommended interventions. Carers can report on various aspects of the patient's well-being, such as:

  # Changes in cognitive function

  # Behavioral and psychological symptoms

  # Physical symptoms

  # Daily activities and patient's independence

  # Emotional and physical health of the carer

  There can be a lot more elements that can be captured; listed above are only a few. Capturing such information is valuable to gain insights about the patient's progress and also the state of the carers. Areas where additional support or adjustments to the care plan are required may also be identifiable.

- **Clinician and Nurse-Reported Outcomes:** Periodic reporting by caring clinicians and nurses is essential for maintaining an accurate and up-to-date model of the patient's health. Healthcare professionals can provide detailed assessments and vital information such as the patient's cognitive and physical status, medication effectiveness and adherence, response to interventions, and more. Some of the elements reported by clinicians and nurses may include the following.

Updated MMSE scores and other cognitive assessments

Medical observations and clinical notes

Treatment adherence, effectiveness, and side effects

Recommendations for further interventions

Again, there can be a lot more elements that can be captured; listed above are only a few. Through the integration of such professional assessments with carer-reported outcomes, the DT solution can ensure a holistic representation of the patient's condition.

- **Evidence Gathering and Continuous Improvement:** The cloud-based system enables the aggregation and analysis of outcome measures from a large number of patients. This data can be used to identify patterns, evaluate the effectiveness of different interventions, refine the DT models, and more. Continuous learning from such allows the DT solution to:

Improve the accuracy of predictions and recommendations

Adapt to new research findings and clinical guidelines

Provide evidence-based insights for personalized care plans

Enhance the overall quality of dementia care

As such, coupling the DT solution with a cloud-based system for continuous learning and outcome reporting converts the solution into a powerful evidence-gathering tool. By incorporating carer-reported and clinician-reported outcomes, the system can continuously refine and improve its models and also incorporate artificial intelligence (AI). Such an approach ensures that dementia care remains precise, personalized, effective, and up to date. This approach not only benefits individual patients but also contributes to the broader

understanding and the body of knowledge about management of dementia.

17.3 Discussion

17.3.1 Summary of the Work Carried Out

In this chapter, we explored the concept of DTs and their potential application to enhance precision and personalization in dementia care. We began by discussing the serious and growing global challenge of dementia, highlighting the complexities in dementia care and the significant burden it places on healthcare systems and family carers. We then discussed precision medicine and how it can help dementia care to provide more targeted and effective interventions.

The target research question of this chapter was "How might the concept of digital twins be used to enhance precision and personalization of dementia care?" We proposed a DT solution as an answer to this question. By leveraging analytics and data, the proposed solution aims to improve the quality of life for individuals with dementia and reduce the burden on caregivers and healthcare systems.

The core of our proposed solution is the use of DTs to create dynamic and virtual models of dementia patients. These models are based on input data about patients, including age, sex, ethnicity, origin of symptoms, and MMSE scores. Through a process of cohort matching and statistical analysis, the DT solution identifies past patients with similar characteristics and cognitive decline trajectories. This allows for precise predictions of the present patient's cognitive decline and personalized recommendations for care.

17.3.2 Strengths, Weaknesses, Opportunities, and Threats

In this section, we have attempted to list down various Strengths, Weaknesses, Opportunities, and Threats associated with the proposed solution.

17.3.2.1 Strengths

- **Precision and Personalization:** The DT solution offers personalized care plans based on patient data and cohort matching. This approach ensures that interventions are tailored to the unique needs of each patient based on evidence, improving outcomes and quality of life.
- **Continuous Learning:** The integration with a cloud-based system for continuous learning and outcome reporting allows the solution to adapt and improve over time. This dynamic approach ensures that care plans remain relevant and effective as new data and research findings emerge.
- **Enhanced Decision-Making:** The solution facilitates shared decision-making between clinicians, patients, and caregivers by

providing personalized information about the patient's condition and potential interventions.

17.3.2.2 Weaknesses

- **Data Privacy and Security:** The collection and storage of sensitive patient data pose significant privacy and security challenges. Ensuring robust data protection measures is crucial to maintaining patient trust and compliance with regulations.
- **Resource Intensive:** Implementing and maintaining the DT system may require substantial resources depending on how rich the DTs are. These include advanced IoT capabilities, data storage facilities, fast computation, personnel with tech literacy to use the DT solution, and substantial data input. These may create some barriers for some healthcare providers and carers, particularly in resource-limited settings.
- **Dependence on Data Quality:** The accuracy and effectiveness of the DT solution depend on the quality and completeness of the input data. Inaccurate or incomplete data can lead to suboptimal predictions and recommendations.

17.3.2.3 Opportunities

- **Scalability:** The DT solution has the potential to be scaled across different healthcare settings and regions, providing personalized dementia care to a broader population. This can be offered in different languages as well and can incorporate AI capabilities like natural language processing.
- **Integration with Other Technologies:** The solution can be integrated with other emerging technologies, such as wearable devices and AI-driven analytics, to enhance data collection and analysis capabilities.
- **Opportunities for Research and Development:** The continuous learning aspect of the solution provides opportunities for ongoing research and development, contributing to the broader understanding and management of dementia.

17.3.2.4 Threats

- **Regulatory Challenges:** Navigating the complex regulations for healthcare technologies can be challenging, particularly with regard to data privacy and security.
- **Resistance to Change/Adoption:** Resistance to change (and adoption) among healthcare providers, carers, and patients may hinder the adoption and implementation of the DT solution.

17.4 Conclusions

In this chapter, we explored the concept of DTs and the potential application to dementia care with the aim of enhancing precision and personalization of dementia care. We discussed the significant challenges posed by dementia, the complexities of care, and the burden on carers, the economy, and healthcare systems alike. By leveraging precision medicine and DT technology, we proposed a solution that creates dynamic virtual models of patients, enabling tailored interventions and improved outcomes.

The proposed DT solution integrates patient data, performs cohort matching, and provides personalized recommendations based on analysis that is real-time (or as fast as it can be). This approach not only enhances the quality of care for individuals with dementia but also supports continuous learning and evidence gathering through a cloud-based system.

While there are challenges to address, such as data privacy and resource requirements, the potential benefits of this solution are substantial. By adopting DT technology, we can move toward a more effective, personalized, and equitable approach to dementia care, ultimately improving the lives of patients and their caregivers.

The proposed solution and the approach followed can have broader applications for other chronic diseases too, not only dementia.

References

1. World Health Organization, 2021. Dementia. https://www.who.int/en/news-room/fact-sheets/detail/dementia. Date of last access: 28/04/2025.
2. Alzheimer's Disease International, 2025. Dementia Statistics. https://www.alzint.org/about/dementia-facts-figures/dementia-statistics/. Date of last access: 28/04/2025.
3. Medical Economics, 2025. Dementia Costs in the US. https://www.medicaleconomics.com/view/u-s-dementia-costs-to-reach-781-billion-in-2025-who-s-really-paying-for-it. Date of last access: 28/04/2025.
4. National Institute of Aging, 2021. What Is Dementia? Symptoms, Types, and Diagnosis. https://www.nia.nih.gov/health/alzheimers-and-dementia/what-dementia-symptoms-types-and-diagnosis. Date of last access: 28/04/2025.
5. Dang, Thu Ha, et al. "'It's too nice': Adapting iSupport lite for ethnically diverse family carers of a person with dementia." Clinical Gerontologist 48.2 (2025): 194–207.
6. Thodis, Antonia, et al. "Improving the lives of ethnically diverse family carers and people living with dementia using digital media resources— protocol for the draw-care randomised controlled trial." Digital Health 9 (2023): 20552076231205733.

7. Ashley, Euan A. "Towards precision medicine." Nature Reviews Genetics 17.9 (2016): 507–522.
8. Barricelli, Barbara Rita, Elena Casiraghi, and Daniela Fogli. "A survey on digital twin: Definitions, characteristics, applications, and design implications." IEEE Access 7 (2019): 167653–167671.
9. Wickramasinghe, Nilmini et al. "Digital Twins for More Precise and Personalized Treatment." MEDINFO 2023—The Future Is Accessible. IOS Press, 2024. 229–233.
10. Wickramasinghe, Nilmini, et al. "A vision for leveraging the concept of digital twins to support the provision of personalized cancer care." IEEE Internet Computing 26.5 (2021): 17–24.
11. Cockrell, Joseph R., and Marshal F. Folstein. "Mini-Mental State Examination." Principles and Practice of Geriatric Psychiatry 24.4 (2002): 689–692.

Epilogue

Key facts noted by the WHO include[1]

- Currently, more than 55 million people have dementia worldwide, over 60% of whom live in low- and middle-income countries. Every year, there are nearly 10 million new cases.

- Dementia results from a variety of diseases and injuries that affect the brain. Alzheimer's disease is the most common form of dementia and may contribute to 60–70% of cases.

- Dementia is currently the seventh leading cause of death and one of the major causes of disability and dependency among older people globally.

- In 2019, dementia cost economies globally US$1.3 trillion, approximately 50% of these costs are attributable to care provided by informal carers (e.g., family members and close friends), who provide on average five hours of care and supervision per day.

- Women are disproportionately affected by dementia, both directly and indirectly. Women experience higher disability-adjusted life years and mortality due to dementia, but also provide 70% of care hours for people living with dementia.

Without a doubt, these facts are alarming. Dementia is indeed a debilitating disease that sadly is affecting many older members of the population and placing a burden on family and caregivers as well as the healthcare system. At present we have no cure for dementia, however advances in digital health most notably empowered with artificial intelligence and machine learning hold the promise and potential of brighter days for people living with dementia, their families and care givers as well as the healthcare community and society at large.

The preceding miscellany of chapters written by international experts has served to capture significant opportunities and the requisite critical success factors to realise the full potential of such digital health solutions. This is indeed the road less travelled but we trust our book has served to take the first step in showing that digital health solutions could hold the key to providing superior diagnosis and care for people living with dementia, their families, caregivers, healthcare professionals and society at large. We trust you enjoyed reading this book at least as much as we did in compiling it. We hope you too will embark on this journey to assist in the provision of superior outcomes for people living with dementia, their family, caregivers, and healthcare professionals for the benefit of society at large.

The Editors
Nilmini Wickramasinghe, Thu Ha Dang, Tuan Nyugen, and Sasan Adibi
Melbourne Feb 2025

Note

1 https://www.who.int/news-room/fact-sheets/detail/dementia

Index

Note: *Italicized* page references refer to figures, **bold** page references refer to tables, and page references with "n" refer to endnotes.

A

Activities of daily living (ADLs), 4–5, 191, 246, 250, 304

Adaptive Synthetic Sampling (ADASYN), 91

Adjusted Rand Index (ARI), 146

Advanced encryption standards (AES), 142, 150

Advanced Neural Networks, 98

Aged Care Quality and Safety (ACRC), 10

Aguirre, G. K., 217

AI-driven simulations, 101

AI-Enhanced Health Monitoring Ecosystem, 64–67
  benefits and impact, 66–67
  cloud-based platform, 66
  components and benefits of, 66–67, **67**
  network of IoT sensors and devices, 66
  notification system, 66
  privacy and security, 66

AI Health Research Assistant, 336

AI-integrated global dementia care framework, 141–145
  data acquisition and management, 142
  data preprocessing and integration, 142
  machine learning models and inference, 142
  user interface and security measures, 142–145

AI Research Assistant tool, 329–331

Alowais, S. A., 131

Alzheimer's disease (AD), 41, 45–48, *62*, 68, 76, **79**, **80**, **81**, *84*, 94, 151, 158
  screening tool for, 215
  spatial navigation, 216–218

Alzheimer's disease and related dementia (ADRD), 246, 307
  caregiving practice gap, 302–303
  in United States (U.S.), 301

Alzheimer's Disease International (ADI), 2

Amazon Echo, 52–53, 62

Ambiguity "rationale capturing," 339

Ambiguous claims
  evaluation and metadata criteria for, 339

American Association of Retired Persons, 306

Amjad, A., 132

Apple Watch, 48, 60, *61*

Artificial intelligence (AI), 3–5, 18, 38, 45–69, 108, 157–169, 171, 303, 304, 311
  AI-Enhanced Health Monitoring Ecosystem, 64–67
  application in dementia care and treatment, 163–164
    drug discovery, 163–164
    socially assistive robots, 163
  application in dementia diagnosis and prognosis, 164–166
    CSF and blood biomarkers, 165
    electroencephalogram (EEG), 166
    genetics, 164
    neuroimaging, 165
    retinal imaging (RI), 166
    speech and language, 164–165
  bias and underrepresentation, 109
  in clinical dementia care, 108–110
  in clinical trial optimization, 101
  commercial tools in healthcare, **107**, 107–108
  in data optimization, 89
  data privacy and security, 108
  defined, 160–161

dementia
  Alzheimer's disease (AD), 158
  defined, 158
  detect earlier, 160
  diagnosed at present, 160
  frontotemporal dementia
    (FTD), 159
  Lewy body dementia (LBD), 159
  mixed dementia (MD), 159
  types of, 158–159
  vascular dementia (VD), 158–159
incorporating with multilingual
    virtual helper, 266–276
integration of, 57
issues in dementia research,
    166–168
  clinical applicability issues, 168
  interpretability of machine
    learning models, 166–167
  reproducibility and replicability,
    167
limitations, 168
in neurological predictive analytics,
    94–98
overview, 157–158
in personalized medicine, 89
real-world data, 161
regulatory challenges, 109
risks from Black-Box models, 109
role in digital twins, 39
underrepresented data, 109–110
Assistive technologies (AT), 1, 3–5, 13,
    189, 243
Atefi, G. L., 310
Australian Human Rights Commission, 9
Australian National Dementia Action
    Plan, 10
Automated fact checking, 330
Autoregressive (AR) Modelling, 91
Aworinde, J., 137

B

Banfield, J., 12
Becker, B., 132
Begum, M., 251
Behavior management, 248, 253
Behaviours that challenge (BtC) in
    dementia, 127–129, 152n1

Bidirectional Long Short-Term Memory
    (BiLSTM), 95
Biomedical model of dementia, 2
Biometric sensors, 40
Bird, M., 293, 296
Black, Asian, and Minority Ethnic
    (BAME), 234
Blood pressure
  brain shrinking, 326
  and dementia, 325–327
  healthy lifestyle, 327
  measurements, 327–328
  sodium intake, 327
Blood pressure monitors and
    glucose monitors, 51–52
Body Area Networks (BANs),
    171–173, 177
Brijnath, B., 237
British Psychological Society—Division
    of Clinical Psychology briefing
    (BPS-DCP), 127–128

C

Cardiovascular health, 325–327, 329
Caregivers
  benefits/challenges of digital
    technology, 315–317
  empowerment of, 336–339
  potential of digital solutions
    for, 301–319
  practice gap, 302–303
  technology support applications,
    307–314
  use of digital technologies
    by, 306–307
Care partners and family members
    (CPFM), 1
Carer-reported outcomes, 354
Cares Framework, 314, **314**
Caring for the Caregiver Network, 309
Case study, 266–276
Cerebrospinal fluid (CSF), 76
ChatGPT, 2, 13, 130, 329
Cheong, Marc, 13
Claims evaluation criteria, **338**
Classification and Regression
    Trees (CART), 91
Classification models, 146

Clinical decision support, 346–358
Clinical Decision Support Systems
  (CDSS), 46
Clinical social work and sociology, 18
Clinicians, 354–355
Clustering and genetic algorithms,
  97–98
Clustering models, 146
Co-designing digital health
  interventions, 279–296
  benefits, issues, and challenges,
    280–283
  Consolidated Framework for
    Implementation Research
    (CFIR), 291–292
  digital health interventions,
    283–289
    accessibility, 284–285
    co-design tools and activities,
      287–288
    communication, 285–287
    developing relationships, 284
    family carer involvement, 285
    overview, 283
  evaluation of, 293–296
  implementation frameworks, 290
  importance of, 279–280
  REAFF framework, 282
  RE-AIM framework, 291
Colbert, Stephen, 26
Commercial AI Chatbots and tools, 139
Communication and language
  support, 249
Complexities in dementia care,
  347–348
Computer-aided diagnosis (CAD), 95
Computer-telephone system (CTIS), 308
Concordance Correlation Coefficient
  (CCC), 147
Consolidated Framework for
  Implementation Research
  (CFIR), 291–292
Continuous glucose monitors
  (CGMs), 51
Continuous learning, 275, 356
Conversational agents in healthcare,
  126–152
  AI-integrated global dementia
    care framework, 141–145

data acquisition and management,
  142
data preprocessing and
  integration, 142
machine learning models
  and inference, 142
user interface and security
  measures, 142–145
commercial AI Chatbots and
  tools, 139
comprehensive AI-powered global
  framework, 140–141
data privacy and security in
  AI applications, 149–151
  compliance with regulatory
    standards, 150
  data access controls and audit
    trails, 150
  data anonymization and
    de-identification, 149
  ethical and legal considerations,
    149
  patient empowerment and
    data control, 150–151
  risks of data breaches and
    mitigation strategies, 150
  secure data storage and
    transmission, 150
essential technological tools,
  141–145
ethical considerations in AI-powered
  healthcare interventions,
  137–139
  challenges in predictive health
    analytics, 138
  general ethical principles in
    AI deployment, 138
  global ethical regulatory
    organization, 139
  impact on patient-physician
    dynamics, 138
  language models, 138–139
integrating AI and ML in dementia
  care, 135–137
  advancing care, 137
  AI-enhanced tools, 136–137
  decision-making, 137
  healthcare connectivity with
    AI, 136

language models, 137
patient-centered digital support,
    135–136
patient engagement through
    AI-driven conversational
    interfaces, 136
structured, non-pharmacological
    interventions, 137
language models and applications in
    patient interaction, 130–133
Natural Language Processing (NLP),
    129–130
overview, 126–127
patient engagement and support,
    135
revolutionizing dementia care, 140–141
standard protocols for patient-centered
    dementia care, 127–129
    advancing care, 128–129
    implementation and practitioner
        insights, 128
    integration with conversational AI
        and NLP in dementia care, 129
    structured, non-pharmacological
        interventions, 128–129
user-friendly conversational
    interfaces, 133–135
    strategies for, 134–135
validation and verification
    framework, 145–149
    classification models, 146
    clustering models, 146
    regression models, 146–147
    responsible and explainable AI
        (XAI), 148–149
    validation metrics for LLMs and
        NLP Models, 147
    validation of models by AI and
        machine learning experts,
        145–147
    verification by physicians, doctors,
        and medical scientists, 147–148
Convolutional Neural Networks
    (CNNs), 95, 99, 106
Crowther, Neil, 15
Culturally and Linguistically Diverse
    (CALD), 234
Cybersecurity, 3, 8, 12
Czaja, S. J., 308, 313

D

Darwin, Charles, 216
Data acquisition and management, 142
Data anonymization, 149
Data preprocessing and integration, 142
Data privacy and security in AI
        applications, 149–151, 357
    compliance with regulatory
        standards, 150
    data access controls and audit
        trails, 150
    data anonymization and
        de-identification, 149
    ethical and legal considerations,
        149
    patient empowerment and data
        control, 150–151
    risks of data breaches and mitigation
        strategies, 150
    secure data storage and transmission,
        150
Data quality, 357
Davies, N., 135
Davies-Bouldin index, 146
D'Cunha, N. M., 251
Deep fakes, 6–7
Deep feedforward neural network
    (DFNN), 167
Deep Learning (DL) Models, 93
De-identification, 149
Dementia, 75–111, 346–347
    AI and ML models for diagnosis
        and drug discovery, 94–107
    AI Research Assistant tool, 329–331
    Alzheimer's disease (AD), 76, 158
    artificial intelligence (AI), 89
    Asia and Pacific, 86–87
    biomedical model of, 2
    and cardiovascular health, 325–327
    commercial AI and ML tools in
        healthcare, 107–108
    data for diagnosis and drug discovery,
        89–94
    defined, 2, 158
    detect earlier, 160
    diagnosed at present, 160
    as disability, 2–3
    Europe, 86

frontotemporal dementia (FTD), 78,
    79, 159
global investment in research
    of, 86–88
Health AI concept, 331–332
identifying genetic biomarkers, 80, **80**
impact of COVID-19 on, 82–85
importance of ethnicity and
    geography, 81–82
improving blood pressure, 325–328
integration of AI in diagnosis and
    management of, 108–110
integration of clinical and
    demographic data, 93–94
intensive health self-management
    support, 327–328
investment figures and
    projections, 87
Lewy body dementia (LBD),
    77, **79**, 159
machine learning (ML), 89
misconceptions, 323–324
mixed dementia (MD), 159
overview, 75, 323–325
participants, 331
research design, 331
social microlearning, 327–328
types of, 76–82, 158–159
United States, 86
user evaluation & data analysis, 332
vascular dementia (VD), 76–77, **79**,
    158–159
Dementia Alliance International, 15
Dementia care
  application in, 163–164
  complexities in, 347–348
  framework, 141–145
    data acquisition and management,
      142
    data preprocessing and
      integration, 142
    machine learning models
      and inference, 142
    user interface and security
      measures, 142–145
  integrating AI and ML in, 135–137
  precision in personalization of care,
    348
  sensor technologies in, 39–41

Dementia Health Management System
    (DHMS), 172
Dementia with Lewy Bodies (DLB), 94
Demiris, G., 252
De-Moraes-Ribeiro, F. E., 310
Describe, investigate, create, evaluate
    (DICE) approach, 311–312
Devices and sensors, IoT, 47–55, *48*
  communication aids, 52–53
    smart speakers and tablets, 52–53
  health monitoring sensors, 51–52
    blood pressure monitors and
      glucose monitors, 51–52
  in-home sensors, 49
    motion sensors, 49
    smart home systems, 49
  location tracking devices, 49–50
    functionality and benefits, 49–50
    GPS trackers, 49
  medication management, 53–55
    smart pill dispensers, 53–55
  wearable devices, 48–49
    smartwatches, 48–49
    wearable sensors, 48–49
Diffusion of Innovation (DOI) theory,
    196
Diffusion Tensor Imaging (DTI), 92
Digital assistants, 304
Digital assistive technologies (DATs),
    250
Digital biomarkers, 236–237, 246–247
Digital cognitive tests, 245–246
Digital dementia, 6
Digital innovation, 235
Digital programs-co-designed, 237–238
Digital solutions, 1, 232–239
  artificial intelligence (AI), 303
  for caregivers of individuals with
    dementia, 301–319
  communication and coordination,
    253–254
  defining diversity, 234
  in dementia treatment, care, and
    support, 243–258
  digital biomarkers, 236–237
  digital innovation, 235
  digital programs-co-designed,
    237–238
  digital solutions, 232–239

early diagnosis and monitoring,
    245–247
  digital biomarkers, 246–247
  digital cognitive tests, 245–246
education and training, 252–253
to empower multicultural families
    impacted by dementia,
    232–239
ethical and practical considerations,
    254–255
ethnically diverse communities in
    research, 235
monitoring technologies, 303
overview, 232–234, 243–244
personalized treatment, 247–249
  behavior management, 248
  communication and language
    support, 249
  engagement and activity
    facilitation, 248–249
  memory stimulation, 248
  reminiscence therapy, 248
platforms, 303–306
promise and challenges of, 307–317
support for people living with
    dementia, 250
use by caregivers, 306–307
web-based platforms, 303
well-being and engagement, 251–252
  experience-based interventions,
    251–252
  reminiscence interventions, 252
  robot-based interventions, 251
Digital technology (DT), 3–5
  artificial intelligence (AI), 303
  for caregivers of individuals with
    dementia, 301–319
  monitoring technologies, 303
  platforms, 303–306
  promise and challenges of, 307–317
  use by caregivers, 306–307
  web-based platforms, 303
Digital tools, 215–224
  immersive virtual reality methods,
    221–222
  screening tool for Alzheimer's
    disease, 215
  spatial navigation, 216–218
    Alzheimer's disease (AD), 216–218

GPS techniques, 222–223
methods for detecting
    impairments in, 218–221
Digital twins (DTs), 38–43, 101
  of dementia patients for clinical
    decision support, 346–358
  ethical considerations and
    challenges, 42–43
  in healthcare, 348–349
  integration of sensor data in, 41–42
  overview, 38–39
  personalized interventions, 42
  predictive analytics, 42
  proposed solution, 350–355
  research question, 349–350
  role of AI in, 39
  sensor technologies in dementia
    care, 39–41
Digital voice assistants, 312–313
Digitization, 303–304
Dimensionality reduction, 97
Dimensionality reduction techniques,
    100
Discrete Wavelet Transform (DWT), 91
DL techniques, 97
Doborjeh, M., 104
Drug-drug interactions (DDIs), 99
Drug-target interactions (DTIs), 99

E

Ecological Momentary Assessment
    (EMA), 314
Electroencephalogram (EEG), 90–91, 180
Electronic health records (EHRs), 54
El Haj, M., 130
ElliQ, 139
EMBED-Care Framework, 137
Embodied conversational agents
    (ECAs), 132–133
Emotional and mental health
    support, 274
Empowerment
  of caregivers, 336–339
  of health professionals, 336–339
  of patients, 336–339
Engagement and activity facilitation,
    248–249
Enhanced decision-making, 356–357

Environmental sensors, 40
Ethical considerations in AI-powered
      healthcare interventions,
      137–139
   challenges in predictive health
      analytics, 138
   general ethical principles in
      AI deployment, 138
   global ethical regulatory
      organization, 139
   impact on patient-physician
      dynamics, 138
   language models, 138–139
Experience-based interventions, 251–252
Explainable AI (XAI) techniques, 96, 100
Extreme Gradient Boosting (XGB), 96

F

FaceTime, 25–26, 35
Fallon, Jimmy, 26
Family carers, 18–37
   activities, 28–30
   carer/advocate/mouthpiece/in-house
      comedian, 23–25
   coping and caring, 30–31, 33–34
   end of home care, 31–32
   family tribe, 18–19
   help, 21–23
   human connections and technology,
      36–37
   people, 25–26
   perplexing oddities, 19–21
   personalized care activities, 32–33
   places, 26–27
   residential care facility-based
      phase, 26
   SRCF placement, 33–34
   system failures, 21
   technology, 34–35
   transition to supported residential
      care facility, 31–32
Family tribe, 18–19
Fast Fourier Transform (FFT), 91
Feature Extraction Battery (FEB), 91
Fernandes, G., 132
Fiddian-Green, A., 238
Finite Impulse Response (FIR), 91
Fitbit, 48, 60, *61*

Ford, E., 236
Fox, S., 284
Frontotemporal dementia (FTD), 78, **79**,
      94, 159
Functional MRI (fMRI) scans, *84*, 92–93,
      140
FUNSAT™, 313
Future Health AI use, 336

G

Gagnon, M.P., 179
Gaugler, J. E., 311
General Data Protection Regulation
      (GDPR), 138, 209
Generative Adversarial Networks
      (GANs), 100, 105–106
Generative models, 105
Genetic risk scores (GRS), 235
Globalization, 347
Global positioning systems (GPS),
      188–189, 216
   feature, 186
   trackers, 49, 62, *63*
   tracking of dementia patients,
      186–187
Google Home, 52–53, 62
Google Scholar, 329
Gradient Boosting Machine (GBM),
      95, 100
Graph-based models, 93
Graph comparison, 352
Graph Neural Networks (GNNs), 100,
      105, 106
Guo, Y. P., 292

H

Health AI
   evaluation and metadata criteria
      for ambiguous claims, 339
   preferences, and information use,
      333, **334**
Health AI Research Assistant, 340
Health AI Tool Concept
   user evaluation on, 332–336
Health and well-being, 18
Healthcare professionals (HCPs),
      126–127, 151

Health Insurance Portability and
Accountability Act (HIPAA),
138, 143, 149, 209
Heart Health AI self-management
support (SMS), 324
Heart rate beats per minute (HR-BPM),
171
Hero Health, 53, 60
Herriot, James, 29, 32, 33
High-throughput screening (HTS)
techniques, 98
Home-based care, 171
Human connections and technology,
36–37
Human Research Ethics Committee
(HREC), 270
Human rights, 8–10
Human rights violation, 10–13
Hung, L., 292
Huq, R., 251
Hybrid intelligence, 330
for ambiguity "rationale capturing,"
339

I

Immersive virtual reality methods,
221–222
Immigration, 347
Independent Component Analysis
(ICA), 90, 92
Integrating AI and ML in dementia
care, 135–137
advancing care, 137
AI-enhanced tools, 136–137
decision-making, 137
healthcare connectivity with AI, 136
language models, 137
patient-centered digital support,
135–136
patient engagement through
AI-driven conversational
interfaces, 136
structured, non-pharmacological
interventions, 137
International Covenant on Civil and
Political Rights (ICCPR), 9
International Organization for
Standardization (ISO), 150

Internet of Things (IoT), 45–69, 173, 274
adaptive IoT systems, 57–58
caregivers, 56
cognitive training, 58–59
commercial IoT tools for dementia
care, **63**
commercial tools, 60–63
comprehensive data analysis, 57
in dementia care, 57
devices and sensors, 47–55, *48*
communication aids, 52–53
health monitoring sensors, 51–52
in-home sensors, 49
location tracking devices, 49–50
medication management, 53–55
wearable devices, 48–49
disease detection, 58
integration of, 57
medical professionals, 56–47
objectives in dementia care using,
58–59
outdoor IoT systems, 57
overview, 46–47
patient assistance, 58
patient localization, 58
patient monitoring, 58
people with dementia, 56

K

Khanna, R., 132
Kimmel, Jimmy, 26
Kiselica, A. M., 314
Kordel, P., 132
Kruse, C. S., 136

L

Language models
and applications in patient
interaction, 130–133
ethical considerations in AI-powered
healthcare interventions,
138–139
integrating AI and ML in dementia
care, 137
Large language models (LLMs), 132
for healthcare, 329
probable-word generators, 330

Lazar, A., 252
Lewy body dementia (LBD), 77,
    79, 159
Life enhancement strategies, 4
Light Gradient Boosting Machine
    (LightGBM), 96
Linear interpolation, 352
Liu, Q., 104–105
Location tracking, 41
Logopenic progressive, non-fluent
    aphasia (LPA), 20
Longino, 2
Long short-term memory (LSTM)
    networks, 98
"Love–hate" relationship, 4
Low- and middle-income countries
    (LMICs), 157, 233

M

Machine learning (ML), 38, 45, 46, **99**,
    102, **106**, 126, 274
    commercial tools in healthcare, **107**,
        107–108
    in data optimization, 89
    defined, 160–161
    innovations for enhanced drug
        discovery, 98–103
    interpretability of, 166–167
    in modern medicine, 104–107
    in neurological predictive analytics,
        94–98
    in personalized medicine, 89
    reinforcement learning, 162–163
    semi-supervised learning, 162
    supervised learning, 161–162
    types of techniques, 161–163
    unsupervised learning, 162
Machine learning models and
    inference, 142
Martire, L. M., 303
Matthews Correlation Coefficient
    (MCC), 146
McCartney, Paul, 33
Mean Absolute Error (MAE), 147
Mean Squared Error (MSE), 147
MedMinder, 53, 60
Memory Lane, 139
Memory stimulation, 248

Metadata criteria for ambiguous
    claims, 339
Mihailidis, A., 251
Mild cognitive impairment (MCI), 313
Mixed dementia (MD), 159
Mobile, 181
Mobile Health Applications
    (mHealth), 280
Molecular dynamics simulations, 101
Mood, memory, thinking, and
    behaviour (MMTB), 171
Motion sensors, 49
Multi-factor authentication (MFA), 150
Multimodal data, 93
Munteanu, D., 130

N

Nabizadeh, A., 133
National Disability Insurance Scheme
    (NDIS), 11
National Institute for Health and Care
    Excellence (NICE), 127, 152n2
National Institute of Standards and
    Technology (NIST), 150
National Institutes of Health (NIH), 86
Natural Language Processing (NLP), 39,
    41, 129–130, 151, 268, 273–274
Neurodegenerative dementia, 1, 159
Neurofilament light (NfL), 76
Niedderer, K., 287
Noel, M. A., 309
Non-governmental organizations
    (NGOs), 141
Normalized Mutual Information
    (NMI), 146
Nurse-reported outcomes, 354–355

O

Olazarán, J., 1
Oliver, Mary, 29
Opportunities for digital health
    solutions, 195–211
    analysis and results, 198–202
        assessment of digital health
            technologies, 200–202
        key drivers for adoption, 202,
            206–207

barriers to digital health adoption, **203–204**
Diffusion of Innovation (DOI), 205, **208–209**
ethical and regulatory considerations, 209–210
methodology, 197–198
overview, 195–197
scoping review, **197**, *198*
"Origin of Certain Instincts" (Darwin), 216
Ornish, Dean, 326

P

Paralympic Games, 13
Patient care, 45–69, 89, 97, 107
artificial intelligence (AI), 45–69, 108
clinical decisionmaking, 129
digital twins in, 43
ethical standards in, 138
individualized simulations for, 210
Internet of Things (IoT), 45–69
potential of chatbots in, 134
sensor technologies, 39
solutions, 145–147
People living with dementia (PLWD), 1–3
alternative perspectives through collaboration with, 13–15
artificial intelligence (AI), 3–5
assistive technology (AT), 3–5
dementia as disability, 2–3
digital technology (DT), 3–5
human rights, 8–10
human rights violation, 10–13
overview, 1–2
pitfalls, 6–8
possibilities, 5–6
post-diagnostic care for, 1
smart technology, 8
Perplexing oddities, 19–21
Personalization, 356
Personalization of care, 348
Personalized care, 34–35
Personalized care activities, 31, 32–33
Personalized treatment, 247–249
behavior management, 248
communication and language support, 249

engagement and activity facilitation, 248–249
memory stimulation, 248
reminiscence therapy, 248
Pham, K. T., 133
"Pill-paradigm," 324
Plans4Care™, 312
Pleasant, M., 310
Positive psychology, 24
Positron emission tomography (PET), 92–93, 95, 97, 110, 140, 165
Precision, 356
medicine, 348
in personalization of care, 348
Predictive analytics, 274
Predictive modelling, 101
Preferred Reporting Items for Systematic Reviews and Meta-Analyses (PRISMA), 198
Principal Component Analysis (PCA), 90–91, 92, 200
Proposed DT solution, 350–355
acquiring precision and personalization, 352–353
cohort matching, 351–352
continuous learning, 354–355
inputs to the solution, 350–351
opportunities, 357
outcomes of the solution, 353–354
strengths, 356–357
summary of the work carried out, 356
threats, 357
weaknesses, 357

Q

Qi, J., 131
Quantitative structure-activity relationship (QSAR) models, 98

R

RE-AIM framework, 291
Real-time health monitoring, 177
Real-world data, 161
Real-World Evidence (RWE) integration, 148
Recurrent Neural Networks (RNNs), 97, 100, 104–105, 165

Redman, Bobby, 280, 282
Regression models, 146–147
Reinforcement learning, 162–163
Reminiscence interventions, 252
Reminiscence therapy, 248
Replicability, 167
Reproducibility, 167
Residential care facility-based phase, 26
Resource intensive, 357
Responsible and explainable AI
      (XAI), 148–149
Retrieval-Augmented Generation
      (RAG) framework, 131
Robot-based interventions, 251
Rodríguez-Domínguez, M. T., 131
Role-based access control (RBAC), 150
Root Mean Squared Error (RMSE), 147
R-squared (Coefficient of
      Determination), 147
Ruggiano, N., 131

S

Sacks, Oliver, 29, 33
SafelyYou, 139
Sakamoto, M., 284
Salvi, M., 137
Scalability, 357
Schmitz, D., 132
Schulz, R., 303
Selek, S., 133
"Self-healing paradigm," 324
Seligman, Martin, 24
Semi-supervised learning, 162
Sensor technologies in dementia
      care, 39–41
   biometric sensors, 40
   environmental sensors, 40
   location tracking, 41
   voice and speech analysis, 41
   wearable sensors, 40
Shawaqfeh, B., 137
Shin, Wonsun, 13
Silhouette score, 146
Smart Dementia Networks
      (SDNs), 171–192
   body area networks (BANs), 177
   dementia data, 174–175
   dementia figures, 174

economic viability, 175–176
extend on smart homes, 178
frameworks and design, 178–183
   context-aware design, 178–179
   context-aware pervasive
      technology, 179
   mobile, smart devices,
      wearables, 181
integration with home health
      systems, 190–191
limitations, 189–190
numeral proportions, 173
objective, 173–176
overview, 171–172
privacy data privacy, 190
security, 190
smart networks, smart homes, 178
use-cases, 183–185
   external environments, 185
   external scenarios, 183
   healthcare (aged care), 183
   healthcare/aged-care centres,
      184–185
   home-based care – internal
      environments, 184
   personalised use-case, 184
   self-health, 183
   universal use case, 184–185
wearable tracking, 186–189
   emergency control equipment,
      187–188
   emergency response handling
      or emergency response
      procedures, 187
   GPS, 188–189
   GPS feature, 186
   GPS tracking of dementia
      patients, 186–187
   precise tracking systems, 188–189
wearable/wireless sensor networks
      (WSNs), 177
Smart devices, 181
Smart healthcare networks, *180*
Smart home technologies, 49, 178, 304
Smart networks, 178
Smart pill dispensers, 53–55
Smart speakers and tablets, 52–53
Smart technology, 8
Smart TV technology, 26, 28

Smartwatches, 48–49
Smart wearable devices, *182*
Socially assistive robots, 163
Socially produced dependency, 2
Social microlearning, 327–328
Soft technologies, 4
Spatial navigation, 216–218
    Alzheimer's disease (AD), 216–218
    classification of, **220**
    GPS techniques, 222–223
    methods for detecting impairments
        in, 218–221
Spiking Neural Networks (SNNs), 96
Spoofing, 6
Stakeholder Advisory Group (SAG), 270
State Department of Health and
    Wellbeing, 18
Statistical matching, 352–353
Subramanian, R. C., 132
Suganthi, S., 131
Suijkerbuijk, S., 281
Summer College Preview Program, 19
Supervised learning, 161–162
Supported Residential Care Facility
    (SRCF), 25, 27, 29–34
Support Vector Machines (SVMs), 97, 98
Sydney Memory and Ageing Study
    (MAS), 96–97

T

Technology Acceptance Model
    (TAM), 330
Thompson, H. J., 252
Time series analysis, 93
Transfer learning, 100
Transport Accident Commission, 18
Transport layer security (TLS), 150
Traumatic brain injury (TBI), 2–3

U

Unified Theory of Acceptance and Use
    of Technology (UTAUT), 330
United Nations Convention on the
    Rights of Persons with
    Disabilities (UNCRPD), 8–10
United States Census Bureau
    International Database (IDB), 4

Universal Declaration of Human
    Rights, 9
Unsupervised learning, 162
User evaluation on Health AI Tool
    Concept, 332–336

V

Validation and verification framework,
    145–149
    classification models, 146
    clustering models, 146
    regression models, 146–147
    responsible and explainable AI
        (XAI), 148–149
    validation metrics for LLMs and
        NLP Models, 147
    validation of models by AI and
        machine learning experts,
        145–147
    verification by physicians, doctors,
        and medical scientists, 147–148
Validation metrics for LLMs and
    NLP Models, 147
Validation of models by AI and machine
    learning experts, 145–147
Variational Autoencoders (VAEs), 100, 105
Vascular dementia (VD), 76–77, **79**, 94,
    158–159
Verification by physicians, doctors, and
    medical scientists, 147–148
Virtual reality (VR), 245
Virtual reality methods, 221–222
Virtual screening, 101
Voice and speech analysis, 41
Voxel-Based Morphometry (VBM), 92, 93

W

Wang, R., 251
Wang, Z., 293, 296
Wearable Devices, 274
Wearables, 181
Wearable sensors, 40, 48–49
Wearable tracking, 186–189
    emergency control equipment, 187–188
    emergency response handling
        or emergency response
        procedures, 187

GPS, 188–189
GPS feature, 186
GPS tracking of dementia patients, 186–187
precise tracking systems, 188–189
Wearable/wireless sensor networks (WSNs), 177
WeCareAdvisor Prescription, 312
Well-being and engagement, 251–252
  experience-based interventions, 251–252
  reminiscence interventions, 252
  robot-based interventions, 251
Winfrey, Oprah, 26

Wireless sensor networks (WSNs), 172–173
World Health Organization (WHO), 2, 10, 158, 195, 235, 269, 270

Y

Yang, D. A., 132
Yeo, L. H., 12
Yin, Robert, 269
Younger onset dementia (YOD), 2

Z

Zhai, S., 310

For Product Safety Concerns and Information please contact our EU
representative GPSR@taylorandfrancis.com
Taylor & Francis Verlag GmbH, Kaufingerstraße 24, 80331 München, Germany